The Surgical Management of Epilepsy

The Surgical Management of Epilepsy

EDITED BY

Allen R. Wyler, M.D.

MEDICAL DIRECTOR, EPILEPSY CENTER, SWEDISH MEDICAL CENTER,
SEATTLE, WASHINGTON

Bruce P. Hermann, Ph.D.

DEPARTMENTS OF PSYCHIATRY AND NEUROSURGERY, UNIVERSITY OF TENNESSEE;
EPI-CARE CENTER, BAPTIST MEMORIAL HOSPITAL; SEMMES-MURPHEY CLINIC,
MEMPHIS, TENNESSEE

WITH 31 CONTRIBUTING AUTHORS

Butterworth–Heinemann

Boston   London   Oxford   Singapore   Sydney   Toronto   Wellington

Every effort has been made to ensure that the drug dosage
schedules within this text are accurate and conform to standards
accepted at time of publication. However, as treatment
recommendations vary in the light of continuing research and
clinical experience, the reader is advised to verify drug dosage
schedules herein with information found on product information
sheets. This is especially true in cases of new or infrequently
used drugs.

Recognizing the importance of preserving what has been written,
it is the policy of Butterworth–Heinemann to have the books it
⊗ publishes printed on acid-free paper, and we exert our best
efforts to that end.

Library of Congress Cataloging-in-Publication Data

The Surgical management of epilepsy / edited by Allen R. Wyler,
    Bruce P. Hermann ; with 31 contributing authors.
        p.   cm.
    Includes bibliographical references and index.
    ISBN 0-7506-9416-5
    I. Wyler, Allen R.   II. Hermann, Bruce P.
    [DNLM: 1. Epilepsy—surgery.   WL 385 S9618 1994]
    RD594.S943   1994
    617.4'81—dc20
    DNLM/DLC
    for Library of Congress   93-15332
                                                          CIP

British Library Cataloguing-in-Publication Data

A catalogue record for this book is available from the British
Library.

Butterworth–Heinemann
80 Montvale Avenue
Stoneham, MA 02180

10   9   8   7   6   5   4   3   2   1

Printed in the United States of America

Contents

PART IV: OUTCOME

APPENDIXES

Index

Contributing Authors

JOHN F. ANNEGERS, PH.D.
Professor, Department of Epidemiology, University of Texas, School of Public Health, Houston, Texas

ISSAM AWAD, M.D., M.SC., F.A.C.S.
Director, Neurovascular Surgery Program, Section of Neurosurgery, Yale University, School of Medicine, New Haven, Connecticut

DIETRICH BLUMER, M.D.
Professor, Department of Psychiatry, University of Tennessee; Director of Neuropsychiatry, Epi-Care Center, Baptist Memorial Hospital, Memphis, Tennessee

WIELAND BURR, PH.D.
University Lecturer, Department of Epileptology, University of Bonn; Physicist, Department of Eileptology, University Hospital, Bonn, Germany

BENJAMIN S. CARSON, M.D.
Director of Neurosurgery, Department of Neurosurgery, Johns Hopkins Hospital, Baltimore, Maryland

GORDON J. CHELUNE, PH.D.
Head, Section of Neuropsychology, Department of Psychiatry and Psychology, Cleveland Clinic Foundation, Cleveland, Ohio

CARL B. DODRILL, PH.D.
Professor, Departments of Neurological Surgery and Psychiatry and Behavioral Sciences, Associate Director, Epilepsy Center, Department of Neurological Surgery, University of Washington, Seattle, Washington

MICHAEL S. DUCHOWNY, M.D.
Clinical Professor, Departments of Neurology and Pediatrics, University of Miami; Director, Seizure Unit and EEG Laboratories, Miami Children's Hospital, Miami, Florida

CHRISTIAN ERICH ELGER, M.D.
Full Professor, Department of Epileptology; Director, Department of Epileptology, University Hospital, University of Bonn, Bonn, Germany

PETER FENWICK, M.B., B CHIR (CANTAB), DPM, FRCPSYCH.
Senior Lecturer, Department of Psychiatry; Consultant, Epilepsy Unit, The Maudsley Hospital, London, England

HERMAN F. FLANIGIN, M.D.
Senior Consultant, Department of Neurosurgery, Medical College of Georgia, Augusta, Georgia

ROBERT T. FRASER, PH.D.
Professor, Neurological Surgery and Rehabilitation Medicine, Harborview Medical Center, University of Washington, Seattle, Washington

JOHN M. FREEMAN, M.D.
Professor of Pediatric Epilepsy, Department of Pediatrics and Neurology, The Johns Hopkins University School of Medicine; Department of Neurology, Johns Hopkins Hospital, Baltimore, Maryland

BRIAN B. GALLAGHER, M.D., PH.D.
Professor, Department of Neurology, Medical College of Georgia, Augusta, Georgia

GREGORY L. HOLMES, M.D.
Associate Professor of Neurology, Department of Neurology, Harvard Medical School; Director of Epilepsy Program, Director of the Clinical Neurophysiology Laboratory, Department of Neurology, Children's Hospital, Boston, Massachusetts

ANDREAS HUFNAGEL, M.D.
Staff Neurologist, Department of Epileptology, University of Bonn, Bonn, Germany

DON W. KING, M.D.
Professor, Department of Neurology, Medical College of Georgia, Augusta, Georgia

GREGORY P. LEE, PH.D.
Associate Professor, Departments of Surgery and Psychiatry; Director of Neuropsychology Service, Medical College of Georgia, Augusta, Georgia

DAVID W. LORING, PH.D.
Associate Professor, Department of Neurology; Director, Adult Neuropsychology Service, Department of Neurology, Medical College of Georgia, Augusta, Georgia

HANS OTTO LÜDERS, M.D., PH.D.
Chairman, Department of Neurology, The Cleveland Clinic Foundation, Cleveland, Ohio

KIMFORD J. MEADOR, M.D.
Associate Professor, Department of Neurology; Director of Behavioral Neurology, Department of Neurology, Medical College of Georgia, Augusta, Georgia

ANTHONY MURRO, M.D.
Associate Professor of Neurology, Medical College of Georgia; Director of EEG Laboratory, Department of Neurology, Veterans' Affairs Medical Center, Augusta, Georgia

GEORGE A. OJEMANN, M.D.
Professor of Neurological Surgery, Department of Neurological Surgery, University of Washington, Seattle, Washington

PHILLIP L. PEARL, M.D.
Clinical Assistant Professor, Departments of Pediatrics and Neurology, George Washington University; Clinical Instructor, Department of Pediatrics, Georgetown University, Washington, District of Columbia

LEONARD SCHÄFFLER, M.D.
Research Fellow, Department of Neurology, Cleveland Clinic Foundation, Cleveland, Ohio

JOSEPH R. SMITH, M.D., F.A.C.S.
Professor, Department of Neurosurgery, Medical College of Georgia, Augusta, Georgia

MICHAEL R. SPERLING, M.D.
Associate Professor, Department of Neurology, University of Pennsylvania; Director, EEG Laboratory, Graduate Hospital, Philadelphia, Pennsylvania

WILLIAM H. THEODORE, M.D.
Chief, Clinical Epilepsy Section, National Institutes of Health, Bethesda, Maryland

EILEEN VINING, M.D.
Associate Professor of Neurology and Pediatrics, The Johns Hopkins University School of Medicine; Department of Neurology, Johns Hopkins Hospital, Baltimore, Maryland

HEINZ GREGOR WIESER, M.D.
Head, Department for EEG and Epileptology, Neurology Clinic, University Hospital, Zurich, Zurich, Switzerland

ELAINE WYLLIE, M.D.
Head, Pediatric Epilepsy Program, Department of Neurology, The Cleveland Clinic Foundation, Cleveland, Ohio

Preface

Renewed interest and remarkable growth has occurred in the surgical treatment of intractable epilepsy. Also, the procedures for preoperative assessment, surgical technique, and effects of the surgery on seizure frequency and psychological and social outcome are undergoing greater scrutiny. An increasing number of texts concerned with epilepsy surgery are available, international conferences are regularly held, a greater proportion of epilepsy-specific scientific meetings are devoted to epilepsy surgery, and an NIH-sponsored Consensus Conference of Epilepsy Surgery was held. Diverse viewpoints and perspectives have been voiced regarding many essential details of the procedure.

The purpose of this book is to add to the ongoing discussions and evaluations of epilepsy surgery. This text provides contributions regarding (1) the multidisciplinary evaluation of potential surgical candidates (including neurophysiological, neuropsychological, and neuropsychiatric viewpoints); (2) operative techniques and procedures; and (3) neurological and psychosocial outcomes. These contributions have been designed to be both of clinical utility and scholarly interest, with an emphasis on critical evaluation of conventional wisdom.

We hope this text will contribute to the knowledge and understanding of those interested in improving the medical and social outcomes of epilepsy surgery for patients with intractable epilepsies.

A.R.W.
B.P.H.

.

PART ONE
THE PROGNOSIS
OF EPILEPSY

Chapter 1

The Natural Course
of Epilepsy: An
Epidemiologic Perspective

J.F. ANNEGERS

This chapter reviews the occurrence and natural history of epilepsy. It addresses the following issues, which relate to the surgical treatment of epilepsy: (a) What is the incidence of epilepsy and of specific seizure types, especially partial epilepsy, which might be considered for surgery? (b) What are the etiologic factors responsible for epilepsy? (c) What are the effects of epilepsy on subsequent mortality? (d) What is the natural history of epilepsy in terms of prospects for remission in patients with epilepsy? (e) What factors are prognostic of seizure remission and seizure intractability?

Frequency of Epilepsy

In order to measure the occurrence of epilepsy or to determine its prognosis, it is first necessary to define epilepsy. Epilepsy is defined here as recurrent seizures that are not due to an acute provoked cause [1]. Since recurrence is a criterion, patients who have experienced only one seizure will not be considered to have epilepsy. Seizures due to acute neurologic insults such as head trauma or ethanol withdrawal and febrile convulsions are considered acute symptomatic seizures rather than epilepsy. However, recurrent seizures that occur after an antecedent neurologic insult such as head trauma, central nervous system insults, or cerebrovascular disease will be considered epilepsy.

Measures of Occurrence

There are three basic measures of disease occurrence—prevalence, cumulative incidence, and inci-

dence rates. Each measures distinct quantities and has different uses in expressing disease occurrence (Fig. 1-1). Prevalence measures the proportion of the population affected with epilepsy at a given time. A *prevalence case* is defined as seizures or use of antiepileptic medication within the past 5 years. Remission is achieved with the successful discontinuation of antiepileptic drugs for 5 years. The total population prevalence of epilepsy is about 7 per 1000 individuals. The age-specific prevalence rises rapidly in childhood and then remains stable from age 15 to 65 years because the occurrence of new cases is balanced by the remission of existing cases and, to a lesser extent, because of the increased mortality rates among people with epilepsy. The prevalence of epilepsy rises to over 1% among the elderly because of the very high incidence of epilepsy associated with cerebrovascular disease.

Cumulative incidence measures the risk of ever having epilepsy to a specific age. The risk of developing epilepsy is about 1% to age 20 years and reaches over 3% over the life span. The age-specific prevalences of epilepsy would be the same as the cumulative incidence if remission of epilepsy did not occur and if mortality were not increased for people with epilepsy. Although less than 1% of the population has epilepsy at a specific point in time, the lifetime risk of ever developing epilepsy is about 3%. It is important to distinguish epilepsy from acute symptomatic seizures because the lifetime cumulative incidence of any type of seizure approaches 10%.

Incidence rates measure the occurrence of new cases of epilepsy and are expressed as cases per 100,000 person-years. Over all age groups the incidence of epilepsy is 45 cases per 100,000 individuals.

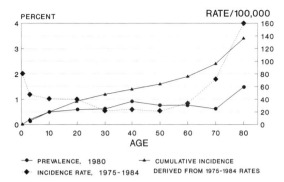

Figure 1-1. Epilepsy: prevalence, cumulative incidence, and incidence rates.

The age-specific incidence rates of epilepsy are highest at the extremes of life, under 1 year and over 75 years, but the rates are over 20 per 100,000 individuals at all ages (Fig. 1-1). If the Rochester, Minnesota experience were extrapolated to the U.S. population, there would be about 112,500 new cases of epilepsy in the country in 1990. About 60,000 of these would be partial seizures, of which about 25% would be intractable and among these about a third might be surgical candidates. If these estimates are reasonable, the total number of new surgical cases each year for partial epilepsy would be about 5000. There would also be a much smaller number of generalized epilepsy cases that could be considered surgical candidates.

Occurrence by Seizure Type

Figure 1-2 presents the age-specific incidence rates of epilepsy by major seizure types. For epidemiologic studies, epilepsy is classified into five broad categories of clinical seizure types that can be applied to population studies—partial, generalized tonic-clonic, myoclonic, absence, and others. During the first year of life myoclonic seizures are the most common but

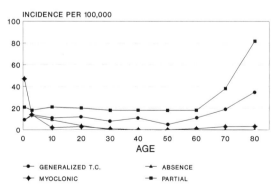

Figure 1-2. Incidence rates of epilepsy by seizure type.

diminish in incidence rapidly thereafter. The incidence of generalized tonic-clonic epilepsy gradually diminishes to age 50 years and increases among the elderly. The incidence of partial-onset seizures, with or without secondary generalization, remains relatively consistent at 20 per 100,000 to age 65 years. The proportion of epilepsy that is of partial onset increases progressively with age.

Etiology

Epidemiologic studies have helped to confirm and define the long-held clinical impression that at least a proportion of epilepsy can be attributed to prior neurologic insults. Nevertheless the proportion of epilepsy that can be attributed to specific causes has apparently been overstated in many clinical series where minor head injuries or vague perinatal insults are considered causes of epilepsy. Only about one third of all cases of epilepsy can be considered secondary to defined insults (Fig. 1-3). Although this proportion is higher for partial-onset epilepsy (36.9%) than for primary generalized epilepsies (24.7%), there is no direct relationship between presumed etiology and seizure type. Some patients with primary generalized seizures have a presumed cause, and most cases of partial-onset epilepsy do not.

The most important known cause of epilepsy in Western countries today is cerebrovascular disease. This fact has implications for the surgical treatment of epilepsy since epilepsy secondary to cerebrovascular disease almost exclusively affects the elderly, a population in which surgical treatment may not be considered appropriate. Developmental epilepsy, the second largest category with a presumed etiology, includes those who have epilepsy in association with neurologic deficits from birth—cerebral palsy and/or mental retardation. About 4% of all cases of epilepsy can be attributed to head trauma, but the proportion is higher among young adult males. Head trauma should be considered the cause of epilepsy only in cases where there is over a 30-min period of loss of consciousness or a depressed skull fracture. The risk of epilepsy after head injury is highest (10–15%) when there has been loss of consciousness of over a day, a brain contusion, or a subdural hematoma [2]. The incidence of epilepsy is greatly elevated after encephalitis and bacterial meningitis although there is no increase after aseptic meningitis. This heightened incidence is maintained for at least 20 years after the central nervous system infection [3]. Epilepsy related to central nervous system infections largely affects children and young adults. Brain tumors are an important cause of partial epilepsy in adults. The

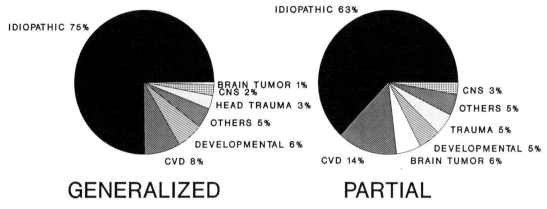

IDIOPATHIC 63%

IDIOPATHIC 75%

BRAIN TUMOR 1%
CNS 2%
HEAD TRAUMA 3%
OTHERS 5%
DEVELOPMENTAL 6%
CVD 8%

CNS 3%
OTHERS 5%
TRAUMA 5%
DEVELOPMENTAL 5%
CVD 14%   BRAIN TUMOR 6%

GENERALIZED

PARTIAL

Figure 1-3. Presumed predisposing causes of epilepsy.

incidence of brain tumors is elevated in patients with epilepsy even many years after the onset of seizures [4,5], and brain tumors are not an uncommon incidental finding at the time of surgery for epilepsy [6].

Most series of partial complex epilepsy report that a substantial proportion of patients have a history of prior febrile seizures that are often prolonged or focal [7]. Children with febrile convulsions have about a 6% risk of developing subsequent epilepsy to age 25 years, but the risk and type of subsequent epilepsy can be differentiated by the characteristics of the febrile convulsion. Children with simple febrile convulsions have only a 2–3% risk of subsequent epilepsy, which usually takes the form of generalized-onset seizures. Children with complex febrile seizures—those that are focal, prolonged, or characterized by repeat episodes with the same illness—have a 6–20% risk of subsequent epilepsy, which usually occurs as complex partial seizures [8]. Febrile convulsions present a special case in the etiology of epilepsy; there is debate over whether the febrile convulsions are a manifestation of a preexisting lesion, or, especially in the case of prolonged febrile convulsions, if they are the cause of a lesion that later leads to complex partial seizures [7–9].

Mortality in Patients with Epilepsy

It has generally been assumed that patients with epilepsy have increased mortality rates [10]. However, some investigators suggest that mortality is not increased for most patients with epilepsy [12,13]. Studies of mortality of epilepsy are of two types—(a) clinical series that give the proportionate mortality by cause of death and (b) cohort studies that compare mortality in patients with epilepsy to that of standard populations.

Proportionate mortality among patients with epilepsy has been presented in a number of clinical series [14–17]. In these studies, 6–19% of deaths were directly related to seizures. The largest proportion of deaths, 20–30%, were attributed to pneumonia. Accidents, especially drowning, accounted for 10–20% of deaths. Most series also report a disproportionately high number of deaths from suicide.

When the mortality experience of patients with epilepsy is compared to the general population a more accurate picture of the effect of epilepsy is obtained [18,19]. These studies show that patients with epilepsy have about twofold increased mortality rates but that the degree of elevation varies greatly by etiology of epilepsy and duration of epilepsy. Among incidence cases of epilepsy in Rochester, Minnesota the mortality rates were increased 57% for patients with idiopathic epilepsy, 276% for those with postnatally acquired epilepsy—for example, head trauma—and 700% for children with epilepsy and neurologic deficits from birth [19].

The increased death rates for individuals with idiopathic epilepsy or postnatally acquired epilepsy occur almost entirely during the first 10 years after diagnosis. Among all patients who have had epilepsy for over 10 years there is little, if any, increased mortality compared to the general population [20]. There are anecdotal reports of death among patients with intractable epilepsy being considered for surgical treatment where death was attributed to the direct or indirect effect of seizures. Unfortunately, an adequate epidemiologic study has not been conducted to determine the magnitude of the excess death rate that may exist in this subgroup of patients with epilepsy. Patients with epilepsy in association with neurologic deficits from birth have greatly increased mortality rates throughout life [20].

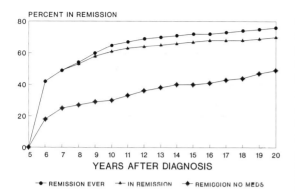

Figure 1-4. Remission of seizures in epilepsy.

Prognosis of Epilepsy

The literature on the prognosis of epilepsy is confusing, since estimates of the prospects for remission range from less than 20% to over 80% [21,22]. Studies conducted at referral centers show poor prognosis because they are weighted toward patients with severe seizures of long duration. Studies that have followed newly diagnosed patients with epilepsy have reported much more favorable prospects for remission [23–28].

The prognosis for all patients with epilepsy is presented in Figure 1-4. Here remission is defined as completing a 5-year period without seizures. The time scale begins at 6 years after diagnosis because remission can occur only after 5 years of follow-up. Among all patients, the probability of achieving remission by 6 years after diagnosis was 42%; after 7 years it was 51%; after 10 years, 65%; and after 20 years, 76%. The net probability of being currently in remission at 10 years after diagnosis was 61% and at 20 years, 70%. The probabilities of ever achieving remission are higher than those for being in remission because some patients experience a relapse of seizures after achieving remission. The curves for remission become relatively stable at 10–15 years after diagnosis.

Prognostic Factors for Remission

The most important prognostic indicator for the eventual remission of seizures is the duration of seizures. The longer one has had seizures the lower the prospects for remission. Other factors are (a) the etiology of epilepsy and (b) seizure type. In considering candidates for surgical treatment of epilepsy the critical question is: How long after the onset of epilepsy, when seizures persist, do the prospects for remission become low? To address this question properly it would be necessary to define an end point of intractability—in terms of seizure frequency and

duration—and then determine the proportion of patients that can be expected to become intractable and factors that are prognostic for that outcome. Unfortunately, such a study has not been done. Nevertheless, studies of the eventual remission of seizures show that, if remission is to occur, it usually begins shortly after the initiation of treatment. Of all patients who achieve a 5-year remission by 15 years after the diagnosis of epilepsy—that is, begin their seizure-free period within 10 years—58% begin their seizure-free period within the first year, 12% during the second year, 20% between 3 and 5 years, and only 10% between 5 and 9 years. Although these figures cannot be extrapolated directly to the pool of potential surgical candidates because of infrequent seizures, seizure type, and other considerations, they suggest that the prospects for "natural remission" or control by medications become very dim within 1–3 years.

Patients with neurologic deficits from birth had only a 46% probability of being in remission 20 years after diagnosis (Fig. 1-5). This finding is similar to that of the Japanese collaborative study where remission was achieved by only 34% of patients with severe intellectual deficits compared to 41% for those with mild deficits and 65% for those without deficits [26].

Patients with remote symptomatic epilepsy have remission probabilities similar to those with idiopathic epilepsy (Fig. 1-5). It must be kept in mind, however, that these probabilities are contingent on survival, which is somewhat reduced in secondary epilepsy. However, those patients with remote symptomatic epilepsy who survive have very good prospects for remission.

Among patients with idiopathic epilepsy, the remission probabilities are slightly higher for generalized seizures than for partial-onset seizures (Fig. 1-6). At 20 years after diagnosis, the probability of being in remission was 85% for those with generalized tonic-clonic seizures and 80% for those with absence seizures,

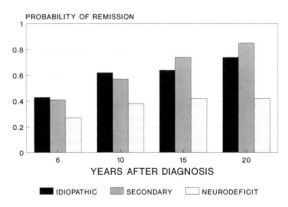

Figure 1-5. Remission of epilepsy by etiology.

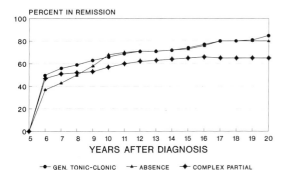

Figure 1-6. Remission by seizure type—idiopathic epilepsy only.

whereas for patients with partial complex seizures the probability for being in remission was only 65%.

References

1. Hauser WA, Kurland LT. The epidemiology of epilepsy in Rochester, Minnesota. *Epilepsia* 1975;16:1–66.
2. Annegers JF, Grabow JD, Groover RV, Laws ER, Elveback LR, Kurland LT. Seizures after head trauma: a population study. *Neurology* 1980;30:683–9.
3. Annegers JF, Hauser WA, Beghi E, Nicolosi A, Kurland LT. The risk of unprovoked seizures after encephalitis and meningitis. *Neurology* 1988;38:1407–10.
4. Clemmesen J, Hjalgrim Jensen S. Brain tumors in children exposed to barbiturates. *J Natl Cancer Inst* 1981;66:215.
5. Shirts SB, Annegers JF, Hauser WA, Kurland LT. Cancer incidence in a cohort of patients with seizure disorders. *J Natl Cancer Inst* 1986;77:83–7.
6. Mathieson G. Pathologic aspects of epilepsy to the surgical pathology of focal cerebral seizures. *Adv Neurol* 1975;8:107–38.
7. Ounsted C, Lindsay J, Norman R. *Biological factors in temporal lobe epilepsy.* Suffolk, England: Lavenham Press, 1966.
8. Annegers JF, Hauser WA, Shirts SB, Kurland LT. Factors prognostic of unprovoked seizures after febrile convulsions. *N Engl J Med* 1987;316:493–8.
9. Nelson KB, and Ellenberg JH. Predictors of epilepsy in children who have experienced febrile seizures. *N Engl J Med* 1976;295:1029–33.
10. Rodin EA, ed. *The prognosis of patients with epilepsy.* Springfield, IL: Charles C Thomas, 1968: 156–71.
11. Heneiksen PB, Juul-Jensen P, Lund M. The mortality of epileptics. *Acta Neurol Scand* 1967;31(Suppl):164–5.
12. Alstrom CH. A study of epilepsy in its clinical, social and genetic aspects. *Acta Psychiatr Neurol Scand* 1950;53 (Suppl).
13. Livingston S. *Living with epileptic seizures.* Springfield, IL: Charles C Thomas, 1963.
14. Steinsiek HD. Über Todesursachen und Lebensdauer bei genuiner Epilepsie. *Arch Psychiatr Zeitsch Neurol* 1950;183:469–80.
15. Iivanainen M, Ldhtinen J. Causes of death in institutionaled epileptics. *Epilepsia* 1979;20:485–92.
16. Loiseau MP, Henry P. Les causes de la mort chez les epileptiques. *Bordeaux Med* 1972;5:2643–8.
17. Krohn W. Causes of death among epileptics. *Epilepsia* 1963;4:315–21.
18. Zielinski JJ. Epilepsy and mortality rate and cause of death. *Epilepsia* 1974;16:191–201.
19. Annegers JF, Hauser WA, Shirts SB. Heart disease mortality and morbidity in patients with epilepsy. *Epilepsia* 1984;25:699–704.
20. Hauser WA, Annegers JF, Elveback LR. Mortality in patients with epilepsy. *Epilepsia* 1980;21:399–412.
21. Gowers WR. *Epilepsy and other chronic convulsive diseases: their causes, symptoms and treatment.* London: William Wood, 1881.
22. Rodin EA. Medical and social prognosis in epilepsy. *Epilepsia* 1972;13:121–31.
23. Annegers JF, Hauser WA, Elveback LR. Remission of seizures and relapse in patients with epilepsy. *Epilepsia* 1979;20:729–39.
24. Elwes RDC, Johnson AL, Shorvon SD, Reynolds EH. The prognosis for seizure control in newly-diagnosed epilepsy. *N Engl J Med* 1984;311:944–7.
25. Goodridge DMG, Shorvon SD. Epilepsy in a population of 6000. 2. Treatment and prognosis. *Br Med J* 1983;297:645–7.
26. Okuma T, Kumashiro H. Natural history and prognosis of epilepsy: report of a multi-institutional study in Japan. *Epilepsia* 1981;22:35–53.
27. Shafer SQ, Hauser WA, Annegers JF, Klass DW. EEG and other predictors of epilepsy remission: a community study. *Epilepsia* 1988;29:590–600.

Chapter 2

Epileptic Syndromes and Their Prognosis

PHILLIP L. PEARL
GREGORY L. HOLMES

Delineation of epileptic syndromes has naturally followed the classification of epileptic seizures. Varying classification schemes of epileptic seizures, based on clinical characteristics, electroencephalographic (EEG) features, and anatomic localization, led eventually to the adoption of the International Classification of Epileptic Seizures (ICES) by the International League Against Epilepsy (ILAE) [1]. The individual seizures, however, are often a component of a constellation of clinical findings customarily occurring together, or epileptic syndrome. Information from the family history, age at onset, and associated neurologic, psychological, and EEG features contribute to the epileptic syndrome. The assignment of a syndrome may imply a particular natural history, choice of therapy, or developmental prognosis. Specific information regarding etiology, structural or genetic, sometimes becomes available when a syndrome diagnosis is established.

The ILAE published a Classification of Epilepsies and Epileptic Syndromes in 1985 [2] and a Proposal for Revised Classification of Epilepsies and Epileptic Syndromes in 1989 [3] (Table 2-1). These divide the syndromes into localization-related and generalized categories, based on whether there is evidence for a localized origin of the seizures. The syndromes are then classified as idiopathic, that is, no underlying cause other than a possible hereditary predisposition; symptomatic, that is, considered the consequence of a central nervous system disorder; or cryptogenic, that is, presumed symptomatic but with unknown etiology. Additionally, allowance is made for syndromes undetermined to be focal or generalized and situation-related seizures.

The classification of epileptic syndromes is in flux and serves as a substrate for enhanced communication, understanding, and research. This chapter describes some of the more widely accepted and recognized pediatric epilepsy syndromes. As the epilepsy syndromes of childhood are largely age-dependent, they are presented in chronological order.

Epileptic Syndromes in Neonates

Benign Neonatal Convulsions

Two syndromes, benign idiopathic neonatal convulsions (BINC) and benign familial neonatal convulsions (BFNC), have been formulated [4] (Table 2-2). The former, also known as "fifth day fits," may occur between days 1 and 7, but with 80% occurring between days 4 and 6 (Fig. 2-1). The seizures are clonic or apneic and frequently evolve into status epilepticus. The interictal electroencephalogram (EEG) has been reported to show a pattern of synchronous and asynchronous sharp theta bursts, the so-called theta pointu alternant. Once the infant recovers from the flurry of seizures, there is no increased risk of epilepsy and the neurologic prognosis is excellent.

In BFNC, the convulsions cluster on the second and third days of life, although exceptions occur, with onset as late as 3 months of age (Fig. 2-2). There are no specific EEG criteria. Although later epilepsy occurs in up to 14% of patients, the developmental outcome is favorable. This syndrome is rare but autosomal dominant, and DNA linkage analysis has recently mapped the responsible gene to the long arm of chromosome 20 [5].

Table 2-1. Overview of Syndromes in the International Classification of the Epilepsies and Epileptic Syndromes

1. Localization-related
   1.1 Idiopathic
       Benign childhood epilepsy with centrotemporal spikes
       Childhood epilepsy with occipital paroxysms
       Primary reading epilepsy
   1.2 Symptomatic
       Chronic progressive epilepsia partialis continua of childhood (Kojewnikow's syndrome)
       Temporal lobe epilepsies
       Frontal lobe epilepsies
       Parietal lobe epilepsies
       Occipital lobe epilepsies
2. Generalized
   2.1 Idiopathic
       Benign neonatal familial convulsions
       Benign neonatal convulsions
       Benign myoclonic epilepsy in infancy
       Childhood absence epilepsy (pyknolepsy)
       Juvenile absence epilepsy
       Juvenile myoclonic epilepsy
       Epilepsy with grand mal on awakening
       Reflex epilepsies
   2.2 Cryptogenic or symptomatic
       West syndrome (infantile spasms)
       Lennox-Gastaut syndrome
       Epilepsy with myoclonic-astatic seizures
       Epilepsy with myoclonic absences
   2.3 Symptomatic
       2.3.1 Nonspecific etiology
             Early myoclonic encephalopathy
             Early infantile epileptic encephalopathy with suppression-burst (Ohtahara)
       2.3.2 Specific syndromes
             Diseases in which seizures are a presenting or predominant feature
3. Epilepsies and syndromes undetermined whether focal or generalized
   3.1 With both generalized and focal seizures
       Neonatal seizures
       Severe myoclonic epilepsy in infancy
       Epilepsy with continuous spike-wave during slow-wave sleep (ESES)
       Acquired epileptic aphasia (Landau-Kleffner syndrome)
   3.2 Without unequivocal generalized or focal features
       All cases with generalized tonic-clonic seizures in which clinical and EEG findings do not permit classification as clearly generalized or localization related
4. Special syndromes
   4.1 Situation-related
       Febrile seizures
       Isolated seizures or isolated status epilepticus
       Metabolic or toxic induced seizures

Adapted from Commission on Classification and Terminology of the International League Against Epilepsy. Proposal for revised classification of epilepsies and epileptic syndromes. *Epilepsia* 1989;30:389–99. With permission from F.E. Driefuss, President ILAE, and the publisher.

Table 2-2. Summary of Clinical and Electroencephalographic Features of Benign Neonatal Convulsions

Clinical Features	BINC	BFNC
Age of onset	First week (typically day 5)	First week (typically day 2–3)
Type of seizure	Clonic	Clonic
EEG	Variable (theta pointu alternant)	Variable
Family history	Negative	Positive
Outcome	Favorable	Favorable

Early Myoclonic Encephalopathy

This devastating syndrome, often familial, has its onset before 3 months of age (Table 2-3). Initially there is fragmentary myoclonus, which may be continuous but often is quite restricted, for example, to a finger or eyebrow [6]. This is followed by erratic partial seizures, massive myoclonus, or infantile spasms [7].

The EEG reveals a suppression-burst pattern. The bursts are characterized by synchronous and asynchronous 1- to 5-s paroxysms of irregular spikes, sharp waves, and slow waves. These paroxysms are separated by 3- to 10-s flattened periods. The bursts are variably synchronous with the clinical myoclonus [6]. The EEG evolves into modified hypsarrhythmia or multifocal discharges.

The clinical course is inexorably progressive, with death occurring within the first 2 years. Although the etiologies are diverse, metabolic disorders compose a large group, especially nonketotic hyperglycin emia and D-glyceric acidemia. Antiepileptic agents, as well as corticosteroids and pyridoxine, are ineffective [6].

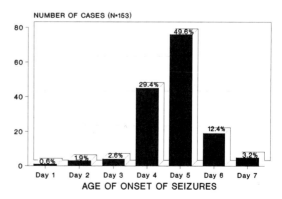

Figure 2-1. Age-related incidence of benign idiopathic neonatal convulsions.

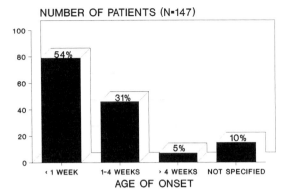

NUMBER OF PATIENTS (N=147)

Figure 2-2. Age-related incidence of benign familial neonatal convulsions.

Ohtahara described a similar syndrome of frequent tonic spasms but rare myoclonic seizures [8,9]. This "early infantile epileptic encephalopathy" has onset before 20 days and a suppression-burst EEG pattern.

Epileptic Syndromes in Infancy and Early Childhood

Infantile Spasms (West Syndrome)

West syndrome consists of a triad of infantile spasms, psychomotor retardation, and hypsarrhythmia. Although one of these elements may be missing, the presence of spasms is generally considered essential [10]. The onset usually occurs within the first 6–8 months of life, with a peak at 5 months.

The spasms are tonic muscle contractions and may be flexor, extensor, head nods, or, most commonly, mixed flexor-extensor [11,12]. The spasms tend to cluster and usually occur on awakening or falling asleep.

The interictal EEG reveals hypsarrhythmia, a pattern originally described by Gibbs and Gibbs [13] and characterized by a continuously abnormal background of high-voltage synchronous and asynchronous shifting sharp and slow waves (Fig. 2-3). This prototypic pattern, when seen, usually occurs in the early stages. More commonly, the EEG shows a variation of this pattern, or modified hypsarrhythmia (Fig. 2-4). Modified hypsarrhythmia, described by Hrachovy et al. [14], manifests as: (a) hypsarrhythmia with increased interhemispheric synchrony; (b) asymmetric or unilateral hypsarrhythmia; (c) hypsarrhythmia with a consistent focus of abnormal discharge; (d) hypsarrhythmia with episodes of generalized, regional, or localized voltage attenuation (suppression-burst variant); or (e) hypsarrhythmia composed primarily of high-voltage, bilaterally asynchronous, slow-wave activity. Additionally, alterations occur during sleep-wake cycling, with normalization of the EEG during rapid eye movement (REM) sleep and maximal expression of the hypsarrhythmia during slow-wave sleep.

The ictal EEG is associated with a transient attenuation of hypsarrhythmia and the appearance of up to 11 different patterns [12]. These consist of generalized slow-wave transients, sharp and slow-wave transients, attenuation episodes, or attenuation episodes with superimposed faster frequencies, either singly or in various combinations. The most common ictal pattern is a high-voltage, generalized, slow-wave transient followed by an abrupt attenuation of background activity, lasting from one to several seconds.

Patients with West syndrome have traditionally been divided into two groups, cryptogenic and symptomatic. Up to 10–15% of patients have been identified as cryptogenic, that is, there are no known historical etiologic explanations, neurodevelopmental status is normal up to the onset of the spasms, and the computed tomography (CT) scan is normal [15–18]. Potential etiologic factors, including a multitude of pre-, peri-, and postnatal conditions, can be identified in 60% of patients [19]. As metabolic studies

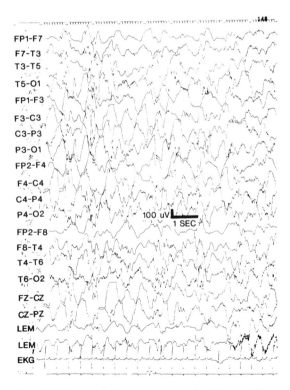

Figure 2-3. Hypsarrhythmia in a 4-month-old boy with West syndrome.

Table 2-3. Comparison of Early and Benign Myoclonic Epilepsies of Infancy

Clinical Features	Early Myoclonic	Benign Myoclonic	Severe Myoclonic
Age of onset	< 3 months	First 2 years	5–6 months
Family history	Frequently positive	Frequently positive	Frequently positive
Seizure type	Myoclonic	Myoclonic	Clonic, myoclonic
EEG	Burst-suppression	Spike-wave	Spike-wave
		Normal background	Focal abnormalities
Outcome	Poor	Favorable	Poor

and neuroimaging techniques have become more sophisticated, etiologic factors will likely be found in an increasing proportion of patients.

The therapy remains controversial, with little consensus on choice of drug, dose, or schedule. Hormonal therapy remains the mainstay of treatment, although the efficacy of adrenocorticotropic hormone (ACTH) versus prednisone remains controversial [20]. One study using high-dosage ACTH (initially 150 U/M^2/day the first week) found that 30 of 30 patients with infantile spasms and hypsarrhythmia responded, versus 8 of 13 patients treated with prednisone (initially 3 mg/kg/day) [21]. Seizures recurred, however, in 14 of the 30 ACTH-treated patients

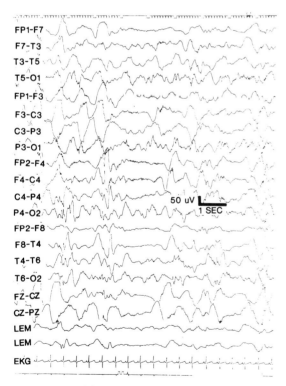

Figure 2-4. Modified hypsarrhythmia (episodes of generalized and lateralized voltage attenuation). This 3-month-old boy with infantile spasms had an aminoaciduria determined to be secondary to cobalamin C deficiency.

within 6 months. This study was not randomized or blinded, and depended on parental report.

In a controlled study comparing low-dosage ACTH and prednisone, utilizing objective video-polygraphic monitoring, the Baylor group [18] found that the response to therapy was all or none only, and that ACTH (20–30 U/day) and prednisone (2 mg/kg/day) shared the same efficacy. About 60–70% of patients responded to either therapy, and this was independent of whether there was a treatment lag over 5 weeks or whether the patient was cryptogenic or symptomatic. Regarding the issue of high-dose versus low-dose ACTH, a retrospective analysis disclosed no difference [22], although a prospective study is currently under way to address this question (RA Hrachovy, personal communication).

A prospective study of 64 treated patients by the Baylor group [15] found that only 5% of the total group had a normal long-term outcome, and the only predictive factor was whether the patient was cryptogenic or symptomatic. Of the cryptogenic group, 38% of patients were normal or only mildly impaired, in contrast to 5% of the symptomatic group. No significant difference in long-term outcome was found between responders and nonresponders to the hormonal therapy. Other seizure types occurred in approximately half of these patients.

Other therapies reportedly effective against infantile spasms are valproic acid [23,24], benzodiazepines including nitrazepam [19,25], and occasionally pyridoxine [26–28].

Benign Myoclonic Epilepsy in Infancy

This rare syndrome is characterized by brief, generalized myoclonic attacks in otherwise normal children during the first 2 years of life [29]. Initially the seizures are very subtle, often described by parents as "spasms" or "head nodding." They become more frequent and intense, and may lead to falls. In contrast to infantile spasms, the attacks are sporadic and occur any time of day. The family history is frequently positive for epilepsy.

The EEG reveals a corresponding generalized 3-Hz spike-wave or multiple spike-wave discharges with an otherwise normal background. Other than simple febrile seizures in some patients, other seizure types are not observed.

The seizures are responsive to valproic acid but tend to persist if left untreated. Generalized tonic-clonic seizures are occasionally seen as late as puberty, and mild neurodevelopmental problems have been described.

This syndrome is distinct from nonepileptic benign myoclonus of early infancy [30]. The latter syndrome has no EEG abnormality, has an earlier onset (4–8 months), and is characterized by spontaneous remission in the second year.

Severe Myoclonic Epilepsy in Infancy

This is a recently defined syndrome, but it appears to be relatively homogeneous and should be distinguished from benign myoclonic epilepsy in infancy (Table 2-3) [31]. The onset usually occurs between 5 and 6 months of age and is heralded by generalized or unilateral febrile clonic seizures, often prolonged and leading to status. Between the ages of 1 and 4 years, myoclonic jerks and complex partial seizures are seen. The family history is positive for epilepsy or febrile seizures in 25% of cases.

The EEG shows generalized fast spike-wave or multiple spike-wave discharges, activated by photic stimulation and sleep. Focal epileptiform abnormalities and rhythmic central theta rhythms are also seen.

Development is normal until the onset, then unfortunately declines and other neurologic signs appear, including ataxia, hyperreflexia, and interictal myoclonus. The seizures are refractory to therapy, and the outcome is poor. This syndrome is distinct from Lennox-Gastaut because of its earlier onset, stereotypical presentation, and absence of slow diffuse spike-waves and multiple spike bursts in sleep on the EEG.

Epilepsy with Myoclonic-Astatic Seizures

This syndrome was described by Doose et al. as centrencephalic myoclonic-astatic petit mal of childhood [32]. The syndrome consists of myoclonic, astatic, and myoclonic-astatic seizures, often in combination with absences, generalized tonic-clonic and tonic seizures, and nonconvulsive status [33]. The status is characterized by apathy or stupor with irregular myoclonus, and tends to occur on awakening.

Onset is between 7 months and 6 years of age and most commonly occurs between 2 and 5 years of age. The first events are febrile seizures in one third of cases. Development is normal until the onset of seizures in 85% of these children. Boys are affected twice as commonly as girls, unless onset is in the first year. The family history is positive for epilepsy or febrile seizures in approximately one third of cases.

The EEG at the onset may show monomorphic rhythmic theta rhythms and irregular spike-waves in sleep. Later, bilateral synchronous irregular 2- to 5-Hz spike-and-wave complexes appear, with an anterior voltage predominance. During status, there are long runs of 2- to 3-Hz spike-and-wave complexes.

The course and prognosis are variable. Valproate is generally considered the treatment of choice. The course may be benign, and spontaneous remissions may occur without any therapy. The prognosis is unfavorable, however, in approximately half of patients, with persistent generalized tonic-clonic seizures, astatic-myoclonic status, and dementia.

Lennox-Gastaut Syndrome

Lennox-Gastaut syndrome is an age-dependent generalized symptomatic or cryptogenic epileptic syndrome. There are three essential features: (a) intractable seizures of multiple types; (b) psychomotor retardation; and (c) generalized slow (less than 2.5 Hz) spike-and-wave interictal EEG pattern (Fig. 2-5). The initial description of this syndrome was made by Gibbs et al. [34] in their identification of the "petit mal variant" on EEG, and Lennox et al. [35] and Gastaut et al. [36] in their descriptions of the associated clinical features.

The syndrome has a prevalence of 3–10% among children with epilepsy [37]. Onset is usually between ages 1 and 6 years, and boys are more frequently affected [38,39]. The most frequently occurring seizures are tonic, tonic-clonic, atonic, myoclonic, and atypical absences. Drop attacks are particularly disabling. Absence status is characteristic, and frank stupor to subtle dullness may persist for weeks or months.

Seizures may occur many times a day, particularly atypical absences and atonic seizures. Myoclonic and myoclonic-astatic seizures can also be frequent, especially on falling asleep or awakening.

The essential EEG feature is the interictal generalized slow spike-and-wave pattern [38]. Other associated patterns include independent multifocal spike discharges [40] and brief runs of generalized,

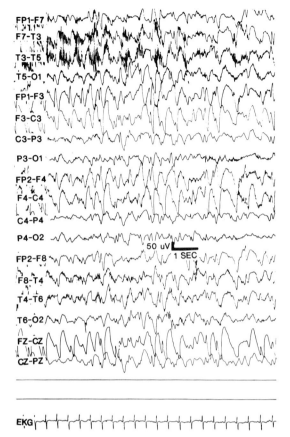

Figure 2-5. A 4-year-old girl with Lennox-Gastaut syndrome. The EEG contains runs of generalized frontocentral dominant 2- to 2.5-Hz spike-and-wave discharges.

paroxysmal fast activity [41]. While the latter resemble the EEG beta discharges accompanying tonic seizures, they tend to occur in sleep without clinical manifestation.

An etiology can be identified in approximately 60% of patients [42,43]. Factors include prenatal, perinatal, and postnatal factors, and both static and, less commonly, progressive disorders. A positive family history has been reported in 2.5–27% of cases [44], but this finding partially reflects the diverse definitions of the syndrome used and the syndrome's role as a component in some inherited disorders, particularly tuberous sclerosis. The evolution of West syndrome to Lennox-Gastaut syndrome is well known, although not constant.

The differential diagnosis of Lennox-Gastaut syndrome includes partial epilepsies, often frontal or mesial hemispheric, or benign generalized syndromes that transiently worsen with atonic or myoclonic

seizures and diffuse slow spike-and-wave pattern on the EEG. This deterioration may be on account of an intercurrent illness or an anticonvulsant overdose [37]. The border zone between Lennox-Gastaut syndrome and myoclonic-astatic epilepsy is blurred. The latter usually occurs in a previously well child with a positive family history for epilepsy, and posterior theta rhythms with fast generalized spike-and-wave pattern on the EEG.

Valproate usually provides the most broad coverage of the various seizure types, although benzodiazepines, particularly clonazepam, have a similar spectrum of action. Although other antiepileptic agents and the ketogenic diet may be helpful, these patients are relatively refractory to therapy. Additionally, atypical absences have been associated with use of carbamazepine [45] and precipitation of tonic status epilepticus with intravenous benzodiazepines [46,47].

Corpus callosotomy is being used increasingly in Lennox-Gastaut syndrome patients, particularly to control the drop attacks. Because disconnection syndromes and long-lasting neurologic sequelae may result from both partial and complete sections, the indications and efficacy of this procedure are currently undergoing evaluation. Patients with prior focal deficits or mixed cerebral dominance for language and handedness seem to be at highest risk for postoperative sequelae [48].

Even with improved seizure control, the prognosis is poor in light of some other neurologic and mental impairment. Risk factors for poor outcome include seizure onset before 2 years of age [43], symptomatic character, evolution from West syndrome, frequent seizures or status epilepticus, and persistently very slow (less than 1.5 Hz) background activity on repeated EEGs [49].

Epileptic Syndromes in Childhood

Childhood Absence Epilepsy (Pyknolepsy)

Childhood absence epilepsy, or pyknolepsy, describes a homogeneous group of children with typical absence seizures who are otherwise normal. Onset occurs between 3 and 12 years of age, with a peak at 6–7 years [50]. There is a strong genetic predisposition, with family histories frequently positive for absence and tonic-clonic seizures. Girls are affected three times more commonly than are boys [51–53].

The absence seizure is characterized by a brief impairment of consciousness with abrupt onset and cessation. Ninety percent of absences have associated

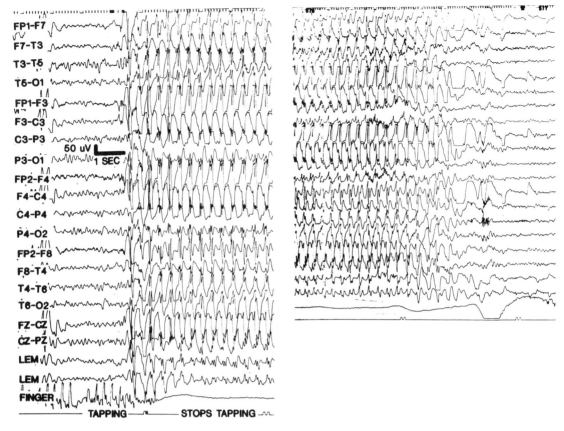

Figure 2-6. Absence seizure in an 8-year-old girl with pyknolepsy. A generalized 3-Hz spike-and-wave paroxysm is elicited during hyperventilation. The complexes are often slightly faster at the onset and slower at the end of the discharge.

automatisms or mild clonic, atonic, tonic, or autonomic components. The seizures cluster and may occur hundreds of times a day. Generalized tonic-clonic seizures occur in 40% of patients [51–55].

Absence seizures must be differentiated from complex partial seizures and daydreaming. Absence seizures are classically induced by hyperventilation but can also be precipitated by boredom, drowsiness, stress, and occasionally eye closure. The EEG is most helpful in helping to differentiate among these seizure types. In childhood absence seizures, the EEG shows paroxysms of synchronous, generalized but frontally predominant, 3-Hz spike-and-wave discharges (Fig. 2-6). These discharges have abrupt onset and cessation in an otherwise normal background. Variations in these discharges include spike-and-wave frequencies at 6 or even 12 Hz, asymmetric discharges that are slight and variable in onset or amplitude, high-amplitude slow waves without spikes, bilaterally independent frontopolar spikes, and irregular patterns

in sleep [57]. A normal EEG that includes several trials of 3–5 min of hyperventilation virtually rules out absence seizures.

Atypical absence seizures would not be expected in childhood absence epilepsy. These usually begin before 5 years of age and are associated with other generalized seizure types and mental retardation. The atypical absence seizure tends to have a longer duration and more change in tone than the typical absence seizure [58]. The EEG reveals background abnormalities and 1.5 to 2.5 Hz slow spike or multiple spike-and-wave ictal discharges, which may be irregular or asymmetric (Fig. 2-7) [59,60].

The first-line therapeutic agents are ethosuximide and valproate. Although both are equally effective [55,56,61–63], most clinicians start with ethosuximide because of the rare but severe hepatotoxicity and pancreatitis associated with valproate [64–67]. Valproate is recommended for patients with generalized tonic-clonic seizures [68,69]. The combination of ethosuximide and valproate may be more effective than either drug alone [62,70], although drug interactions require careful monitoring [71]. Clonazepam is also efficacious but has limited use because of sedation, behavioral side effects, and tolerance [72,73]. The combination of valproate and clonazepam has been associated with precipitation of absence status [66].

Most clinicians taper the medication after 2 or 3 seizure-free years, as long as the EEG contains no more than fragmentary discharges during drowsiness and sleep. A more epileptiform EEG usually means that the child is having continuing absences that have been missed.

Childhood absence epilepsy responds well to medical therapy and has an overall favorable prognosis. Risk factors for persistent seizures include onset of tonic-clonic seizures prior to absences, absences with prominent myoclonic or atonic components, a positive family history, and mental or neurologic deficits. Ninety percent of patients with none of these risk factors remit [74].

A related but probably distinct syndrome is myoclonic absence epilepsy [75]. These absences are characterized by severe bilateral rhythmic myoclonic jerks. The average age of onset is 7 years, and there is a male preponderance. The seizures occur several times every day and do not cluster like those of pyknolepsy. The EEG is the same as in childhood absence epilepsy. Although associated tonic-clonic seizures are unusual, the prognosis is worse than that of pyknolepsy. The seizures are difficult to control, and mental deterioration and evolution of the Lennox-Gastaut syndrome occur.

Still another variant syndrome is eyelid myoclonia with absences [76]. This is characterized by marked myoclonic jerks of the eyelids with upward deviation of the eyes. The EEG shows paroxysmal discharges on eye closure and a photoconvulsive response. The age of onset is 6 ± 2 years, and spontaneous absences and tonic-clonic seizures occur. The response to therapy and prognosis are not as good as in pyknolepsy.

Benign Partial Epilepsies

Benign Rolandic Epilepsy

Also known as benign childhood epilepsy with centrotemporal spikes, sylvian epilepsy, or benign focal epilepsy of childhood, this common syndrome is seen in 15–20% of children with epilepsy [77]. Age of onset ranges between 2 and 13 years but is usually

between 5 and 10 years, with a peak at 9 years [78]. There is a slight male predominance. As in absence seizures, genetic studies indicate that the EEG trait is inherited, probably as an autosomal-dominant gene with age-dependent penetrance [79]. Only 25% of persons with this EEG trait, however, actually experience seizures [80].

The hallmark seizure type is a brief hemifacial tonic or clonic contraction, associated with oropharyngeal symptoms and homolateral sensorimotor phenomena. Oropharyngeal symptoms include excessive salivation with difficulty in swallowing, guttural sounds, involuntary tongue or jaw movements, numbness or paresthesias of the tongue, gum, and cheek, or speech arrest [81].

Three fourths of patients have seizures only during sleep [82]. Typically, a child awakens and comes to his parents unable to speak, with his mouth twisted and drooling. Hemifacial twitches may be seen, and the

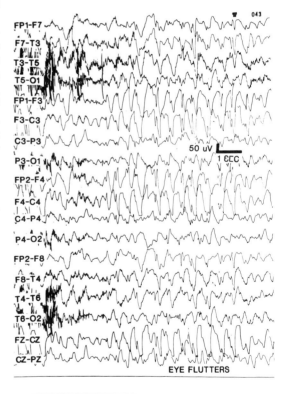

Figure 2-7. Atypical absence seizure in a 4-year-old girl with Lennox-Gastaut syndrome. A paroxysm of generalized slow spike-and-wave (1½- to 2-Hz) activity is accompanied by eyelid flutters.

spell is over within a couple of minutes. Loss of consciousness and even generalized tonic-clonic convulsions can occur. In the latter case, a postictal paralysis after a nocturnal seizure may be the only clue as to the nature of the syndrome. Somatosensory oral and pharyngeal auras are probably common but underreported [83].

The classic EEG contains interictal high-amplitude, broad centrotemporal spike discharges on an otherwise normal background (Fig. 2-8). The spikes may be unilateral or bilateral or shift from side to side in serial recordings of the same patient. They tend to exhibit an electrical horizontal dipole with maximum temporal negativity and frontal positivity (Fig. 2-9). The spikes tend to occur in runs and are activated by drowsiness and sleep (Fig. 2-10).

Associated paroxysmal abnormalities, including multiple spike foci, occipital foci, and bilateral synchronous 3-Hz spike-and-wave discharges with absence seizures, have been reported [78,82,84].

The prognosis is excellent, and the most important point regarding surgical evaluation is to not mistake

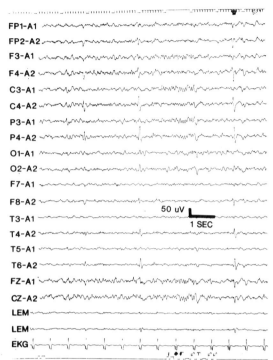

Figure 2-9. Benign rolandic epilepsy. Same patient as in Figure 2-8. The referential montage assists in demonstrating the horizontal electrical dipole, with maximal right frontopolar positivity and temporal negativity. The voltage of the temporal discharges is affected by the "contaminated" ear reference.

the EEG finding as supportive of temporal lobe epilepsy. The visceral aura, clouding of consciousness, and automatisms or psychic phenomena of complex partial seizures are absent [77].

One fifth of patients with benign rolandic epilepsy have a single seizure, and another one fifth may have seizures in clusters but with long seizure-free intervals [82]. Although serial or prolonged seizures have been reported in up to 25% of patients [85], complete remission occurs in almost all cases, and associated neuropsychological difficulties are absent assuming the benign nature of the syndrome is emphasized and overly vigorous use of pharmaceuticals is avoided.

Benign Epilepsy with Occipital Paroxysms

This is another familial, school-age, benign epileptic syndrome but is quite uncommon. The seizures are characterized by visual illusions or blindness, followed by hemiclonic seizures or automatisms [86].

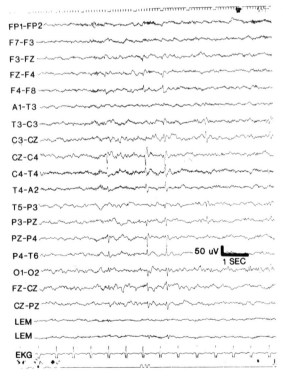

Figure 2-8. Benign rolandic epilepsy. This 9-year-old boy presented with a single left tonic seizure on awakening. The EEG reveals frequent right centrotemporal spikes in drowsiness.

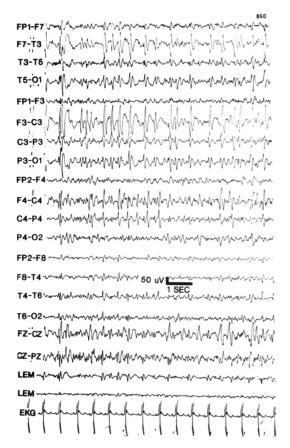

Figure 2-10. A 6-year-old girl with benign rolandic epilepsy. Note the activation of the discharges during drowsiness.

There is a postictal headache in up to one third of patients. The headache is usually diffuse, but sometimes is hemicranial, and often is associated with nausea and vomiting.

The interictal EEG reveals unilateral or bilateral posterior high-amplitude spike-and-wave semirhythmic paroxysms that occur on eye closure. The background is otherwise normal. During seizures, these occipital discharges spread to the central or temporal areas, corresponding to the clinical ictal manifestations.

The classic anticonvulsant medications are effective, with complete seizure control in 60% of 53 patients in one study [86]. Remission of epilepsy occurs in adolescence in 95%. There are cases of benign childhood partial epilepsy with both occipital paroxysms and centrotemporal spikes.

Benign Partial Epilepsy with Affective Symptoms (Benign Psychomotor Epilepsy)

This rare syndrome consists of frequent affective seizures with a benign outcome. Age of onset is between 2 and 9 years, and there is a family history for epilepsy in over one third of patients [87]. The seizures are characterized by sudden fright or terror, sometimes associated with oropharyngeal or autonomic symptoms. The attacks are stereotypical and occur in both waking and sleep states, particularly when falling asleep. The EEG reveals broad frontotemporal or parietotemporal spike discharges that are activated by sleep. The background is otherwise normal. The seizures respond to the first-line antiepileptic agents.

Although behavioral and psychological problems have been reported at the time of frequent seizures, the prognosis for complete recovery without neurologic abnormalities is excellent. As in the other benign pediatric epilepsy syndromes, the distinction between these attacks and lesion-associated complex partial seizures is paramount. The latter may have affective symptomatology but usually occurs in the setting of an aura with more polymorphous seizures and prominent motor activity.

Landau-Kleffner Syndrome

First described by Landau and Kleffner [88], this syndrome is also known as acquired epileptic aphasia. There is an insidious deterioration of language, taking the form of a verbal auditory agnosia, associated with paroxysmal epileptiform EEG abnormalities. Seizures are seen in two thirds of patients, and psychomotor disturbances are common.

This rare nonfamilial disorder of early childhood has a male predominance of 2:1. Early language development is most often normal, but progressive loss of comprehension for words and even for familiar noises follows. Verbal expression is also affected, with stereotypies, perseverations, paraphasic errors, and loss of speech. Other intellectual functions, including writing, may be preserved. Personality and psychomotor disturbances, particularly hyperkinesis, are frequent [89].

The EEG shows high-amplitude diffuse spike and spike-and-wave discharges, often with a temporal (one half of cases) or parieto-occipital (one third of cases) predominance (Fig. 2-11). Focal discharges also occur. Sleep activates the discharges, and the pattern

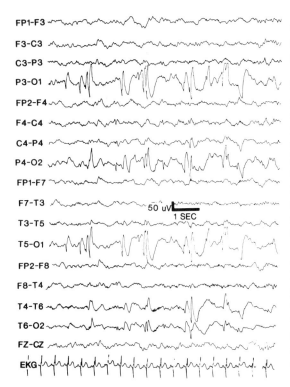

Figure 2-11. A 4-year-old boy with Landau-Kleffner syndrome. The EEG reveals high-amplitude posterior spike-and-wave complexes with right posterior temporal extension. There was no history of seizures.

may be identical to epilepsy with continuous spike-and-wave during slow-wave sleep (see Epilepsy with Continuous Spike-and-Wave During Slow-Wave Sleep).

Seizures are absent in 30% of patients. In one third, there is a single convulsion or bout of status epilepticus at approximately the beginning of the disorder. When later seizures do occur, they are mainly nocturnal, generalized, or simply partial, and responsive to anticonvulsant therapy. The seizures remit in adolescence, and the aphasia improves to a variable extent. Hormonal therapy with steroids has been advocated [90].

Epilepsy with Continuous Spike-and-Wave During Slow-Wave Sleep

This rare pediatric syndrome, first described in 1971 [91], is also known as epilepsy with electrical status epilepticus during slow sleep (ESES). The mean age of seizure onset is 4 years and 6 months [92]. The epilepsy is characterized by rare partial or generalized

motor attacks (not tonic) in sleep and atypical absences in wakefulness. The seizures remit spontaneously in adolescence.

The hallmark EEG finding is continuous generalized spike-and-wave during slow-wave sleep and appears 1–2 years after the onset of seizures. An index of 85% has been used as a guideline for the affected time of slow-wave sleep [91,92], although other authors have used a minimum index of 50% [93]. Normal non-rapid eye movement (NREM) sleep features, for example, spindles and vertex sharp transients, may not be identifiable. Waking and REM records reveal rare diffuse or focal paroxysmal abnormalities. The electrographic status disappears at an average age of 12.5 years.

The overall prognosis is not optimistic. Neuropsychological deterioration occurs during the time of ESES with decrease in intelligence quotient (IQ), impairment of language, memory, and temporospatial orientation, disturbances of personality and attention, and occasionally psychosis. Hence, there is considerable overlap with the Landau-Kleffner syndrome. Antiepileptic therapy is largely ineffective, except for some partial success with ACTH [93,94].

Epilepsia Partialis Continua

Two particular types of epilepsia partialis continua, or Kojewnikow's syndrome, can be distinguished. One is a focal nonprogressive form seen in both adults and children [95]; the other is a diffuse unilateral chronic encephalitis of childhood and adolescence, or Rasmussen's encephalitis [96].

The focal form is characterized by continuous, well-localized partial motor seizures, followed in time by myoclonic jerks. The jerks tend to be quite distal, although jacksonian spread and even generalization may occur [97]. The jerks may increase with emotion, attempts at movement, or proprioceptive input. The EEG shows corresponding focal epileptiform discharges, which rarely are periodic lateralized discharges time-locked to the jerks [98]. The background is otherwise normal.

These seizures are the result of fixed rolandic cortical lesions, including vascular, neoplastic, and, most commonly in children, atrophic processes. Metabolic dysfunction, including nonketotic hyperglycinemia and mitochondrial encephalopathy (e.g., mitochondrial encephalomyopathy, lactic acidosis, stroke-like episodes [MELAS]), has also been associated with this syndrome [3,99].

The seizures may persist for hours to months to years, or reappear intermittently [97,100]. They are notoriously resistant to medical treatment, and limited cortical excision, when feasible, is curative [95].

The chronic progressive form, or Rasmussen's encephalitis, has onset between 2 and 10 years and includes other seizure types, especially complex partial. The myoclonus becomes erratic and diffuse, and associated neurologic dysfunction, including mental deterioration, aphasia, hemiplegia, and abnormal movements, occurs [97]. Neuroimaging shows progressive atrophy of the frontotemporal region, whole hemisphere, or even the whole cerebrum. The EEG ranges from focal spike discharges in the corresponding brain area to multifocal discharges or even unilateral or diffuse slowing without focal or epileptiform features. Although a viral etiology is suspected, the cerebrospinal fluid (CSF) examination is normal in over half of patients [101], and pathologic studies reveal nonspecific inflammatory changes.

The prognosis is grave with continued seizures and progressive encephalopathy. Control with antiepileptic drugs cannot be expected. Modified hemispherectomy is advocated once the focal paresis is disabling and the diagnosis firm [102].

Epileptic Syndromes in Adolescence

Juvenile Myoclonic Epilepsy

Although reported since the nineteenth century, the syndrome of juvenile myoclonic epilepsy (JME) or impulsive petit mal was delineated by Janz in the 1950s and subsequently named after him [103]. This syndrome appears between 12 and 18 years of age with early morning mild to moderate myoclonia, predominantly of the neck, shoulders, and arms. The intensity may range from a subjective feeling of shakiness or mild electric shocks to violent flinging of

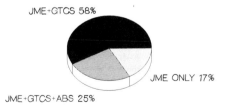

Figure 2-12. Proportion of seizure types in 275 patients with JME. From Asconape J, Penry JK: Some clinical and EEG aspects of benign juvenile myoclonic epilepsy. *Epilepsia* 1984;25:108–14. With permission from the authors and publisher.

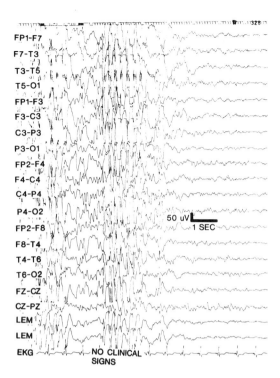

Figure 2-13. Generalized fast-spike or polyspike-and-wave paroxysms in an 11-year-old girl with JME.

objects and rarely falling. Consciousness is unaffected. Generalized tonic-clonic seizures occur in almost all patients and are often the reason for seeking medical advice [104]. The myoclonic jerks may culminate into a generalized tonic-clonic seizure. Multiple environmental factors, including sleep deprivation, fatigue, stress, menses, alcohol, and recreational drugs, are well known to exacerbate the seizures [104,105]. Absences occur in a significant proportion of patients (Fig. 2-12) [104,106].

The interictal EEG abnormality is a fast (3.5- to 6-Hz), irregular spike-and-wave or multiple spike-and-wave complex (Fig. 2-13). Photic stimulation and sleep deprivation activate the discharges. During the myoclonias, rapid multiple spike discharges followed by irregular slow waves can be seen.

It may be difficult to predict whether a patient with absences will develop JME. Absences may begin up to 9 years prior to the onset of myoclonic and tonic-clonic seizures [106]. The distinction between childhood absence and JME is important, as lifelong antiepileptic therapy is recommended for the latter. Recent comparative EEG studies have identified characteristic differences between the absence syndromes [106,107]. The ictal EEG discharge is briefer in JME (mean 6.6 ± 4.2 s) than in pyknolepsy (12.4 ± 2.1 s) or in juvenile absence epilepsy (16.3 ± 7.1 s). JME tends to be characterized by more multiple spikes and fragmented discharges.

Differential diagnosis between JME and the Lennox-Gastaut syndrome, epilepsy with myoclonic astatic seizures, and epilepsy with myoclonic absences essentially lies in the earlier age of onset of the latter syndromes, as well as more severe seizures and mental impairment. Differentiation must be made from the progressive myoclonus epilepsies, in which nonepileptic myoclonus and epileptic seizures coexist. These tend to be degenerative disorders associated with variable degrees of cerebellar ataxia and dementia. Although these disorders run a gamut from familial syndromes with or without neuronal storage products to metabolic and mitochondrial disorders, in general the myoclonus is more sporadic, focal, and refractory to treatment than that of JME.

Since the epileptic components of JME include myoclonic, tonic-clonic, and absence seizures, valproate is recommended as the antiepileptic agent of choice for its spectrum of efficacy. Between 80 and 90% of patients can be controlled with valproate, alone or in combination with other medicines [108]. As stated, relapses can be expected if antiepileptic therapy is discontinued. The environmental triggers alluded to earlier are the areas on which to concentrate in order to achieve the greatest yield in seizure control.

The genetic inheritance of JME has been recently intensely studied, and the gene has been mapped to chromosome locus 6p21.3 [109]. Using both epileptic and asymptomatic "EEG-positive" relatives of 68 JME patients, deoxyribonucleic acid (DNA) linkage analysis showed the JME gene is tightly linked to the properdin factor B (Bf)-HLA (human leukocyte antigen) loci on chromosome 6. Some of the affected family members had different seizure types than their JME probands, including tonic-clonic, absence, and febrile seizures. The challenge of molecular biology in epilepsy will be to explain the genetic diversity of the inherited epilepsies, as well as the genetic susceptibility to acquired epilepsy.

Juvenile Absence Epilepsy

Juvenile absence epilepsy begins around the time of puberty and differs from pyknolepsy in that the seizures are more sporadic and the sex distribution is equal. Retropulsive movements have been reported much less commonly than in pyknolepsy [110,111]. This syndrome blurs with JME, as generalized tonic-clonic seizures and myoclonias may be seen on awakening (Table 2-4). Generalized tonic-clonic seizures have been reported in up to 83% of patients [110].

The EEG spike-waves during absences are often slightly faster than 3 Hz (3.5–4 Hz). Sleep deprivation and hyperventilation are potent activators. Photic stimulation, alternatively, is much less of an activator in juvenile absence epilepsy than in childhood absence epilepsy, JME, or the syndrome of generalized tonic-clonic seizures on awakening [110] (see Photosensitive Epilepsy, below). The response to therapy is good, although those patients with incomplete absence control tend to have poor control of the generalized tonic-clonic seizures as well [110].

There is a tendency toward absence status in juvenile absence epilepsy. This is a nonconvulsive status epilepticus characterized by persistent impairment of consciousness associated with generalized, irregular, approximately 3-Hz spike-and-wave EEG discharges. Most patients appear dull and confused but are partially responsive and able to carry out routine tasks [112]. Facial twitching, eye blinking, staring, and automatisms may be noted [113–116]. The EEG may also show multiple spike-and-wave discharges, prolonged bursts of generalized spike discharges, or irregular slow spike-and-wave discharges [112]. Intravenous diazepam is effective [116], although

Table 2-4. Comparison of Childhood Absence, Juvenile Absence, and Juvenile Myoclonic Epilepsy

Clinical Features	Childhood	Juvenile	JME
Age of onset	3–12 years	Puberty	Puberty
Frequency	Multiple daily	Rarely daily	Variable
EEG epileptiform activity	3-Hz spike-wave	3.5- to 4-Hz spike-wave	3.5- to 6-Hz spike-wave
Generalized tonic-clonic	40–60% (during adolescence)	80% (often before adolescence)	80–85%
Medications	Ethosuximide	Valproic acid	Valproic acid
	Valproic acid	Ethosuximide	
Prognosis	Favorable	Favorable	Favorable

intravenous acetazolamide (500 mg, or 250 mg for children weighing less than 35 kg) has been advocated [117]. The usual antiabsence drugs may be effective if oral or rectal administration is feasible.

Photosensitive Epilepsy

Photic stimulation is a potent activator of seizures, particularly in the childhood and juvenile absence, juvenile myoclonic, and progressive myoclonus epilepsies. An estimated 3% of epileptics are susceptible to visually induced seizures, including photic, pattern, eye-closure, and color-evoked spells [118,119]. Photic sensitivity is familial and has a female predominance of 1.7:1. The median age of onset is 14 years.

The associated seizures are generalized, usually tonic-clonic but also absences or myoclonic, and rarely partial. The EEG reveals a diffuse spike or multiple spike-and-wave discharge during the stimulus, to be distinguished from anterior photomyoclonus and regional posterior discharges, or occipital spikes. The photoparoxysmal response is most liable to occur at stimulation rates between 15 and 20 Hz and on eye closure. Discharges that outlast the stimulus are considered more epileptogenic.

The most homogeneous syndrome of photosensitive epilepsy is a pure form of induced seizures with no spontaneous convulsions. Television viewing, flickering sunlight as seen from a moving vehicle, stroboscopic light, and video games are the usual precipitants. The EEG is often normal except for a generalized photoparoxysmal response. While valproate and clonazepam are effective, simple precautions such as covering one eye with the palm on approaching a television, watching television from some distance in a well-lit room, and wearing sunglasses may be sufficient. Photosensitivity can persist in adulthood.

Epilepsy with Grand Mal on Awakening

This is a rare generalized idiopathic epilepsy with generalized tonic-clonic seizures that occur shortly after awakening or occasionally during drowsiness [120]. The age of onset is in the second decade of life in the majority of cases. The family history is positive in 10–12% of cases. The EEG reveals disorganized background activity, increased slowing, and generalized spike-and-wave paroxysms.

Many patients also have absences, myoclonic seizures, and photosensitivity. Thus, the overlap between this syndrome, JME, and juvenile absence epilepsy is considerable. The grand mal seizures of JME tend to develop from antecedent myoclonias.

Similar environmental triggers seen in JME have been described in epilepsy with grand mal on awakening. While the majority of patients can be controlled with antiepileptic therapy, the relapse rate following drug withdrawal is high.

Summary and Conclusions

Just as a seizure is a symptom and not a diagnosis, an epileptic syndrome is a framework to assemble relevant clinical data, as the underlying pathologic disturbance remains unknown. Identification of a syndrome, however, provides anticipatory guidance regarding the natural evolution and role of therapy for a given patient.

The most recent classification of epileptic syndromes [3] addresses whether the seizures appear focal or generalized, and then whether the etiology is idiopathic, symptomatic, or cryptogenic. This logical approach helps to organize the syndromes in terms of patient evaluation and treatment. In general, the idiopathic epilepsies fare the best, regardless of whether focal or generalized.

There is considerable overlap between some of the syndromes. JME, juvenile absence epilepsy, and epilepsy with grand mal on awakening share common clinical and EEG characteristics and probably represent a spectrum of disorders rather than discrete entities. Landau-Kleffner syndrome and epilepsy with continuous spike-and-wave during slow-wave sleep may be indistinguishable.

Only a certain amount of splitting is possible, and not all syndromes can be categorized. Some patients do not fit any described syndrome or straddle two or more entities. But as the classification of the syndromes evolves, the pathophysiologic understanding and rational management of the epilepsies will progress.

References

1. Dreifuss FE. Proposal for revised clinical and electroencephalographic classification of epileptic seizures. *Epilepsia* 1981;20:489–501.

2. Commission on Classification and Terminology of the International League Against Epilepsy. Proposal for classification of epilepsies and epileptic syndromes. *Epilepsia* 1985;26:268–78.

3. Commission on Classification and Terminology of the International League Against Epilepsy. Proposal for revised classification of epilepsies and epileptic syndromes. *Epilepsia* 1989;30:389–99.

4. Plouin P. Benign neonatal convulsions (familial and non-familial). In: Roger J, Dravet C, Bureau M, Dreifuss FE, Wolf P, eds. *Epileptic syndromes in infancy, childhood and adolescence.* London: John Libbey, 1985:2–11.

5. Leppert M, Anderson VE, Quattlebaum T, et al. Benign familial neonatal convulsions linked to genetic monkeys on chromosome 20. *Nature* 1989;337:647–8.

6. Aicardi J. Early myoclonic encephalopathy. In: Roger J, Dravet C, Bureau M, Dreifuss FE, Wolf P, eds. *Epileptic syndromes in infancy, childhood and adolescence.* London: John Libbey, 1985:12–23.

7. Dalla Bernardina B, Dulac O, Fejerman N, et al. Early myoclonic encephalopathy (E.M.E.E.). *Eur J Pediatr* 1983;140:248–52.

8. Ohtahara S. Clinico-electrical delineation of epileptic encephalopathies in childhood. *Asian Med J* 1978;21:7–17.

9. Ohtahara S, Ishida T, Oka E, et al. On the age-dependent epileptic syndromes: the early infantile encephalopathy with suppression–burst. *Brain Dev* 1976;8:270–88.

10. Jeavons PM. West syndrome: infantile spasms. In: Roger J, Dravet C, Bureau M, Dreifuss FE, Wolf P, eds. *Epileptic syndromes in infancy, childhood and adolescence.* London: John Libbey, 1985:42–50.

11. Frost JD Jr, Hrachovy RA, Kellaway P, Zion T. Quantitative analysis and characterization of infantile spasms. *Epilepsia* 1978;19:273–82.

12. Kellaway P, Hrachovy RA, Frost JD Jr, Zion T. Precise characterization and quantification of infantile spasms. *Ann Neurol* 1979;6:214–8.

13. Gibbs FA, Gibbs EL. *Atlas of electroencephalography*, vol. 2, *epilepsy.* Cambridge, MA: Addison-Wesley, 1952.

14. Hrachovy RA, Frost JD Jr, Kellaway P. Hypsarrhythmia: variations on the theme. *Epilepsia* 1984;25:317–25.

15. Glaze DG, Hrachovy RA, Frost JD Jr, et al. Prospective study of outcome of infants with infantile spasms treated during controlled studies of ACTH and prednisone. *J Pediatr* 1988;112:389–96.

16. Hrachovy RA, Frost JD Jr, Kellaway P, Zion T. A controlled study of prednisone therapy in infantile spasms. *Epilepsia* 1979;20:403–7.

17. Hrachovy RA, Frost JD Jr, Kellaway P, Zion T. A controlled study of ACTH therapy in infantile spasms. *Epilepsia* 1980;21:631–6.

18. Hrachovy RA, Frost JD Jr, Kellaway P, Zion T. Double-blind study of ACTH vs. prednisone therapy in infantile spasms. *J Pediatr* 1983;103:641–5.

19. Lacy RJ, Penry JK. *Infantile spasms.* New York: Raven Press, 1976.

20. Hrachovy RA, Frost JD Jr. Infantile spasms. *Cleve Clin J Med* 1988;56(Suppl):S10–6.

21. Snead OC III, Benton JW, Myers GJ. ACTH and prednisone in childhood seizure disorders. *Neurology* 1983;33:966–70.

22. Riikonen R. A long-term follow-up study of 214 children with the syndrome of infantile spasms. *Neuropediatrics* 1982;13:14–23.

23. Bachman DS. Use of valproic acid in treatment of infantile spasms. *Arch Neurol* 1982;39:49–52.

24. Dyken PR, DuRant RH, Minden DB, King DW. Short-term effects of valproate on infantile spasms. *Pediatr Neurol* 1985;1:34–7.

25. Dreifuss F, Farwell J, Holmes G, et al. Infantile spasms: comparative trial of nitrazepam and corticotropin. *Arch Neurol* 1986;43:1107–10.

26. Bankier A, Turner M, Hopkins IJ. Pyridoxine dependent seizures—a wide clinical spectrum. *Arch Dis Child* 1983;58:415–8.

27. Blennow G, Starck L. *High-dose B_6 treatment in infantile spasms.* Neuropediatrics 1986;17:7–10.

28. French JH, Grueter BB, Druckman R, O'Brien D. Pyridoxine and infantile myoclonic seizures. *Neurology* 1965;15:101–13.

29. Dravet C, Bureau M, Roger J. Benign myoclonic epilepsy in infants. In: Roger J, Dravet C, Bureau M, Dreifuss FE, Wolf P, eds. *Epileptic syndromes in infancy, childhood and adolescence.* London: John Libbey, 1985:51–8.

30. Lombroso C, Fejerman N. Benign myoclonus of early infancy. *Ann Neurol* 1977;1:138–43.

31. Dravet C, Bureau M, Roger J. Severe myoclonic epilepsy in infants. In: Roger J, Dravet C, Bureau M, Dreifuss FE, Wolf P, eds. *Epileptic syndromes in infancy, childhood and adolescence.* London: John Libbey, 1985:58–67.

32. Doose H, Gerken H, Leonhardt R, et al. Centrencephalic myoclonic-astatic petit mal. *Neuropediatrics* 1970;2:59–78.

33. Doose H. Myoclonic-astatic epilepsy in childhood. In: Roger J, Dravet C, Bureau M, Dreifuss FE, Wolf P, eds. *Epileptic syndromes in infancy, childhood and adolescence.* London: John Libbey, 1985:78–88.

34. Gibbs FA, Gibbs EL, Lennox WG. The influence of blood sugar level on the wave and spike formation in petit mal epilepsy. *Arch Neurol Psychiatry* 1939;41:1111–6.

35. Lennox WG, Davis JP. Clinical correlates of the fast and slow spike-wave electroencephalogram. *Pediatrics* 1950;5:626–44.

36. Gastaut H, Roger J, Soulayrol R, et al. Childhood epileptic encephalopathy with diffuse slow spike-waves

(otherwise known as "petit mal variant") or Lennox syndrome. *Epilepsia* 1966;7:139–79.

37. Beaumonoir A. The Lennox-Gastaut syndrome. In: Roger J, Dravet C, Bureau M, Dreifuss FE, Wolf P, eds. *Epileptic syndromes in infancy, childhood and adolescence.* London: John Libbey, 1985:89–99.

38. Aicardi J. The problem of the Lennox syndrome. *Dev Med Child Neurol* 1973;15:77–81.

39. Aicardi J, Chevrie JJ. Myoclonic epilepsies of childhood. *Neuropediatrics* 1971;3:177–90.

40. Noriega-Sanchez A, Markand ON. Clinical and electroencephalographic correlation of independent multifocal spike discharges. *Neurology* 1976;26:667–72.

41. Brenner RP, Atkinson R. Generalized paroxysmal fast activity: electroencephalographic and clinical features. *Medicine* 1982;299:812–6.

42. Markand ON. Slow spike-wave activity in EEG and associated clinical features: often called "Lennox" or "Lennox-Gastaut" syndrome. *Neurology* 1977;27:746–57.

43. Chevrie JJ, Aicardi J. Childhood epileptic encephalopathy with slow spike-wave. A statistical study of 80 cases. *Epilepsia* 1972;13:259–71.

44. Erba G, Browne TR. Atypical absence, myoclonic, atonic, and tonic seizures, and the "Lennox-Gastaut syndrome." In: Browne TR, Feldman RG, eds. *Epilepsy, diagnosis and management.* Boston: Little, Brown, 1983:75–94.

45. Snead OC, Hosey LC. Exacerbation of seizures in children by carbamazepine. *N Engl J Med* 1985;313:916–21.

46. Bittencourt PRM, Richens A. Anticonvulsant-induced status epilepticus in Lennox-Gastaut syndrome. *Epilepsia* 1981;22:129–34.

47. Tassinari CA, Dravet C, Roger J, Cano JP, Gastaut H. Tonic status epilepticus precipitated by intravenous benzodiazepines in five patients with Lennox-Gastaut syndrome. *Epilepsia* 1972;13:421–35.

48. Spencer S. Corpus callosum section and other disconnection procedures for medically intractable epilepsy. *Epilepsia* 1988;29(Suppl 2):S85–99.

49. Blume WT, David RB, Gomez MR. Generalized sharp and slow wave complexes. Associated clinical features and long-term follow-up. *Brain* 1973;96:289–306.

50. Loiseau P. Childhood absence epilepsy. In: Roger J, Dravet C, Bureau M, Dreifuss FE, Wolf P, eds. *Epileptic syndromes in infancy, childhood and adolescence.* London: John Libbey, 1985:106–20.

51. Hertoft P. The clinical, electroencephalographic, and social prognosis in petit mal epilepsy. *Epilepsia* 1963;4:298–314.

52. Gibberd FB. The prognosis of petit mal. *Brain* 1968;89:531–8.

53. Dalby MA. Epilepsy and 3 per second spike and wave rhythms. A clinical, electroencephalographic and prognostic analysis of 346 patients. *Acta Neurol Scand* 1969;45(Suppl 40):1–183.

54. Charlton MY, Yahr MD. Long-term follow-up of patients with petit mal. *Arch Neurol* 1967;16:595–8.

55. Sato S, Dreifuss FE, Penry JK, et al. Long-term followup of absence seizures. *Neurology* 1983;33:1590–5.

56. Sato S, White BG, Penry JK, et al. Valproic acid versus ethosuximide in the treatment of absence seizures. *Neurology* 1982;32:157–63.

57. Engel J Jr. *Seizures and epilepsy.* Philadelphia: F.A. Davis, 1989.

58. Holmes GL, McKeever M, Adamson M. Absence seizures in children: clinical and electrographic features. *Ann Neurol* 1987;21:268–73.

59. Blume WT. Abnormal EEG: epileptiform potentials. In: Blume WT, ed. *Atlas of pediatric EEG.* New York: Raven Press, 1982:139–48.

60. Blume WT, David RB, Gomez MR. Generalized sharp and slow wave complexes. Associated clinical features and long-term follow up. *Brain* 1973;96:289–306.

61. Callaghan N, O'Hare J, O'Driscoll D, et al. Comparative study of ethosuximide and sodium valproate in the treatment of typical absence seizures (petit mal). *Dev Med Child Neurol* 1982;24:830–6.

62. Santavuori P. Absence seizures: valproate or ethosuximide? *Acta Neurol Scand* 1983;68(Suppl 97):41–8.

63. Suzuki M, Maruyama H, Ishibashi Y, et al. A double-blind comparative trial of sodium dipropylacetate and ethosuximide in epilepsy in children with special emphasis on pure petit mal seizures. *Med Prog* 1972;82:470–88.

64. Committee on Drugs. Valproic acid: benefits and risks. *Pediatrics* 1982;70:316–9.

65. Dreifuss FE. How to use valproate. In: Morselli PL, Pippenger CE, Penry JK, eds. *Antiepileptic drug therapy in pediatrics.* New York: Raven Press, 1983:219–27.

66. Jeavons PM. Non-dose-related side effects of valproate. *Epilepsia* 1984;25(Suppl 1):S50–5.

67. Schmidt D. Adverse effects of valproate. *Epilepsia* 1984;25(Suppl 1):S44–9.

68. Turnbull DM, Rawling MD, Weightman D, et al. A comparison of phenytoin and valproate in previously untreated adult epileptic patients. *J Neurol Neurosurg Psychiatry* 1982;45:55–9.

69. Wilder BJ, Ramsay RE, Murphy JV, et al. Comparison of valproic acid and phenytoin in newly diagnosed tonic–clonic seizures. *Neurology* 1983;33:1474–6.

70. Rowan AJ, Meijer JW, deBeer-Pawlikowski NKB, et al. Sodium valproate: serial monitoring of EEG and serum levels. *Neurology* 1979;29:1450–9.

71. Mattson RH, Cramer JA. Valproic acid and ethosuximide interaction. *Ann Neurol* 1980;7:583–4.

72. Browne TR. Clonazepam: a review of a new anticonvulsant drug. *Arch Neurol* 1976;33:326–32.

73. Browne TR. Clonazepam. *N Engl J Med* 1978;299:812–6.

74. Loiseau P, Pestre M, Dartigues JF, Commenges D, Barberger-Gateau C, Cohadon S. Long-term prognosis

in two forms of childhood epilepsy: typical absence seizures and epilepsy with rolandic (centrotemporal) EEG foci. *Ann Neurol* 1983;13:642–8.

75. Tassinari CA, Bureau M. Epilepsy with myoclonic absences. In: Roger J, Dravet C, Bureau M, Dreifuss FE, Wolf P, eds. *Epileptic syndromes of infancy, childhood and adolescence*. London: John Libbey, 1985:121–9.

76. Jeavons PM. Nosological problems of myoclonic epilepsies in childhood and adolescence. *Dev Med Child Neurol* 1977;19:3–8.

77. Lerman P. Benign partial epilepsy with centrotemporal spikes. In: Roger J, Dravet C, Bureau M, Dreifuss FE, Wolf P, eds. *Epileptic syndromes of infancy, childhood and adolescence*. London: John Libbey, 1985:150–8.

78. Beaussart M. Benign epilepsy of children with rolandic (centrotemporal) paroxysmal foci. *Epilepsia* 1972; 13:795–811.

79. Heijbel J, Blom S, Rasmuson M. Benign epilepsy of childhood with centrotemporal EEG foci: a genetic study. *Epilepsia* 1975;16:285–93.

80. Bray PF, Wiser WL. The relation of focal to diffuse epileptifom EEG discharges in genetic epilepsy. *Arch Neurol* 1965;13:223–7.

81. Loiseau P, Duche B. Benign childhood epilepsy with centrotemporal spikes. *Cleve Clin J Med* 1989; 56(Suppl 1):S17–22.

82. Lerman P, Kivity S. Benign focal epilepsy of childhood. A follow-up study of 100 recovered patients. *Arch Neurol* 1975;32:261–4.

83. Lombroso CT. Sylvian seizures and mid-temporal spike foci in children. *Arch Neurol* 1967;17:52–9.

84. Petersen J, Nielsen CJ, Gulann NC. Atypical EEG abnormalities in children with benign partial (rolandic) epilepsy. *Acta Neurol Scand* 1983;94(Suppl):57–62.

85. Deonna T, Ziegler AL, Desplan DPA, Van Melle G. Partial epilepsy in neurologically normal children: clinical syndromes and prognosis. *Epilepsia* 1986; 27:241–7.

86. Gastaut H. Benign epilepsy of childhood with occipital paroxysms. In: Roger J, Dravet C, Bureau M, Dreifuss FE, Wolf P, eds. *Epileptic syndromes in infancy, childhood and adolescence*. London: John Libbey, 1985: 159–70.

87. Dalla Bernardina B, Chiamenti C, Capovilla G, Trevisan E, Tassinari CA. Benign partial epilepsy with affective symptoms ("benign psycho-motor epilepsy"). In: Roger J, Dravet C, Bureau M, Dreifuss FE, Wolf P, eds. *Epileptic syndromes in infancy, childhood and adolescence*. London: John Libbey, 1985:171–5.

88. Landau WM, Kleffner FR. Syndrome of acquired aphasia with convulsive disorder in children. *Neurology* 1957;7:523–30.

89. Beaumanoir A. The Landau-Kleffner syndrome. In: Roger J, Dravet C, Bureau M, Dreifuss FE, Wolf P, eds. *Epileptic syndromes in infancy, childhood and adolescence*. London: John Libbey, 1985:181–91.

90. Lerman P. Discussion of benign partial epilepsies. In: Roger J, Dravet C, Bureau M, Dreifuss FE, Wolf P, eds. *Epileptic syndromes in infancy, childhood and adolescence*. London: John Libbey, 1985:213–5.

91. Patry G, Lyagoubi S, Tassinari CA. Subclinical "electrical status epilepticus" induced by sleep in children. *Arch Neurol* 1971;24:242–52.

92. Tassinari CA, Bureau M, Dravet C, Dalla Bernardina B, Roger J. Epilepsy with continuous spikes and waves during slow sleep. In: Roger J, Dravet C, Bureau M, Dreifuss FE, Wolf P, eds. *Epileptic syndromes in infancy, childhood and adolescence*. London: John Libbey, 1985:194–204.

93. Billard C, Autret A, Laffont F, Lucas B, Degiovanni E. Electrical status epilepticus during sleep in children: a reappraisal from eight new cases. In: Sterman MB, Shouse MN, Passouant P, eds. *Sleep and epilepsy*. London: Academic Press, 1982:481–94.

94. Kellerman K. Recurrent aphasia with subclinical bioelectric status epilepticus during sleep. *Eur J Pediatr* 1978;128:207–12.

95. Bancaud J. Kojewnikow's syndrome (epilepsia partialis continua in children). In: Roger J, Dravet C, Bureau M, Dreifuss FE, Wolf P, eds. *Epileptic syndromes in infancy, childhood and adolescence*. London: John Libbey, 1985:286–98.

96. Aguilar MJ, Rasmussen T. Role of encephalitis in pathogenesis of epilepsy. *Arch Neurol* 1960;2:663–76.

97. Aicardi J. *Epilepsy in children*. New York: Raven Press, 1986.

98. PeBenito R, Cracco JB. Periodic lateralized epileptiform discharges in children. *Ann Neurol* 1979; 37:47–8.

99. Singh BJ, Strobos RJ. Epilepsia partialis continua associated with nonketotic hyperglycemia: clinical and biological profile in 21 patients. *Ann Neurol* 1980;8: 155–60.

100. Thomas JE, Reagan TJ, Klass DW. Epilepsia partialis continua. *Arch Neurol* 1977;34:266–75.

101. Rasmussen T. Further observations on the syndrome of chronic encephalitis and epilepsy. *Appl Neurophysiol* 1978;41:1–12.

102. Rasmussen T. Commentary: extratemporal cortical excisions and hemispherectomy. In: Engel J Jr, ed. *Surgical treatment of the epilepsies*. New York: Raven Press, 1987:417–24.

103. Delgado-Escueta AV, Enrile-Bascal F. Juvenile myoclonic epilepsy of Janz. *Neurology* 1984;34:285–94.

104. Asconape J, Penry JK. Some clinical and EEG aspects of benign juvenile myoclonic epilepsy. *Epilepsia* 1984; 25:108–14.

105. Dreifuss FE. Juvenile myoclonic epilepsy: characteristics of a primary generalized epilepsy. *Epilepsia* 1989;30(S4):S1–7.

106. Panayiotopoulos CP, Obeid T, Waheed G. Juvenile myoclonic epilepsy: a clinical and video-electroencephalographic study. *Ann Neurol* 1989; 25:391–7.

107. Panayiotopoulos CP, Obeid T, Waheed G. Differentiation of typical absence seizures in epileptic syndromes. *Brain* 1989;112:1039–56.

108. Penry JK, Dean JL, Riela AR. Juvenile myoclonic epilepsy: long-term response to therapy. *Epilepsia* 1989;30(S4):S19–23.

109. Delgado-Escueta AV, Greenberg DA, Treiman L, et al. Mapping the gene for juvenile myoclonic epilepsy. *Epilepsia* 1989;30(S4):S8–18.

110. Wolf P. Juvenile absence epilepsy. In: Roger J, Dravet C, Bureau M, Dreifuss FE, Wolf P, eds. *Epileptic syndromes in infancy, childhood and adolescence*. London: John Libbey, 1985:242–6.

111. Wolf P, Inoue Y. Therapeutic response of absence seizures in patients of an epilepsy clinic for adolescents and adults. *J Neurol* 1984;231:225–9.

112. Porter RJ, Penry JK. Petit mal status. In: Delgado-Escueta AV, Wasterlain CG, Treiman DM, Porter RJ, eds. *Status epilepticus: mechanisms of brain damage and treatment*. New York: Raven Press, 1983:61–7. (Advances in neurology; vol 34.)

113. Andermann F, Roble JP. Absence status: a reappraisal following review of thirty-eight patients. *Epilepsia* 1972;31:177–87.

114. Belafsky MA, Carwille S, Miller P, et al. Prolonged epileptic twilight states: continuous recordings with nasopharyngeal electrodes and videotape analysis. *Neurology* 1978;28:239–45.

115. Geier S. Prolonged psychic absence seizures: a study of the absence status. *Epilepsia* 1978;19:431–45.

116. Moe PG. Spike-wave stupor. *Am J Dis Child* 1971; 121:307–13.

117. Browne TR. Status epilepticus. In: Browne TR, Feldman RG, eds. *Epilepsy. Diagnosis and management*. Boston: Little, Brown. 1983:341–54.

118. Jeavons PM. Photosensitive epilepsies. In: Roger J, Dravet C, Bureau M, Dreifuss FE, Wolf P, eds. *Epileptic syndromes in infancy, childhood and adolescence*. London: John Libbey, 1985:232–6.

119. Jeavons PM, Harding GFA. Photosensitive epilepsy: a review of the literature and a study of 460 patients. In: *Clinics in Developmental Medicine*, no. 56. Philadelphia: J.B. Lippincott, 1975:121.

120. Wolf P. Epilepsy with grand mal on awakening. In: Roger J, Dravet C, Bureau M, Dreifuss FE, Wolf P, eds. *Epileptic syndromes in infancy, childhood and adolescence*. London: John Libbey, 1985:259–70.

Chapter 3

Who Should Consider Epilepsy Surgery? Medical Failure in the Treatment of Epilepsy

MICHAEL R. SPERLING

The goal of medical therapy for epilepsy is to enable patients to live as normal a life as possible. This is best accomplished by eliminating seizures. If seizures persist despite drug therapy and lower the quality of life, medical therapy has failed. When this occurs, surgical therapy may be considered [1,2]. This chapter reviews the causes and components of medical failure and the reasons that patients seek surgical treatment for their epilepsy.

What Types of Seizures Merit Surgical Consideration?

Seizures that impair well-being, either by posing a medical risk or by causing cognitive, psychological, or social impairment, lead to surgical consideration. A variety of factors render seizures more or less tolerable and influence how well patients adjust to their disorder (Table 3-1).

Whether seizures alter consciousness largely determines their impact on social and psychological function. Seizures that impair consciousness, including complex partial, secondarily generalized, and generalized seizures (except for myoclonus) [3], are disabling and often leave patients dissatisfied, imposing social and psychological burdens [4,5]. These seizures restrict employment opportunities, inhibit social interactions, and limit independence, particularly in societies where operation of a motor vehicle is important. In contrast, simple partial seizures, which do not alter consciousness, rarely interfere substantially with daily life and permit essentially normal function. Affected patients suffer little social stigma or restriction. However, some simple partial seizures, particu-

larly those with prominent motor, autonomic, or psychic effects, may be quite disturbing.

How frequently should seizures occur for doctor and patient to consider surgical treatment? There is no simple answer. There is wide variability in patient acceptance of seizures. One individual with several seizures per year may believe that the quality of life is significantly impaired, whereas another with daily seizures may not find them constraining. Establishing rigid criteria that a certain number of seizures must occur per year to consider surgical therapy is arbitrary and unrealistic and does not allow for individual variation in tolerance of seizures. In practice, few individuals whose seizures occur less frequently than monthly contemplate the surgical option; those whose seizures occur monthly or more frequently are more likely to be dissatisfied and receptive to alternatives. This demarcation is reasonable and has the practical advantage of suiting modern assessment protocols that require the monitoring of seizures. However, less frequent seizures occasionally warrant surgical treatment, and future advances in evaluation methods and surgical technique may further expand the pool of patients for whom surgery is advisable.

Timing and predictability of seizures are also critical factors influencing the severity of epilepsy. Nocturnal seizures rarely affect daytime function, so most of the social and psychological consequences of epilepsy are avoided. Some patients can predict when their seizures will occur with remarkable accuracy. They can then structure their schedules to minimize the effect of seizures. Other individuals have seizures preceded by prolonged auras and can use that warning to minimize the adverse impact of epilepsy on their lives.

Table 3-1. Factors Influencing Patient Tolerance of Seizures

Better Tolerated	Poorly Tolerated
No physical injury	Repeated trauma
Preserved consciousness	Impaired consciousness
Rare	Frequent or continuous
Predictable	Erratic
Brief duration	Long duration
Warning (aura)	No warning
Socially tolerable ictal behavior	Socially stigmatizing ictal behavior
Brief postictal state	Prolonged postictal state

Ictal behavior and duration of a seizure also influence the degree to which patients are willing to tolerate their seizures. Seizures with socially stigmatizing ictal behaviors such as disrobing, urinary incontinence, and agitation or reactive violence are more disabling and less well tolerated than are seizures that do not attract public attention. Brief seizures, lasting seconds, cause less disruption than seizures lasting minutes.

Behavioral abnormalities related to the postictal state may at times be disruptive or incapacitating. Some patients have prolonged periods of postictal stupor or confusion, which may last for days [6]. Others may suffer transient postictal psychoses [7,8]. Although the ictal behavior itself may cause little trouble, these patients can have severe functional disabilities due to the postictal state.

Other seizures lead to consideration of surgery because they pose direct medical risk. Repeated injuries such as bone fractures, lacerations, loss of teeth, and hematomas may result from the trauma associated with tonic-clonic, atonic, complex partial, and tonic seizures. Recurrent prolonged seizures or status epilepticus may necessitate frequent hospitalizations, expose patients to the danger of iatrogenic complications, and cause brain injury, either from anoxia or trauma [9,10].

Epilepsy Syndromes

Consideration must be given to underlying epileptic syndromes when planning therapy [11]. Partial and generalized seizures may be acquired or inherited and can be progressive, static, or remitting, so accurate diagnosis is essential. The inherited partial epilepsies, for example, benign rolandic epilepsy [12] or occipital epilepsy [13], usually remit in adolescence, and it would be inappropriate to perform focal excisions in patients with those conditions. Similarly, inherited generalized epilepsy syndromes, for example, juvenile myoclonic epilepsy [14] or childhood absence epilepsy [15], are usually treated effectively with medication, and surgery is not indicated. In certain progressive epilepsy syndromes, for example, progressive myoclonus epilepsy [16] and chronic encephalitis [17], the usual course of the disease and projected life span dictate whether or not surgical treatment is an option.

What Constitutes Adequate Anticonvulsant Therapy?

Rational treatment with anticonvulsants does not guarantee success, since 20–30% of patients do not respond fully to maximal anticonvulsant therapy [18–20]. If seizures persist, the following measures should be taken:

1. Confirm the diagnosis. Epileptic seizures must be distinguished from nonepileptic events, such as psychogenic seizures, parasomnias, or cardiac syncope. This may require intensive video-electroencephalogram (EEG) monitoring in some patients.

2. Confirm the classification. Partial epilepsy must be differentiated from generalized epilepsy. Complex partial and complex absence seizures may be similar in appearance, and tonic-clonic seizures may have either focal or generalized origin. Combining the interictal and ictal EEG with the history is the best way to make this distinction.

3. Confirm that the medication chosen is appropriate for the syndrome. Some drugs suited for partial epilepsy are not effective in generalized epilepsy, and the converse is also true. Lack of response to medication may simply be due to inappropriate therapy.

4. Ensure that adequate serum anticonvulsant levels have been achieved. Obstacles to therapeutic levels include absorption abnormalities, interactions with other medications (especially other anticonvulsants), and rapid metabolic inactivation.

5. Ascertain that the patient properly complies with the medical regimen. Medication must be taken to be effective, and the patient must understand the need for and the basic pharmacology of the drug.

6. Eliminate any extraneous precipitating factors. Alcohol ingestion and sleep deprivation may provoke seizures that are otherwise suppressed by medication.

What medications should be tried before concluding that drug therapy is ineffective? Unfortunately, no studies definitively answer this question. With the large number of anticonvulsants available, a variety of possibilities for treatment exist, and most patients are happy to try new treatment regimens. Moreover, to conclude that drug therapy is ineffective requires that the treating physician concede failure, which is not readily done. These interrelated factors may conspire to leave patients on an unsatisfactory therapeutic course for many years. For partial epilepsy, one drug from each of the primary classes of anticonvulsants, hydantoin (phenytoin or mephenytoin), barbiturate (phenobarbital or primidone), and iminostilbine (carbamazepine) should be tried. Each of these medications should be administered in monotherapy before being abandoned as ineffective. Sodium valproate may be effective in treating partial seizures [21] and should be tried prior to surgical referral. For symptomatic generalized epilepsy, sodium valproate should be prescribed in monotherapy in addition to the primary agents mentioned above. Although combination therapy (polytherapy) with two drugs is usually detrimental [22,23], seizure frequency occasionally diminishes [23–25]. Polytherapy may be attempted either with the previously mentioned agents or by adding secondary agents such as benzodiazepines (clonazepam, clorazepate, clobazepam), acetazolamide, methsuximide, or phenacemide to one of the primary drugs. After serial trials of three single medications and one or two trials with two agents in combination, further trials are fruitless, and treatment should resume with the single agent that proved most effective and was best tolerated. Far too often, patients are maintained on polytherapy at the expense of significant side effects, despite a lack of benefit from the added medication. Simplification of therapy to a single drug should always be attempted, although the transition is at times unsuccessful.

Although serum anticonvulsant levels are useful in planning therapy, one cannot insist that the upper limit of the standard therapeutic range be achieved before acknowledging treatment failure for any particular agent. Therapeutic ranges are simply guidelines that apply to populations, not to individuals. When a patient experiences persistent unacceptable side effects from a drug, that drug has failed, irrespective of its serum level. For that reason, an agent may be regarded as ineffective even though serum levels in the usual therapeutic range have not been achieved. Conversely, a medication has not failed until it has produced undesirable side effects, so that treatment should proceed beyond the usual upper limit of the therapeutic range if the agent is well tolerated and seizures persist. An allergic reaction to a medication, such as persistent rash or fever, constitutes adequate grounds for treatment failure.

Deciding that side effects have become unacceptable means that a particular medication has failed. However, defining "unacceptable" is like defining obscenity; individual standards vary and are highly subjective. While patients or their families are usually the best judges of significant toxicity, the physician must at times make this decision, especially when a medication may have impaired the patient's judgment. Common anticonvulsant side effects are somnolence, cognitive impairment, personality and mood changes, gait imbalance, cosmetic or gingival abnormalities, and gastrointestinal disturbances [26]. These side effects may impair school or job performance, restrict activity, hamper interpersonal relationships, and, in the case of gingival hyperplasia, cause loss of teeth and require dental surgery. When a medication produces these effects, therapy should be altered. An anticonvulsant is not beneficial when it causes as many problems as the epilepsy.

How long should medical therapy be continued and at what age should surgery be considered? Once medical therapy has proved ineffective and it is known that remission will not occur, surgical therapy should be considered. There is no reason to pursue ineffective medical therapy. In conditions such as epilepsia partialis continua, surgical intervention may be warranted within the first year of onset of disease. Similarly, infants or small children whose normal development halts or is markedly delayed because of frequent seizures are candidates for early intervention. For less serious conditions such as temporal lobe epilepsy, surgical treatment can be considered if seizures remain refractory for at least 2 years [2]. This reflects the time required for adequate drug trials and allows for the possibility of remission. Beyond this point, further delay is detrimental. Younger patients have a better psychosocial prognosis after surgery than do older patients [27–29]. Seizures during adolescence impose significant medical and psychological morbidity [30], which might be averted with earlier operation. Consequently, surgical therapy should be considered in childhood, to avoid some of the long-term adverse consequences of intractable epilepsy.

Is there an upper age limit for epilepsy surgery? Epilepsy surgery is infrequently counseled for people over 50 years of age. Older people are thought to be less able to adapt to new circumstances than are young people, and they might not obtain full psychosocial benefit. Coexisting ailments may lessen the benefit by raising surgical morbidity or reducing life expectancy. However, surgery should be considered at any age if relief from seizures has a high probability of enhancing the quality of life and anticipated morbidity is relatively low.

Psychosocial Considerations

The persistence of seizures at tolerable doses of medication does not necessarily constitute medical failure. Many patients continue to experience seizures while taking anticonvulsant medication, yet they do not judge their therapy as ineffective. Anticonvulsant treatment may have adequately diminished the frequency and severity of their seizures, and they may have learned to compensate for any inconveniences [31]. It is only when seizures lead to significant psychosocial impairment or discontent that therapy has failed.

The importance of these psychosocial consequences cannot be underestimated. Ultimately, they determine how well seizures are tolerated and whether medical therapy is satisfactory. The fear of public embarrassment and loss of "self-control" may restrict social contact and lead to agoraphobia. Feelings of dependence and loss of freedom are troubling emotions. People with epilepsy may find that employment opportunities are limited, chances for promotion are reduced, and training programs may be unavailable. These and other reasons for discontent [32] lead patients to consider surgical treatment for their epilepsy.

Personality dictates the degree to which impairments are tolerated. For example, inability to drive may lead one individual to feel socially isolated and dependent, whereas another individual with the same limitation may function normally. External factors can have enormous influence. Family relationships, lifestyle, environment (rural vs. urban), and availability of public transportation may either magnify or diminish adversity. This complicated interplay of internal and external factors makes every case unique. The application of standard psychological measurements, such as the Minnesota Multiphasic Personality Inventory or Washington Psychosocial Seizure Inventory, can assist in objectively measuring function and disability [33].

Epilepsy also disturbs family relationships [34], so the elimination of seizures may help restore a more normal family life. Parents of children with epilepsy experience feelings of guilt, resentfulness, isolation, and disappointment. Relations with siblings and spouses may be abnormal. Psychological development may not progress normally, and excessive dependence or rebellion may take place. These consequences may be further exacerbated by neurologic handicaps common to the brain injured, such as learning disabilities, impulsivity, and emotional lability [35].

Cognitive Considerations

Do seizures cause ongoing cognitive impairment and neuronal death? The evidence suggests that surgery should be advocated early for uncontrolled epilepsy. Some studies suggest that progressive cognitive deficits occur in children [36,37] and animals [38] with uncontrolled seizures. The anatomic substrate for this may be the hippocampus, which is important for acquisition of new memory and learning. The hippocampus commonly displays pathologic damage in epilepsy [39,40], and cell death might be caused by recurrent seizures [41–43], possibly from release of excitatory amino acid transmitters [44,45]. But although cell loss has been convincingly demonstrated after status epilepticus [9], it has not been confirmed after intermittent brief seizures. Bertram et al. [46] recently were unable to demonstrate hippocampal cell loss consequent to intermittent seizures in a rat model. Further study is needed to clarify the effect of repeated intermittent seizures on cognitive function and to determine if early surgical intervention forestalls the cognitive impairment and decline associated with uncontrolled seizures.

Goals of Surgery

Surgery is an option only when medical therapy has failed. However, concluding that medical therapy has failed does not mean that a patient should consider surgery. Such a recommendation can be made only if surgery offers a realistic chance of attaining the desired objectives. Surgical therapy and medical therapy share the same goal: to offer as normal a life as possible, by restoring well-being, alleviating disability, and eliminating risk of injury. Abolishing or limiting seizures is the means to achieve that goal but is not the ultimate objective.

It is important to determine that a particular patient's disabilities and dissatisfactions associated with persistent seizures are largely the result of the seizures themselves and do not stem from coexisting cognitive or psychosocial impairments. This is because surgery can only relieve seizures and the limitations they impose, but it does not eliminate coexisting neurologic or psychiatric disabilities [4,5,47]. If severe, these latter disabilities can prevent meaningful improvement and social rehabilitation [48] even though surgical treatment may have cured the seizures. For example, interictal psychoses and personality disorders are usually not affected by epilepsy surgery, so that the profound psychosocial disability is retained postoperatively. Specific attributes have been identified that predict psychosocial outcome, and these can be used to aid in the selection of candidates for surgery [28,48,49].

Complete seizure relief need not occur for surgery to be beneficial. Changing the ictal behavior or pattern of occurrence may be sufficient to produce a dramatic improvement in the quality of life. It is worthwhile to eliminate seizures that impair consciousness or cause bodily injury, even though other seizure types might persist. Similarly, eradication of daytime seizures can greatly improve the quality of daytime life, even if nocturnal seizures continue.

Conclusion

This chapter has avoided discussion of specific features, such as EEG findings, imaging studies, historical details, and so forth, which determine whether epilepsy surgery is feasible or potentially successful for a particular patient. While these factors are crucial, they are irrelevant to the primary question—Has medical therapy failed? If the answer is yes, then referral for surgical evaluation is indicated. Suitability for surgery, its risks, and its benefits can be determined at a specialized center. Once these are known, the patient and the family can decide with professional guidance on the appropriate course of action.

Acknowledgment

The author gratefully acknowledges the helpful comments of H. Hurtig, D. Glosser, and M. Morrell in preparing the manuscript.

References

1. McNaughton FL, Rasmussen T. Criteria for selection of patients for neurosurgical treatment. In: Purpura DP, Penry JK, Walter RD, eds. *Advances in neurology.* New York: Raven Press, 1975:37–48.

2. Walter RD. Principles of clinical investigation of surgical candidates. In: Purpura DP, Penry JK, Walter RD, eds. *Advances in neurology.* New York: Raven Press, 1975:49–58.

3. Commission of Classification and Terminology of the International League Against Epilepsy. Proposal for revised clinical and electroencephalographic classification of epileptic seizures. *Epilepsia* 1981;22:489–501.

4. Flor-Henry P. Ictal and interictal psychiatric manifestations in epilepsy: specific or non-specific? A critical review of some of the evidence. *Epilepsia* 1972; 13:767–72.

5. Kaminer Y, Apter A, Aviv A, et al. Psychopathology and temporal lobe epilepsy in children. *Acta Psychiatr Scand* 1988;77:640–4.

6. Sperling MR, Cahan LD, Brown WJ. Relief of seizures from a predominantly posterior temporal tumor with anterior temporal lobectomy. *Epilepsia* 1989;30: 559–63.

7. Serafetinides EA. Psychosocial aspects of neurosurgical management of epilepsy. In: Purpura DP, Penry JK, Walter RD, eds. *Advances in neurology.* New York: Raven Press, 1975:323–332.

8. Serafetinides EA, Falconer MA. The effects of temporal lobectomy in epileptic patients with psychosis. *J Ment Sci* 1962;108:584–93.

9. Meldrum BS. Metabolic factors during prolonged seizures and their relation to nerve cell death. In: Delgado-Escueta AV, Wasterlain CG, Treiman D, Porter RJ, eds. *Status epilepticus: mechanisms of brain damage and treatment.* New York: Raven Press, 1983:261–76. (Advances in neurology, vol 34.)

10. Siesjo BK, Wieloch T. Epileptic brain damage: pathophysiology and neurochemical pathology. In: Delgado-Escueta AV, Ward AA Jr., Woodbury DM, Porter RJ, eds. *Basic mechanisms of the epilepsies: molecular and cellular approaches.* New York: Raven Press, 1986: 813–47. (Advances in neurology; vol 44.)

11. Commission on Classification and Terminology of the International League Against Epilepsy. Proposal for revised classification of epilepsies and epileptic syndromes. *Epilepsia* 1989;30:389–99.

12. Loiseau P, Duche B, Cordova S, et al. Prognosis of benign childhood epilepsy with centrotemporal spikes: a follow-up study of 168 patients. *Epilepsia* 1988; 29:229–35.

13. Panayiotopoulos CP. Benign childhood epilepsy with occipital paroxysms: a 15-year prospective study. *Ann Neurol* 1989;26:51–6.

14. Janz D. Epilepsy with impulsive petit mal (juvenile myoclonic epilepsy). *Acta Neurol Scand* 1985;72:339–59.

15. Holmes GL, McKeever M, Adamson M. Absence seizures in children: clinical and electroencephalographic features. *Ann Neurol* 1987;21:268–73.

16. Berkovic SF, Andermann F, Carpenter S, Wolfe LS. Progressive myoclonus epilepsies: specific causes and diagnosis. *N Engl J Med* 1986;315:295–305.

17. Rasmussen T, Andermann F. Update on the syndrome of "chronic encephalitis" and epilepsy. *Cleve Clin J Med* 1989;56(Suppl):S181–4.

18. Callaghan N, Kenny RA, O'Neill B, et al. A prospective study between carbamazepine, phenytoin and sodium valproate as monotherapy in previously untreated and recently diagnosed patients with epilepsy. *J Neurol Neurosurg Psychiatry* 1985;48:639–44.

19. Annegers JF, Hauser WA, Elveback LR. Remission of seizures and relapse in patients with epilepsy. *Epilepsia* 1979;20:729–37.

20. Goodridge DMG, Shorvon SD. Epilepsy in a population of 6000. 1. Demography, diagnosis, and classification, and the role of the hospital services. 2. Treatment and prognosis. *Br Med J [Clin Res]* 1983;287:641–7.

21. Loiseau P, Cohadon S, Jogiex M, et al. Efficacy of sodium valproate in partial epilepsies. *Rev Neurol* 1984;140:434–7.

22. Reynolds EH. Mental effects of antiepileptic medication. *Epilepsia* 1983;24(Suppl 2):S85–95.

23. Callaghan N, Goggin T. Adjunctive therapy in resistant epilepsy. *Epilepsia* 1988;29(Suppl 1):S29–35.

24. Schmidt D. Two antiepileptic drugs for intractable epilepsy with complex partial seizures. *J Neurol Neurosurg Psychiatry* 1982;45:1119–24.

25. Mattson RH, Cramer JA, Collins JF, et al. Comparison of carbamazepine, phenobarbital, phenytoin, and primidone in partial and secondarily generalized tonic–clonic seizures. *N Engl J Med* 1985;313:145–51.

26. Dam M. Adverse reactions to antiepileptic drugs. In: Laidlaw J, Richens A, eds. *A textbook of epilepsy*. Edinburgh, Churchill Livingstone, 1982:348–58.

27. Rausch R, Crandall PH. Psychological status related to surgical control of temporal lobe seizures. *Epilepsia* 1982;23:191–202.

28. Jensen I. Temporal lobe epilepsy. Social conditions and rehabilitation after surgery. *Acta Neurol Scand* 1976;54:22–44.

29. Jensen I, Vaernet K. Temporal lobe epilepsy. Follow-up investigation of 74 resected patients. *Acta Neurochir (Wien)* 1977;37:173–200.

30. Lindsay J, Ounsted C, Richards P. Long-term outcome in children with temporal lobe seizures. V: Indications and contraindications for neurosurgery. *Dev Med Child Neurol* 1984;26:25–32.

31. Levin R, Banks S, Berg B. Psychosocial dimensions of epilepsy: a review of the literature. *Epilepsia* 1988;29:805–16.

32. Sands H. *Epilepsy. A handbook for the mental health professional*. New York: Brunner/Mazel, 1982.

33. Dodrill CB. A neuropsychological battery for epilepsy. *Epilepsia* 1978;19:611–23.

34. Ziegler RG. The child with epilepsy: psychotherapy and counseling. In: Sands H, ed. *Epilepsy. A handbook for the mental health professional*. New York: Brunner/Mazel, 1982:158–88.

35. Lezak M. Living with the characterologically altered brain-injured patient. *J Clin Psychiatry* 1977;12:592–8.

36. Bourgeois BF, Prensky AL, Palkes HS, et al. Intelligence in epilepsy: a prospective study in children. *Ann Neurol* 1983;14:438–44.

37. Rodin EA, Schmaltz S, Twitty G. Intellectual functions of patients with childhood-onset epilepsy. *Dev Med Child Neurol* 1986;28:25–33.

38. Holmes GL, Thompson JL, Marchi TA, et al. Effects of seizures on learning, memory, and behavior in the genetically epilepsy-prone rat. *Ann Neurol* 1990;27:24–32.

39. Babb TL, Brown WJ. Pathological findings in epilepsy. In: Engel J Jr, ed. *Surgical treatment of the epilepsies*. New York: Raven Press, 1987:511–40.

40. Brown WJ. Structural substrates of seizure foci in the human temporal lobe. In: Brazier MAB, ed. *Epilepsy: its phenomena in man*. New York: Academic Press, 1973:339–74.

41. Dikmen S, Matthews CG, Harley JP. Effect of early versus late onset of major motor epilepsy on cognitive-intellectual performance: further considerations. *Epilepsia* 1977;18:31–6.

42. Mouritzen-Dam A. Hippocampal neuron loss in epilepsy and after experimental seizures. *Acta Neurol Scand* 1982;66:601–42.

43. O'Leary DS, Lovell MR, Sackellares JC, et al. Effects of age on onset of partial and generalized seizures on neuropsychological performance in children. *J Nerv Ment Dis* 1983;171:624–9.

44. Sloviter RS, Dempster DW. "Epileptic" brain damage is replicated qualitatively in the rat hippocampus by central injection of glutamate or aspartate but not by GABA or acetylcholine. *Brain Res Bull* 1985;15:39–60.

45. Dichter MA, Choi, DW. Excitatory amino acid neurotransmitters and excitotoxins. In: Appel SH, ed. *Current neurology*. Chicago: Year Book Medical Publishers, 1989:1–26.

46. Bertram EH, Lothman EW, Lenn NJ. The hippocampus in experimental chronic epilepsy: a morphometric analysis. *Ann Neurol* 1990;27:43–8.

47. Taylor DC, Falconer MA. Clinical, socio-economic, and psychological changes after temporal lobectomy. *Br J Psychiatry* 1968;114:1247–61.

48. Fraser RT. Improving functional rehabilitation outcome following epilepsy surgery. *Acta Neurol Scand* 1988;117(Suppl):122–8.

49. Augustine EA, Novelly RA, Mattson RH, et al. Occupational adjustment following neurosurgical treatment of epilepsy. *Ann Neurol* 1984;15:68–72.

PART TWO

PREOPERATIVE EVALUATION

Chapter 4

Physical and Chemical Methods to Activate the Epileptic Focus

CHRISTIAN ERICH ELGER
ANDREAS HUFNAGEL

The central objective of presurgical evaluation of epileptic patients is the localization and delineation of the epileptic focus. There appears to be widespread agreement on the point that electrophysiologic and clinical measures of ictal events and quantification of interictal epileptiform activity contribute the most valuable data [1–3]. Although in some patients extracranial electroencephalographic (EEG) recordings, in conjunction with imaging techniques of the brain morphology or metabolism, may suffice to determine the epileptogenic area to be resected, most centers usually or even generally employ long-term intracranial recording techniques [1]. Clinical experience has shown, however, that recording of seizures quite often is a difficult and time-consuming process and the characterization of the interictal epileptogenic situation may turn out to be complex. To save recording time, in particular when intracranial electrodes have been implanted, and to contribute complementary information about the location and the extent of the (primary) epileptogenic area, methods of activation of the epileptic focus have been devised. These methods offer the chance to induce interictal epileptiform activity or seizures under controlled circumstances, that is, when the situation is appropriate, for example, when a high recording capacity is available or when time is limited such as intraoperatively. In principle, an activation of the epileptic focus may be achieved by physical or chemical methods.

Physical Activation Methods

Intracranial Electrical Stimulation

Electrical stimulation of the exposed primate motor cortex was first performed in 1870 [4]. Bartholow in 1874 and Horsley in 1887 may be credited as the first to have performed electrical stimulation of the exposed cortex in humans [5,6]. Widespread recognition of the clinical applicability of the method was gained only after Cushing in 1909, Foerster in 1936, and, in particular, Penfield and Jasper during the late 1930s to 1950s used electrical stimulation in the operating theater, either to induce epileptiform activity prior to epilepsy surgery or to carry out functional anatomical mapping of the human cortex [7–9]. In the decades that followed, electrical cortical stimulation has been integrated into many presurgical work-up programs. Its significance, however, has often been questioned. During the presurgical work-up, several goals are to be achieved by electrical stimulation: (a) the localization of the area where stimulation reproduces the patient's habitual aura or seizure [9–15], (b) the determination of the threshold stimulation intensity to evoke epileptiform afterdischarges [9,13,15,16], and (c) the delineation of the cortical areas of functional importance (17–23) that must be spared in resective surgery.

Method

Technical Devices. Electrical cortical stimulation may be performed acutely in the operating theater or via chronically implanted intracranial electrodes (subdural electrodes, depth electrodes). The protocols followed vary considerably among the different centers. Most centers apply stimuli with a biphasic waveform generated by a constant current stimulator through bipolar electrodes. The stimulation parameters vary as follows: frequency, 0.1–300 Hz; intensity, 0.5–30 V or 0.5–10 mA; duration of pulse, 0.1–10 ms; and duration of stimulus train, 3–20 s [24].

Activation of Epileptogenic Cortical Areas. The identification of the (primary) epileptogenic cortical area by means of induction of seizures or epileptiform afterdischarges may be best carried out via chronically implanted electrodes. There is no time constraint, and examinations may be extended to include a wide range of psychometric or electrophysiologic parameters or they may be repeated under altered circumstances, for example, altered levels of anticonvulsant medication. When attempting to induce seizures, mainly intensity, frequency, or duration of stimulus trains is varied at each electrode tested. Care should be taken to proceed symmetrically and to allow sufficient time between stimulation series to reduce facilitation of epileptiform afterdischarge. To test cortical threshold intensities, the stimulation intensity is increased from a subthreshold level until epileptiform afterdischarge potentials are elicited.

Functional Mapping. Acute electrical stimulation at the exposed cortex at present is mainly performed for precise localization of functionally important brain areas, such as the sensorimotor cortex or language areas or their associated memory zones. Tests of memory function require conduction of the operation under local anesthesia. A current suitable to block or excite the underlying brain function is passed through the electrode (e.g., sensorimotor cortex: bipolar electrodes 5 mm apart, 60 Hz, 6 mA) [18]. Impairment of language or failure during a specific memory task indicates that the underlying cortical area is essential for language or recent memory. Muscular twitches or sensations evoked at the contralateral limb determine the primary motor or sensory area. The identification of the pre- and postcentral gyrus can also be achieved by use of the evoked potential technique. A reversal of phases may be observed when recording anterior and posterior to the central sulcus. The main advantage of acute stimulation is that the stimulating electrodes can easily be moved and adjusted to the topography of the brain.

Functional mapping through chronically implanted subdural electrodes is more satisfactory when the subdural electrode strips are closely spaced or of the grid type [20]. Single subdural strip electrodes enable testing of only a few cortical sites.

Histologic alterations caused by continuous electrical cortical stimulation have not been demonstrated unless a charge/phase of more than 0.5 μC/phase or a charge density of more than 7.5 μC/cm/phase was applied [25–27]. Ample data have been published on the kindling of epileptic foci by repeated daily electrical stimulation in animals [28]. A *de novo* generation of epileptic foci in humans by cortical electrical stimulation has never been documented.

Two examples may serve to illustrate the induction of seizures by electrical stimulation and at the same time point out the controversial issue of inducing habitual or "artificial" seizures. Figure 4-1 shows the induction of a habitual seizure in a 30-year-old patient who suffered from drug-resistant complex partial seizures of left frontal origin since the age of 4 years. The patient did not have any neurologic deficit or memory impairment. A gliotic lesion could be demonstrated in the left frontal lobe by magnetic resonance imaging (MRI). His seizures started with an unspecific strange feeling and continued with restlessness followed by screaming and a clonic-like vocalization for 10–30 s. He did not lose consciousness throughout the seizure. The origin of the seizure activity could not be localized adequately by extracranial EEG. Electrocorticographic (ECoG) recordings via ten subdural electrode strips implanted bilaterally in frontal and temporal positions (Fig. 4-1A) depicted ictal onset in a circumscribed left lateral frontal area located approximately 2.5 cm anterior to the Broca's area. Electrical stimulation of the same area repeatedly induced the patient's habitual seizure. The stimulation parameters were 15 Hz, 20 V, 0.25 ms stimulus duration, and a stimulus train of 6 s duration. Electrical stimulation outside the "focal area" did not result in the induction of epileptiform afterdischarges.

A second case is an example of a patient with a bitemporal epilepsy in whom complex partial seizures not resembling the habitual seizures could be induced (Fig. 4-2). The 27-year-old man had medically intractable complex partial seizures since the age of 8 years. Neurologic examination and MRI scan were normal. He had had two episodes of epileptic psychosis 2 and 6 years prior to the presurgical evaluation. Psychometric testing revealed severe verbal and visual memory deficits. The ECoG recordings via subdural electrodes exhibited persistent bitemporal interictal epileptiform activity and bilateral but predominantly left temporal lobe ictal onset (Fig. 4-2B). Electrical stimulation applied to the right mesiotemporal

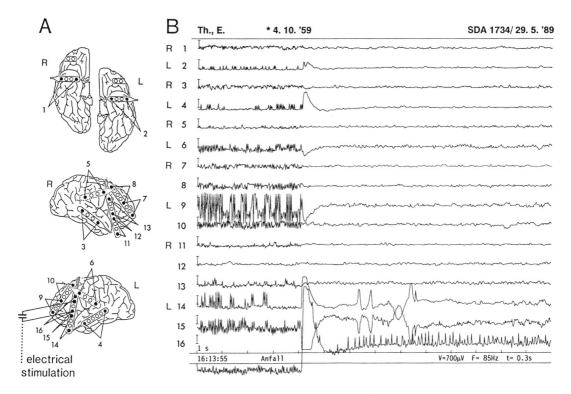

Figure 4-1. Induction of a habitual complex partial seizure by electrical cortical stimulation. ECoG registration via subdural electrodes. (*A*) Schematic drawing of the implanted subdural electrode strips. The numbers in the drawing refer to the numbers of the tracings (L = left, R = right). (*B*) A bipolar stimulation train of 5 s duration, 30 V, 2.5 ms stimulus duration, and 15 Hz is passed onto a circumscribed area of the left lateral frontal cortex (close to channel 16 assumed to be the site of ictal onset. Multiple afterdischarge spiking, which outlasts the stimulus train, provokes the patient's habitual seizure. The electrical seizure activity remains confined to electrode 16 and does not spread. Filter = 85 Hz, time constant = 0.3 s, amplitude: 1 cm = 700 μV.

area next to the amygdaloid nucleus induced a complex partial seizure that resembled neither the clinical nor the electrophysiologic features of the patient's habitual seizure (Fig. 4-2C). The stimulation parameters were 10 Hz, 25 V, 0.25 ms stimulus duration, and a stimulus train of 5 s prior to the induction of the seizure.

Comment. The effect of electrical stimulation on the epileptogenic area varies considerably in an individual as well as among individuals. Seizures are easy to induce in some patients and difficult to induce in others [9]. The reproduction of a seizure with the patient's typical initial clinical symptoms was presumed by Penfield et al. to be the most reliable criterion of localization of the epileptic focus [9]. This assumption, however, could not be confirmed later by Halgren and coworkers [29]. Electrically induced seizures have been compared with spontaneous seizures and the location of the epileptic focus as determined throughout presurgical evaluation. The observed correlations vary extremely from 0% to 97% [24,29].

Wieser saw concordances of 77% [3] when only one side of the brain but not the exact site of ictal onset was taken into consideration. Consequently, a high localizational value is attributed to electrical stimulation in one center [24] and denied in another [29]. Virtually all stimulation parameters such as frequency, current density, stimulus duration, stimulus polarity, stimulus train duration, and waveform and other factors such as electrode configuration and orientation, the degree of spontaneous epileptiform activity present, the levels of anticonvulsant medication, and many more may alter the response of the epileptic focus to electrical stimulation. Such differences in the technique of stimulation or patient selection, however, may suffice to explain some of the observed differences but hardly all of them. In particular, in bitemporal epilepsy, where distinction of the primary epileptic focus from the secondary is the prime interest [30,31], correlations between spontaneous and induced seizures are low [3]. Two explanations may contribute to the understanding of these discrepancies. First, it is a known fact that not only

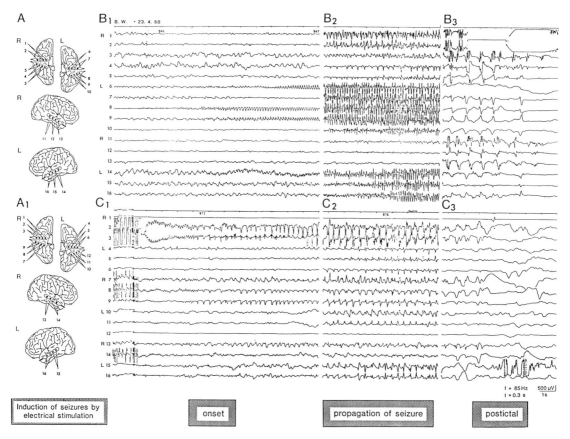

Figure 4-2. Induction of an "artificial" seizure by electrical cortical stimulation. ECoG registration via subdural electrodes. The numbers in the drawing refer to the numbers of the tracings (L = left, R = right). (A) and (A₁) Schematic drawing of the implanted electrodes and montages. (B) Spontaneous habitual seizure. (C) Electrically induced seizure. (B₁) Onset of the spontaneous seizure in the left temporal lobe (channel 8). (B₂) Propagation of the seizure to the anterior mesial (channels 6, 7, 9, 10) and lateral aspects (channels 14–16) of the left temporal lobe and the anterior mesiobasal aspects of the right temporal lobe (channels 1 and 2). (B₃) A generalized postictal suppression of electrical brain activity may be seen. (C₁) A train of bipolar electrical stimuli of 4 s duration, 15 Hz, 2.5 ms stimulus duration, and 30 V is passed through electrode No. 1 at the anterior mesiobasal aspects of the right temporal lobe. During the stimulation the patient reported an aura different from the habitual one. Immediately after the stimulation the onset of a complex partial seizure was noted, which started in the right temporal lobe (channels 2 and 3). (C₂) Generalization of the seizure. (C₃) Postictally there is a generalized suppression of electrical brain activity. Filter = 85 Hz, time constant = 0.3 s, amplitude.

the epileptogenic brain is able to react to electrical stimulation with the evolution of a seizure but also perifocal or even nonepileptogenic tissues can do so. Second, the electrical stimulus or the induced afterdischarges may propagate from the site of stimulation to an even distant epileptogenic area via anatomical interconnections. Limbic pathways particularly have been found to be considerably facilitated in epileptic patients and as such may transmit the inducing current even to the contralateral hemisphere [32]. Most centers regard the area with the lowest threshold to induce afterdischarges as the site of epileptogenicity. However, the opposite may well be true when a

sclerotic hippocampus is stimulated [16]. According to Gloor [13], afterdischarge thresholds provide only suggestive evidence as to the location of the epileptogenic area. Only long-lasting afterdischarges associated with the patient's initial ictal symptoms may reconfirm the location of the epileptic focus derived from spontaneous ictal activity arising in the same area [13].

In summary, seizures or epileptiform afterdischarges elicited by electrical stimulation may be an aid in localizing the primary site of epileptogenicity. The method, however, does not stand on its own, and the induced activity must be compared to the spontaneous epileptiform discharges.

Transcranial Magnetic Stimulation

Transcranial magnetic stimulation (TMS) applied to the intact skull was introduced in 1985 as a method of monitoring central and peripheral motor pathways [33]. It has rapidly gained recognition as a reliable, safe, and painless technique [34–38]. Apart from the induction of epileptic seizures in very rare cases, no adverse effects have been reported [39–43]. The capability of TMS to induce epileptiform afterdischarges in epileptic foci could be demonstrated in a considerable proportion of 48 patients during the presurgical work-up [42]. TMS works on a magneto-electrical principle and generates a large electrical current of low charge density in the brain [34]. The hypothetical concept that cortical excitation of this kind may be capable of activating epileptic foci was derived from observations made in animal experiments. These studies indicate that a diffuse electrical, epicortical stimulation can induce epileptiform afterdischarges in epileptic foci even when these are located remote from the site of stimulation [44,45].

Method

The stimulation was performed with a Magstim 200/Novametrix (produced in Wallingford, CT, U.S.A.) using a circular coil with a 14-cm or a 7-cm outer diameter. Stimulation intensities were set 5–30% above the cortical threshold to evoke motor potentials in the abductor pollicis brevis. The coil was held tangentially to the skull and centered over various positions according to the international 10/20 system of EEG. In practical terms, the first 50 stimuli were always applied to the vertex. The coil was then lateralized to the temporal or parietal regions starting with the hemisphere that contained the (primary) epileptic focus. Sides were alternated after each series of 25 stimuli. The total number of stimuli applied was limited to 350. There was a break of at least 30 s after each series of 25 stimuli. The stimulation frequencies varied from 0.1 Hz to 0.3 Hz. Since the system requires time to recharge, 0.3 Hz was the highest stimulation frequency possible. All patients had medically intractable, complex partial seizures of mainly temporal lobe origin. None of the patients had neurologic deficits or a history of psychosis or severe depression. In most patients the anticonvulsant medication was reduced rapidly and substantially or it was discontinued completely during the invasive phase of presurgical evaluation. The stimulus artifact created with each stimulus may be reduced by carefully moving wirings out of reach of the magnetic field, avoiding central common references, decreasing stimula-tion intensities, alternating current flow within the coil, or using the smaller coil.

Stimulation Effects: Induction of Epileptiform After-discharges. The induction of epileptiform afterdischarges (EAD) was possible in approximately 55% of the patients and generally selective of the epileptic focus (or foci). The induction of EAD was inconsistent and varied from just single spikes or sharp waves to longer series of spikes and sharp waves that usually started within 0.5–5 s after the stimulus had been applied and lasted 2–10 s and rarely even longer. Whereas only one in 10–20 stimuli induced EAD in about 50% of the patients, it increased to 60% of the applied stimuli in a few. In about one third of the patients a stimulus could also interrupt spontaneous paroxysms of epileptiform activity. A facilitation of EAD was seen in more than half of the patients during serial TMS (Fig 4-3). The term "facilitation" implies that repetitive application of stimuli increased either the spike frequency or the duration of an afterdischarge series or that induction of EAD started at one or a few electrodes and extended to neighboring or distant electrodes or to other epileptic foci. In most patients the induction of EAD in the epileptic focus could be observed during application of stimuli over the epileptic focus as well as to other ipsilateral sites but also to the contralateral hemisphere. In patients with several foci as determined by other methods, the primary epileptic focus appeared to be exclusively or preferentially activated. A more focal TMS by use of the small (7-cm) coil was superior to a more widespread stimulation with the large (14-cm) coil when stimulating above the temporal lobe because artifacts were grossly reduced and the induction of EAD was equivalent. Usually, TMS-induced effects ceased within a few seconds after the end of the stimulation.

Stimulation Effects: Seizures. With stimulation intensities and frequencies applied, two complex partial seizures and one aura occurred during TMS after application of a total of 56, 71 and 174 stimuli, respectively (Fig. 4-4). Two more complex partial seizures and one aura occurred after a lapse of 2–4 min after cessation of the stimulation and may be associated with TMS. When judged by all electrophysiologic and clinical means the seizures were identical to those observed spontaneously. In summary, seizures may only rarely be induced by TMS. The value of the method in the process of presurgical evaluation is therefore limited.

Comment. In conclusion, according to the data accumulated so far, TMS is able to activate the epileptic focus (or foci). Rarely suppression of focal epileptic

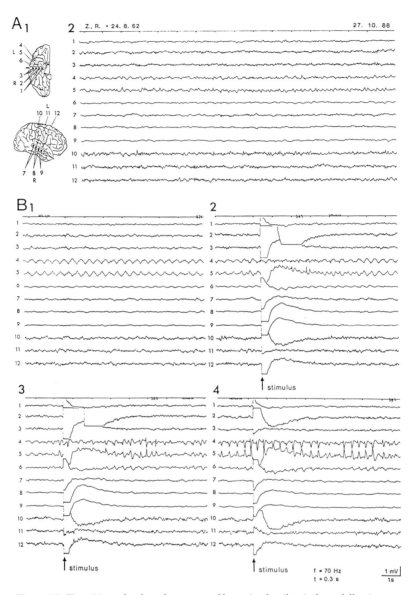

Figure 4-3. Transition of a theta-focus to a self-sustained epileptic focus following transcranial magnetic stimulation. (A_1) Schematic drawing of the location of the implanted subdural electrodes. The numbers in the drawing refer to the numbers of the tracings (L = left, R = right). (A_2) A left mesio-temporo-basal theta-focus (channels 4 and 5) could be observed before stimulation commenced. (*B*) ECoG recordings during TMS. (B_1) Gradual development of a regular 2–2.5/s delta activity with the application of 20–60 stimuli to the vertex. (B_2) First epileptiform afterdischarges after application of 60 stimuli to the vertex. (B_3) Acceleration of background activity and increase of epileptiform afterdischarge after a total of 60–70 stimuli to the vertex. (B_4) Transition to a self-sustained continuous pattern of sharp wave potentials formed with the application of 70–90 stimuli to the vertex. Filter = 70 Hz, time constant = 0.3 s, amplitude: 1 cm = 700 μV. From Hufnagel A, Elger CE, Durwen HF, et al. Activation of the epileptic focus by transcranial magnetic stimulation of the human brain. *Ann Neurol* 1990; 27:49–60, with permission.

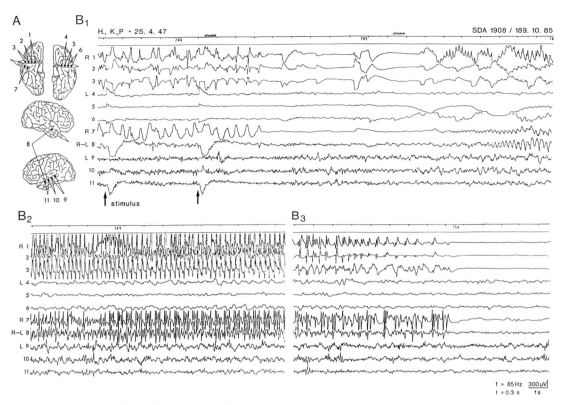

Figure 4-4. ECoG recording of the induction of a complex partial seizure by transcranial magnetic stimulation. (*A*) Schematic drawing of the implanted subdural electrodes. The numbers in the drawing refer to the numbers of the tracings (L = left; R = right). (*B₁*) Onset of the seizure during serial transcranial magnetic stimulation in the anterior mesiobasal aspects of the right temporal lobe as indicated by flattening of the ECoG (channels 1–3 and 7). Consecutive appearance of miniature spikes that turn into multiple spiking of higher amplitude but lower frequency. (*B₂*) The seizure remained confined to the right temporal lobe. (*B₃*) Termination of the seizure and focal postictal isoelectric line. Filter = 85 Hz, time constant = 0.3 s, amplitude: 1 cm = 700 μV. From Hufnagel A, Elger CE. Responses of the epileptic focus to transcranial magnetic stimulation. *Electroencephalogr Clin Neurophysiol Suppl* 1990; 86–99, with permission.

activity was seen in the same patients. Excitatory as well as inhibitory TMS-induced cortical responses have also been documented during other studies [38]. The activation is selective of the epileptogenic brain area (or areas), and the primary epileptic focus appears to be exclusively or preferentially activated. These characteristics of TMS-induced activation of epileptic foci would favor a further clinical utilization of the technique in the process of presurgical evaluation. The clinical use of the method, however, is limited by the fact that induction of EAD is not possible in approximately 45% of the patients and is subtle in about half of the remaining patients. Furthermore, the induction of seizures with stimulation intensities and frequencies currently utilized here is scarce but may be more likely when higher stimulation frequencies become available [43].

Chemical Activation

Methohexital-Induced Activation of Epileptic Foci

The properties of methohexital that act on epileptic foci were first described by Pampiglione in 1965 [46] and later confirmed by others [47–54]. At present methohexital is used mainly as an aid in the delineation of the epileptic focus during long-term presurgical ECoG recordings. It may be of help intraoperatively in determining the limits of the epileptogenic area to be resected [53]. Ample clinical experience with methohexital has been accumulated during use of the drug as an induction agent of anesthesia. From the data gathered during clinical use, the drug has been characterized as a substance of rapid onset, short duration, and safe clinical use [51]. Cumulation of effects following repeated administrations of the drug is thought to be minimal [51]. During ECoG, as little as 20 mg of methohexital may suffice to abruptly induce or increase spiking in the epileptogenic area [53]. Selective induction of epileptiform potentials in the epileptogenic area occurred in approximately 85% of the cases during acute ECoG [53] or scalp-derived EEG, including with the use of sphenoidal electrodes [52]. The activating properties of methohexital appear to be superior to those of other barbiturates such as thiopentone [55–57] or other induction agents of anesthesia such as propofol [58]. The induction of seizures has been reported but appears to be a rare event even in epileptic patients [59,60]. Application of as much as 1000 mg of methohexital within 5 min under controlled circumstances has shown that the focal generation of spikes may be refractory to the suppressive effects. Whereas the electrical brain activity of nonepileptogenic areas or the background activity in the epileptic focus is suppressed to an almost isoelectric line with large doses of methohexital, the spiking continues [54]. A second feature, namely the loss or reduction of drug-induced beta-activity over the epileptogenic area, may contribute additional information [55].

Our own experiences were derived from 112 high-dose intravenous applications of methohexital in 56 patients who suffered from medically intractable complex partial seizures of temporal lobe ($n = 43$) or frontal lobe ($n = 8$) or temporal + extratemporal ($n = 5$) origin. During all of the tests ECoG recordings were performed using bilaterally implanted subdural electrodes. Doses of 50 mg and 100 mg were applied to induce a short narcosis to allow painless percutaneous extraction of the subdural strip electrodes at the end of the presurgical evaluation. The analysis of the electrophysiologic data was visual. Informed consent was obtained from each patient.

The major conclusions to be emphasized from our data [54] are: (a) the procedure is simple, quick, and safe; (b) an activation of the epileptic focus was possible in 41 of 43 patients with temporal lobe epilepsy following application of 100 mg; (c) no activation was seen in 5 of 8 patients with frontal lobe epilepsy, and in the remaining 3 patients the activation was subtle; (d) the observed patterns of activation were congruent with areas of spontaneous ictal onset or interictal spike-predominance; (e) the patterns of activation have a high prognostic relevance; and (f) loss or reduction of drug-induced beta-activity over the epileptic focus is an additional localizing feature.

The application of low (50-mg) and high (100-mg) doses of methohexital in the same patient may prove to be of importance in the distinction of primary from secondary epileptic foci. Figure 4-5 is an example of a 46-year-old man who presented with a history of complex partial seizures since the age of 28 years. He did not have secondary generalized seizures. Long-term ECoG recordings exhibited monotypic ictal onset in the left mesiobasal temporal lobe but persistent bitemporal interictal epileptiform activity at a left-to-right temporal lobe ratio of 1:1. A low dose of 50 mg of methohexital induced a spike-burst-suppression pattern only in the left temporal focus, which was assumed to be the primary one. In contrast, a high dose of 100 mg of methohexital induced an enhanced focal spike-burst-suppression pattern mainly in the primary epileptic focus but also in the right-sided epileptic focus regarded as the secondary focus.

The induction of a clinical seizure is rare. We observed the induction of a seizure within 3 min after the injection of methohexital in only two patients. Figure 4-6 is an example of the induction of a short complex partial seizure. The 33-year-old woman was under consideration for resective surgery of a left temporal lobe epileptic focus. She had complex partial seizures since the age of 13 years. The patient reported her habitual aura 40 seconds after intravenous injection of 20 mg of methohexital. Thereafter the initial clinical symptoms of her habitual seizure were observed, paralleled by the electrophysiologic characteristics of a seizure that remained confined to the left temporal lobe and thus had a high localizing value.

Comment

Methohexital is a safe drug for the induction of interictal epileptiform afterdischarges and occasionally an ictal event. A dose of 20 mg of methohexital may suffice to activate epileptic foci. A focal spike-burst-suppression pattern, which is clear-cut activation and delineation of the primary epileptic focus, may be induced in the large majority of patients with temporal lobe foci after application of 100 mg of methohexital. The focal spike-burst-suppression pattern has a high diagnostic and prognostic relevance.

Activation of the Epileptic Focus by Amobarbital

Since its introduction in 1949 [61], intracarotid amobarbital tests have gained recognition as fairly safe and reliable procedures to establish the lateralization of cerebral speech dominance and to determine memory function [62,63]. Compared to the number of patients investigated by the intracarotid

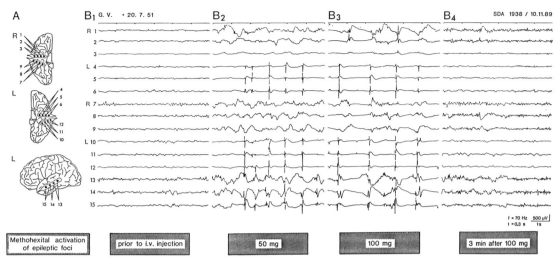

Figure 4-5. Localization of the primary epileptic focus by application of different doses of methohexital in a patient with persistent bitemporal interictal epileptiform activity but unilateral left temporal ictal onset. ECoG registration via subdural electrodes. *(A)* Schematic drawing of the implanted subdural electrode strips. The numbers in the drawing refer to the numbers of the tracings (L = left, R = right). *(B$_1$)* Prior to the injection only scarcely interspersed epileptiform activity was seen. *(B$_2$)* Induction of a focal spike-burst-suppression pattern in the area of the primary epileptic focus (left temporal lobe; channels 4–6 and 10–15) following intravenous administration of 50 mg of methohexital. *(B$_3$)* Induction of a focal spike-burst-suppression pattern in the primary left temporal lobe (channel 4–6 and 10–15) but also in the secondary epileptic focus (right temporal lobe; channels 1–3) following intravenous application of 100 mg of methohexital. *(B$_4$)* Three minutes after the injection of 100 mg of methohexital a loss of drug-induced beta-activity can be noted only over the primary left temporobasal focus. Filter = 70 Hz, time constant = 0.3 s, amplitude: 1 cm = 500 μV.

amobarbital test during the more than 40 years of its existence, electrophysiologic data, derived from invasive or noninvasive recordings during the investigation, have been utilized only scarcely to act as a means of delineation of the epileptic focus [64–69]. Gloor et al. were able to localize the (primary) epileptic focus in a group of patients with secondary bilateral synchrony by use of the intracarotid amobarbital-pentylenetetrazol EEG test [70,71]. The postoperative test results in this group, however, were not different from another group, where the test had indicated a diffuse or multifocal epileptogenic condition. They considered the test to be unrewarding and not optimally suited especially in temporal lobe epilepsy [71]. Scalp-derived EEG recorded during testing of speech and memory function is grossly impaired by artifacts of motion as well as arousal of the patient, which, to a large extent, masks the underlying electrical brain activity. To avoid these confounding circumstances, separate intracarotid amobarbital tests have been devised in the past merely for the sake of acquisition of electrophysiologic data [70,71]. In addition, skull and scalp act as a low-pass filter, which handicaps identification of beta-activity induced by barbiturates over unaffected cortex [55–57]. Data derived from depth electrodes are limited to a smaller

number of circumscribed recording sites [72]. In our experience ECoG recordings via subdural electrodes remain artifact-free even during speech or intensive movements of the patient, which renders this method applicable during the intracarotid amobarbital test [73]. ECoG recordings during the test may contribute complementary information about the location of the (primary) epileptic focus. The method and main use of the intracarotid amobarbital test, namely identification of the side of cerebral speech dominance or the testing of memory function, have been described and discussed in detail in another chapter in this volume. In this chapter we describe electrophysiologic findings observed during the procedure.

Our own experiences with the intracarotid amobarbital test were derived from observations in 34 patients (68 tests). All patients had drug-resistant temporal lobe (*n* = 31) or frontal lobe (*n* = 3) epilepsy with complex partial seizures. In 19 patients the anticonvulsant medication was maintained at levels considered to be therapeutic. Eleven patients had one or several drugs below therapeutic level. Anticonvulsant medication was completely discontinued in four patients. ECoG recordings were performed via bilaterally implanted subdural electrodes for a period of approximately 10 minutes prior to and following

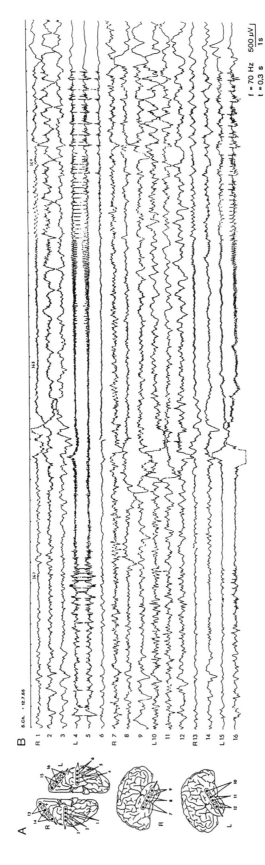

Figure 4-6. ECoG recording of a complex partial seizure induced by methohexital. (*A*) Schematic drawing of the implanted subdural electrode strips. The numbers in the drawing refer to the numbers of the tracings (L = left, R = right). (*B*) Forty seconds after an intravenous injection of 20 mg of methohexital the patient reported her habitual aura. The seizure started and remained confined to the mesiobasal aspects of the left temporal lobe. The postictal isoelectric suppression in the focal area (channels 4–6) is of additional localizing value. Filter = 70 Hz, time constant = 0.3 s, amplitude: 1 cm = 500 μV.

the injection. The subdural electrodes generally covered the basal, mesiobasal, and lateral aspects of both temporal lobes and additional areas according to the assumed location of the epileptic focus. Between 16 and 64 electrode contacts were available on 4 to 10 subdural electrode strips. Prior to the intracarotid amobarbital test, the location of the epileptic focus (foci) had been identified by ECoG registration of 4 to 26 seizures in each patient. The analysis of the data was visual. A standard dose of 200 mg of amobarbital was injected into first one and then the other internal carotid artery on consecutive days via a catheter advanced from the femoral artery. Vascular anomalies or a crossover flow via the anterior communicating artery had been excluded by routine angiography of both carotid arteries prior to the examination.

No adverse effects were observed by the investigators or reported by the patients. The ECoG recordings via subdural strip electrodes remained almost free of artifacts even during testing speech and memory function. No seizure was induced. The effects of amobarbital on the nonepileptogenic tissues followed fairly regular patterns. An isoelectric line could be observed in a few patients at the point of maximum suppression of electrical brain activity. From there recovery back to baseline passed through intermittent phases of burst-suppression, polyphasic waves, high-amplitude beta-activity (>300 μV), and low-amplitude beta-activity (<300 μV). The response of the epileptic focus was specific and may be characterized as follows: (a) induction of a focal spike-burst-suppression pattern in the primary epileptic focus following injection of amobarbital into the ipsilateral carotid artery ($n = 16$) (Fig. 4-7), (b) induction of epileptiform potentials in the primary epileptic focus following injection into the contralateral carotid artery ($n = 10$), (c) loss or reduction of drug-induced beta-activity over the epileptic focus ($n = 18$), and (d) suppression of preexistent epileptiform activity ($n = 5$).

The most conspicuous feature was the induction of a focal spike-burst-suppression pattern in the area of the epileptic focus (or foci). The spike-burst-suppression pattern appeared at the end of the inductional phase as an unequivocal induction of spikes (Fig. 4-7). The pattern persisted for approximately 0.5–5 min. The cessation of the pattern was paralleled by recovering function of the nonepileptogenic tissues (transition from polyphasic waves to high-amplitude beta-activity). In 13 patients of the group with a well-defined unilateral temporal epileptic focus, induction of a mesiobasal spike-burst-suppression

pattern served to confirm the location of the epileptic focus, determined through ECoG presurgical evaluation. So far 10 of these 13 patients postoperatively have remained free from seizures and auras. However, the observational period is limited to 9–20 months (mean = 14 months). Loss or reduction of drug-induced beta-activity over the epileptic focus yielded additional information about the location of the epileptic focus. However, this could be observed over the primary as well as over secondary foci.

The induction of a focal spike-burst-suppression pattern may be an aid in determining the location of the primary epileptic focus in patients with bitemporal epilepsy. Figure 4-8 is an example of a 46-year-old man with persistent bitemporal interictal epileptiform activity but monotype left mesiobasal temporal ictal onset. A focal spike-burst-suppression pattern was induced in each temporal lobe following application of amobarbital through the ipsilateral carotid artery. However, the spike-burst-suppression pattern was more pronounced on the left side and lasted approximately 5 min, whereas it ceased after 2–3 min in the right temporal lobe, which contained the secondary epileptic focus.

Comment

The unilateral induction of a spike-burst-suppression pattern in the mesiobasal aspects of the temporal lobe may be an aid in determining the location of the primary epileptic focus. It seems to indicate a limbic origin of the epilepsy and a good outcome from surgery. For explanation of this phenomenon, evidence may be derived from monkey and cat experiments, which clearly indicate that spontaneous epileptiform potentials are consistently suppressed wherever the epileptic focus is completely perfused by amobarbital but that, in contrast, epileptic foci situated outside, but near the border of, the brain area perfused by amobarbital may be activated [74]. With regard to this, epileptic foci located in the mesiobasal temporal structures may be activated since the amobarbital injected into the internal carotid artery reaches only the lateral temporal cortex and not the mesial part that receives its blood supply from the posterior cerebral artery.

In conclusion, ECoG recordings during the intracarotid amobarbital test yield important information about the primary epileptic focus in a high proportion of patients. Results are sufficiently favorable to encourage utilization of these data in the process of presurgical evaluation of medically intractable epilepsy.

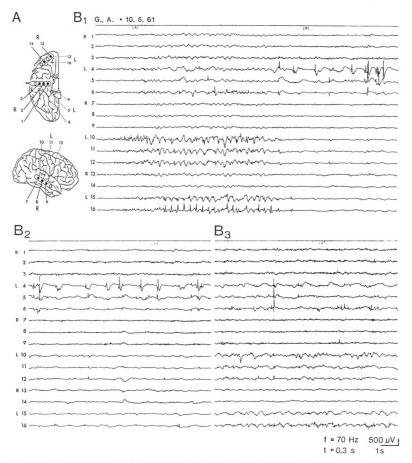

Figure 4-7. Activation of a left temporal epileptic focus by amobarbital. (*A*) Schematic drawing of the implanted subdural electrode strips. The numbers in the drawing refer to the numbers of the tracings (L = left, R = right). (*B₁*) Inductional phase: The first ECoG alterations become visible 10 seconds after the injection of 200 mg of amobarbital into the left carotid artery. After another 10 seconds the maximum of effect is reached. Note the induction of a spike-burst-suppression pattern in the mesiobasal aspects of the left temporal lobe (channels 4–6). (*B₂*) One minute later the spike-burst-suppression pattern still persists in the "focal" left temporal lobe. (*B₃*) The cessation of the spike-burst-suppression pattern is paralleled by recovering function of the nonepileptogenic tissues. Filter = 70 Hz, time constant = 0.3 s, amplitude: 1 cm = 500 μV. From Hufnagel A, Elger CE. Responses of the epileptic focus to transcranial magnetic stimulation. *Electroencephalogr Clin Neurophysiol Suppl* 1990; 86–99, with permission.

Other Substances

Artificial induction of seizures by convulsant drugs such as pentylentetrazol [75–79] or bemegride [80–82] has been almost completely abandoned. The major reasons for doing so were (a) induced seizures frequently showed quick generalization, which implies that a focal onset of the ictal discharge could not be determined; (b) the drug-induced seizures frequently did not represent the patient's habitual seizure pattern; and (c) injections of pentylenetetrazol often caused an anxiety reaction in the patient [13].

Concluding Remarks

The aforementioned physical and chemical methods of activation of the epileptic focus exhibit a wide variation as to the inducibility of seizures and to the concordance of induced seizures with spontaneous seizures or interictal epileptiform activity. Other methods such as the application of megimide and pentylenetetrazol are no longer in use. Of the described methods the deep methohexital-induced narcosis appears to combine the highest capability to induce epileptiform discharges with an exclusive or preferential activation of the (primary) epileptogenic area. Methohexital may activate temporal lobe foci in > 90%. A clear-cut delineation of the primary epileptic focus may be achieved in patients who exhibit a focal

spike-burst-suppression pattern following application of 100 mg of methohexital. In addition, the method allows estimation of outcome from temporal lobectomy. Electrically induced afterdischarges or seizures in most patients may easily be obtained but can be misleading because they do not necessarily represent the patient's spontaneous epileptiform activity. TMS-induced seizures were identical to spontaneous ones, and epileptiform afterdischarges were selectively induced in spontaneously epileptogenic brain areas. However, the induction of a seizure by TMS is rare, and a marked activation of the epileptic focus takes place in only 30–40% of the patients. Clinical experience with the method is limited at present. The intracarotid amobarbital test offers the unique opportunity of unilateral pharmacologic testing of the

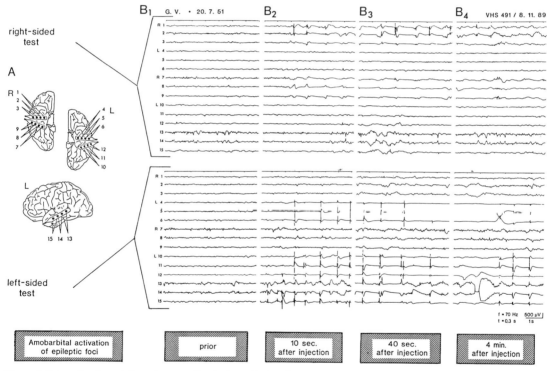

Figure 4-8. Localization of the primary epileptic focus during the intracarotid amobarbital test. (*A*) Schematic drawing of the implanted subdural electrode strips. The numbers in the drawing refer to the numbers of the tracings (L = left, R = right). *Lower traces 1–15:* Investigation of the primary (left temporal) focus. *Upper traces 1–15:* Investigation of the secondary (right) focus the next day. (*B₁*) Prior to either examination, none or only scarce spontaneous epileptiform activity was seen. (*B₂*) Ten seconds after the injection of 200 mg of amobarbital into the right (*upper traces*) or left (*lower traces*) internal carotid artery a spike-burst-suppression pattern was induced in both the primary (lower channels 4–6, 10–12, and 15) and the secondary (upper channels 1–3) epileptic focus. (*B₃*) Forty seconds after each injection the spike-burst-suppression pattern persists in the primary epileptic focus as well as in the secondary epileptic focus. (*B₄*) Four minutes after the injection the spike-burst-suppression pattern still persists in the primary (left temporal) focus (lower channels 4–6 and 10–15) but has ceased in the (right temporal) secondary focus (upper channels 1 and 2). Filter = 70 Hz, time constant = 0.3 s, amplitude: 1 cm = 500 μV.

epileptic focus (or foci). ECoG recordings during the test provide valuable data about the location of the (primary) epileptic focus and should generally be performed.

Acknowledgement

This work was supported by the Ministry of Social Affairs of the Federal Republic of Germany. The authors wish to thank Maria Schruff, Karin Schmidt, and Mathias Dümpelmann for their technical assistance.

References

1. Engel J. Approaches to localization of the epileptogenic lesion. In: Engel J, ed. *Surgical treatment of the epilepsies.* New York: Raven Press, 1987:75–95.

2. Lüders H, Lesser RP, Dinner DS, et al. Commentary: chronic intracranial recording and stimulation with subdural electrodes. In: Engel J, ed. *Surgical treatment of the epilepsies.* New York: Raven Press, 1987:297–321.

3. Wieser HG, Bancaud J, Talairach J, Bonis A, Szikla G. Comparative value of spontaneous and electrically induced seizures in establishing the lateralization of temporal lobe seizures. *Epilepsia* 1979;20:47–59.

4. Fritsch R, Hitzig E. Über die elektrische Erregbarkeit des Grosshirns. *Arch Anat Physiol Wissensch Med* 1870;37:300–32.

5. Bartholow R. Experimental investigation into the functions of the human brain. *Am J Med Sci* 1874;67:305–13.

6. Horsley V: A note on the means of topographical diagnosis of focal disease affecting the so-called motor region of the cerebral cortex. *Am J Med Sci* 1987;93: 342–69.

7. Cushing H. A note upon faradic stimulation of the postcentral gyrus in conscious patients. *Brain* 1909; 32:44–54.

8. Foerster O. The motor cortex in man in light of Hughlings Jackson's doctrines. *Brain* 1936;59:135–59.

9. Penfield W, Jasper H. *Epilepsy and the functional anatomy of the human brain.* Boston: Little, Brown, 1954.

10. Ajmone-Marsan C. Focal electrical stimulation. In: Purpura DP, et al, eds. *Experimental Models of Epilepsy.* New York: Raven Press, 1972:147–72.

11. Bancaud J, Talairach J. Méthodologie de l'exploration SEEG et de l'intervention chirurgicale dans l'épilepsie. *Rev Otoneuroophthalmol* 1973;45:315–28.

12. Bancaud J, Talairach J, Morel P, Bresson M, Bonis A, Geier S, Hemon E, Buser P. Generalized epileptic seizures elicited by electrical stimulation of the frontal lobe in man. *Electroencephalogr Clin Neurophysiol* 1974;37:275–82.

13. Gloor P. Contributions of electroencephalography and electrocorticography to the neurosurgical treatment of the epilepsies. In: Purpura DP, Penry JK, Walter RD, eds. *Neurosurgical management of the epilepsies.* New York: Raven Press, 1975;59–105. (Advances in neurology, vol. 34.)

14. Gloor P, Olivier A, Ives J. Loss of consciousness in temporal lobe seizures: observtions obtained with stereotaxic depth electrode recordings and stimulation. In: Canger R, Angeleri F, Penry JF, eds. *Advances in epileptology: XIth Epilepsy International Symposium.* New York: Raven Press, 1980:349–53.

15. Olivier A, Gloor P, Anderman F, Ives J. Occipitotemporal epilepsy studied with stereotaxically implanted depth electrodes and successfully treated by temporal resection. *Ann Neurol* 1982;11:428–32.

16. Cherlow D, Dymond A, Crandall PH, Watter RD, Serafetinides EA. Evoked responses and afterdischarge thresholds to electrical stimulation in temporal lobe epileptics. *Arch Neurol* 1977;34:527–31.

17. Fedio P, Van Buren J. Memory deficits during electrical stimulation of the speech cortex in conscious man. *Brain Lang* 1974;1:29–42.

18. Ojemann GA. Intraoperative functional mapping at the University of Washington, Seattle. In: Engel J, ed. *Surgical treament of the epilepsies.* New York: Raven Press, 1987:635–9.

19. Ojemann GA, Ojemann J, Lettich E, Berger M. Cortical language localization in left, dominant hemisphere. An electrical stimulation mapping investigation in 117 patients. *J Neurosurg* 1989; 71:316–26.

20. Ojemann GA, Engle J. Acute and chronic intracranial recording and stimulation. In: Engle J, ed. *Surgical treatment of the epilepsies.* New York: Raven Press, 1987:263–88.

21. Burchiel KJ, Clarke H, Ojemann GA, Dacey RG, Winn HR. Use of stimulation mapping and corticography in the excision of arteriovenous malformations in sensorimotor and language-related neocortex. *Neurosurgery* 1989;24:322–7.

22. Lesser RP, Lüder H, Klein G, Dinner DS, Morris HH, Hahn J. Cortical afterdischarge and functional response thresholds: results of extra-operative testing. *Epilepsia* 1984;25:615–21.

23. Lüders H, Lesser RP, Dinner DS, Morris HH, Wyllie E, Godoy J. Localization of cortical function: new information from extraoperative monitoring of patients with epilepsy. *Epilepsia* 1988;29(Suppl 2):56–65.

24. Bernier GP, Saint-Hilaire JM, Giard N, Bouvier G, Mercier M. Commentary: intracranial electrical stimulation. In: Engel J, ed. *Surgical treatment of the epilepsies.* New York: Raven Press, 1987:323–34.

25. Babb TL, Soper HV, Lieb JP, Brown WJ, Ottino CA, Crandall PH. Electrophysiological studies of long-term electrical stimulation of the cerebellum in monkeys. *J Neurosurg* 1977;47:353–65.

26. Brown WJ, Babb TL, Soper HV, Lieb JPO, Ottino CA, Crandall PH. Tissue reaction to long term electrical

stimulation of the cerebellum in monkeys. *J Neurosurg* 1977;47:366–79.

27. Yuen TGH, Agnew WF, Bullara LA, Jacques S, McCreery DB. A histological evaluation of neural damage from electrical stimulation: considerations for the selection of parameters for clinical application. *Neurosurgery* 1981;9:292–9.

28. Goddard GV, McIntyre DC, Leech GK. A permanent change in brain function resulting from daily electrical stimulation. *Exp Neurol* 1969;25:295–330.

29. Halgren E, Walter RD, Cherlow DG, Crandall PH. Mental phenomena evoked by electrical stimulation of the human hippocampal formation and amygdala. *Brain* 1978;101:83–117.

30. Rasmussen T, Jasper H. Temporal lobe epilepsy: indication for operation and surgical technique. In: Baldwin M., Bailey P, eds. *Temporal lobe epilepsy.* Springfield, IL: Charles C Thomas, 1958:440–60.

31. VanBuren JM, Ajmone-Marsan C, Matsuga N, Sadowsky D. Surgery of temporal lobe epilepsy. In: Purpura DP, Penry JK, Walter RD, eds. *Neurosurgical management of the epilepsies.* New York: Raven Press, 1975:155–96. (Advances in neurology, vol. 8.)

32. Buser P, Bancaud J, Talairach J. Depth recordings in man in temporal lobe epilepsy. In: Brazier MAB, ed. *Epilepsy, its phenomena in man.* New York: Academic Press, 1973:67–97.

33. Barker AT, Freeston IL, Jalinous R, Merton PA, Morton HB. Magnetic stimulation of the human brain. *J Physiol* 1985;369:3.

34. Barker AT, Freeston IL, Jalinous R, Jarratt JA. Magnetic stimulation of the human brain and peripheral nervous system: an introduction and the results of an initial clinical evaluation. *Neurosurgery* 1987;20:100–9.

35. Agnew WF, McCreery DB. Consideration for safety in the use of extracranial stimulation for motor evoked potentials. *Neurosurgery* 1987;20:143–7.

36. Amassian VE, Stewart M, Quirk GJ. Physiological basis of motor effects of transient stimulus to cerebral cortex. *Neurosurgery* 1987;20:74–93.

37. Cracco RQ. Evaluation of conduction in central motor pathways: techniques, pathophysiology and clinical interpretation. *Neurosurgery* 1987;20:199–203.

38. Cracco RQ, Amassian VE, Maccabee PJ, Cracco JB. Excitatory and inhibitory effects of magnetic coil stimulation of human cortex. In: Rossini PM, Mauguiere F, eds. New trends and advanced techniques in clinical neurophysiology. *Electroencephalogr Clin Neurophysiol Suppl* 1990;41:134–9.

39. Tassinari CA, Michelucci R, Forti A, et al. Transcranial magnetic stimulation of the cerebral cortex in epilepsy: usefulness and safety. *Neurology* 1990;40:1132–3.

40. Hömberg V, Netz J. Generalised seizure induced by transcranial magnetic stimulation of the motor cortex. *Lancet* 1989;II:1223.

41. Hufnagel A, Elger CE, Durwen HF, Böker DK, Entzian W. Activation of the epileptic focus by transcranial

magnetic stimulation of the human brain. *Ann Neurol* 1990;27:49–60.

42. Hufnagel A, Elger CE. Responses of the epileptic focus to transcranial magnetic stimulation. *Electroencephalogr Clin Neurophysiol Suppl.* 1990;Suppl 43 86–99.

43. Dhuna A, Gates J, Pascual-Leone A. Transcranial magnetic stimulation in patients with epilepsy. *Neurology* 1991;41:1067–71.

44. Elger CE, Speckmann EJ. Focal interictal epileptiform discharges (FIED) in the epicortical EEG and their relations to spinal field potentials in the rat. *Electroencephalogr Clin Neurophysiol* 1980;48:447–60.

45. Purpura DP, Penry JK, Tower DB, et al. *Experimental models of epilepsy.* New York: Raven Press, 1972.

46. Pampiglione G. Very short acting barbiturate (methohexital) in the detection of cortical lesions. *Electroencephalogr Clin Neurophysiol* 1965;19:314–6.

47. Harris R, Paul R. The use of methohexitone in electrocorticography. *Electroencephalogr Clin Neurophysiol* 1969;27:333–4.

48. Musella L, Wilder BJ, Schmidt RP. EEG activation with intravenous Brevital in psychomotor epilepsy. *Neurology* 1969;19:278.

49. Wilder BJ. EEG activation in medically intractable epileptic patients. Activation techniques including surgical follow-up. *Arch Neurol* 1971;25:415–26.

50. Celesia GG, Paulsen RE. Electroencephalographic activation with sleep and methohexital. *Arch Neurol* 1972; 27:361–3.

51. Whitwam JG. The pharmacology of brietal sodium (methohexitone). Das Ultrakurznarkotikum Methohexital. *Anaesth Resuscitation* 1972;57:2–8.

52. Hardiman O, Coughlan A, O'Moore B, Phillips J, Staunton H. Interictal spike localisation with methohexitone: preoperative activation and surgical follow up. *Epilepsia* 1987;28:35–39.

53. Wyler AR, Richey ET, Atkinson RA, Hermann BP. Methohexital activation of epileptogenic foci during acute electroencephalography. *Epilepsia* 1987;28(5):490–4.

54. Hufnagel A, Burr W, Elger CE, Nadstawek J, Hefner G. Localization of the epileptic focus during methohexital-induced anesthesia. *Epilepsia* 1992;33:271–84.

55. Pampiglione G. Induced fast activity in the EEG as an aid in the location of cerebral lesions. *EEG Clin Neurophysiol* 1952;1:79–82.

56. Kennedy WA, Hill D. The surgical prognostic significance of the electroencephalographic prediction of Ammon's horn sclerosis in epileptics. *J Neurol Neurosurg Psychiatry* 1958;21:24–36.

57. Engel J, Driver MV, Falconer MA. Electrophysiological correlates of pathology and surgical results in temporal lobe epilepsy. *Brain* 1975;98:129–56.

58. Hufnagel A, Elger CE, Nadstawek J, Stoeckel H, Böker DK. Specific response of the epileptic focus to anaesthesia with propofol. *J Epilepsy* 1990;3:37–45.

59. Rockoff MA, Goudsouzian NG. Seizures induced by methohexital. *Anesthesiology* 1981;54:333–5.

60. Galley AH. Methohexitone. Proc R Soc Med (Section of anesthetics) 1963;56:377–8.
61. Wada J. A new method for the determination of the side of cerebral speech dominance. A preliminary report on the intracarotid injection of sodium amytal in man. *Igaku to Seibutssugaku* 1949;14:1221–2 .
62. Milner B, Branch C, Rasmussen T. Study of short term memory after intracarotid injection of sodium amytal. *Trans Am Neurol Assoc* 1962;87:224–6.
63. Silvenius H, Christianson SA, Nilsson LG, Saisa J. Preoperative investigation of cerebral hemisphere speech and memory with the bilateral amytal test. *Acta Neurol Scand Suppl* 1988;117:79–83.
64. Rovit R, Gloor P, Rasmussen T. Intracarotid amobarbital in epileptic patients. *Arch Neurol* 1961;5:606–26.
65. Perez-Borja C, Rivers MH. Some scalp and depth electrographic observations on the action of intracarotid sodium amytal injections on epileptic discharges in man. *Electroencephalogr Clin Neurophysiol* 1963;15:588–98.
66. Serafetinides EA, Driver MV, Hoare RD. EEG patterns induced by intracarotid injection of sodium amytal. *Electroencephalogr Clin Neurophysiol* 1965;18:170–5.
67. Ricci GB, Silipo P, Gagliardi F. Paradoxical activating EEG responses to the intracarotid amytal test in focal and multifocal epilepsies. *Electroencephalogr Clin Neurophysiol* 1969;27:707.
68. Aasly J, Blom S, Silvenius H, Zetterlund B. Effects of amobarbital and methohexital on epileptic activity in mesial temporal structures in epileptic patients. An EEG study with depth electrodes. *Acta Neurol Scand* 1984;70:423–31.
69. Aasly J, Silfvenius H, Zetterlund B. Barbiturate effects on EEG in complex partial epilepsy. *J Neurol* 1989;236:15–20.
70. Garretson H, Gloor P, Rasmussen T. Intracarotid amobarbital and metrazol test for the study of epileptiform discharges in man: a note on its technique. *Electroencephalogr Clin Neurophysiol* 1966;21:607–10.
71. Gloor P, Rasmussen T, Altuzarra A, Garretson H. Role of the intracarotid amobarbital-metrazol EEG test in the diagnosis and surgical treatment of patients with complex seizure problems. *Epilepsia* 1976;17:15–31.
72. Gloor P. Volume conductor principles: their application to the surface and depth electroencephalogram. In: Wieser HG, Elger CE, eds. *Presurgical evaluation of epileptics.* New York: Springer, 1987:59–68.
73. Wyler AR, Ojemann GA, Lettich E, Ward AA. Subdural strip electrodes for localizing epileptogenic foci. *J Neurosurg* 1984;60:1195–2000.
74. Coceani F, Libman I, Gloor P. The effects of intracarotid amobarbital injections upon experimentally induced epileptiform activity. *Electroencephalogr Clin Neurophysiol* 1966;20:542–558.
75. Langeluddeke A. Ueber Cardiazolkraempfe. *Ztschr Neurol Psychiat* 1938;161:347–8.
76. Janz HW. Zur diagnostischen Verwertbarkeit der Cardiazolkrämpfe. *München Med Wchschr* 1937;84:471.
77. Cure C, Rasmussen T, Jasper H. Activation of seizures and electroencephalographic disturbances in epileptic and in control subjects with "Metrazol." *Arch Neurol Psychiatry* (Chicago) 1948;59:691–717.
78. Gastaut H. Techniques, indications and results of Metrazol activation. *Electroencephalogr Clin Neurophysiol Suppl* 1955;4:120–36.
79. Friedlander WJ. Clinical evaluation of metrazol activation in electroencephalography. *Neurology* (Minneap) 1954;4:264–70.
80. Bingle J. Bemegride as an activator in electroencephalography. *Br Med J* 1958;1:923–6.
81. Delay J, Verdeaux G, Verdeaux J, Drossopoulo G, Schuller E, Chanoit P. Un neuro-stimulant epileptogene, la megimide. *Presse Med* 1965;64:1525–7.
82. Bancaud J. EEG activation by metrazol and megimide in the diagnosis of epilepsy. In: Naquet R, ed. *Handbook of EEG Clinical Neurophysiology.* Amsterdam: Elsevier, 1974:105–20. (Activation and provocation methods in clinical neurophysiology, Vol 3D).

Chapter 5

Long-Term Monitoring with Scalp and Sphenoidal Electrodes

CHRISTIAN ERICH ELGER
WIELAND BURR

The recording of brain electrical activity plays one of the most important diagnostic roles in the presurgical evaluation of candidates for epilepsy surgical intervention. Not only is it regarded as the only specific investigation to prove the suspected epileptic nature of a malfunction, but it is also essential in the differentiation between types of seizures and the localization of their origin. Among the various kinds of brain electrical signals (others are registered by corticography and depth recordings [1]) the surface electroencephalogram (EEG) is relatively simple to register and yet is capable of providing essential diagnostic information. As demonstrated in this chapter, the surface EEG might either in itself be sufficient to establish the exact location of the epileptic focus or—more often—be the basis of further, more invasive steps, such as planning electrode implantation. In either case, along with clinical, psychological, radiologic, or other morphologic and functioning imaging diagnostics, it is an indispensable step within the presurgical evaluation scheme.

Methods of Recording

In the diagnosis of epilepsy mainly four different kinds of electrographic information are distinguished: (a) nonspecific abnormalities (e.g., low-frequency focal activity), (b) interictal epileptiform discharges (e.g., spikes, sharp waves), (c) ictal patterns (initial flattening, onset and maximum of spiking), and (d) postictal abnormalities. The general problem is to obtain unbiased data, both with regard to temporal as well as local coverage of the relevant signal sources. The former problem, that is, temporal resolution (or to warrant a sufficient length of registration), is of particular relevance with respect to the ictal patterns, namely to record seizures that are typical for the specific patient. This can be achieved by using various techniques of long-term monitoring. The problem of good local resolution, or of the coverage of all relevant brain areas, demands the use of a sufficient number of electrodes and their appropriate location. This implies the extension of the classical scheme of electrode montage to the anterior temporal scalp (11,12) and/or sphenoidal electrodes, particularly when mesiotemporal structures possibly are involved. If neotemporal or extratemporal foci are likely, closely spaced electrodes (according to the so-called 10–20 system) or even additional electrodes should be used (Fig. 5-1). Even long-term recordings may not contain an adequate number of ictal events. Therefore, special conditions that make use of either patient-dependent precipitating factors (e.g., situational factors, self-inducing mechanisms) or of generally seizure-provoking methods (reduction of antiepileptic medication, emotional stress) may be indicated.

Electrodes

Scalp Electrodes

Most epilepsy centers use cup-shaped electrodes (0.5–1 cm in diameter) consisting of silver chloride, impregnated silver–silver chloride, or gold-plated silver. The electrodes are held in place either by a cap

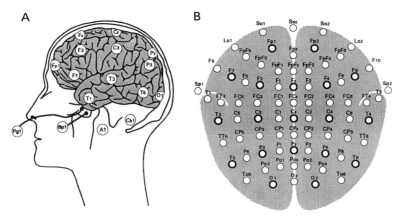

Figure 5-1. Schematic drawing of the electrode positions of the 10–20 system together with the anterior temporal (T1), sphenoidal (Sp1), and pharyngeal (Pg1) electrodes in relation to the brain (*A*) and the closely spaced (10–20) electrode positions (*B*).

(Beckmann cap), by adhesive paste, or—for prolonged recording for up to several days—by collodion. When using the paste, which has limited-duration fixation, on the one hand drying out of the paste must be avoided, on the other hand there must not be any bridging between electrodes. Even when using collodion, electrode gel is needed, which means that bridging must be prevented. Electrode impedance must not exceed 5 kΩ.

Electrode positions should generally follow the standard 10–20 system. According to the specific question under consideration and the capacity of the amplifier and recording system, additional scalp electrodes may be useful. Especially extratemporal foci require closely spaced electrodes following the 10–20 system. The anterior temporal electrode position (T1,2) is particularly recommended to investigate the temporal lobe. Others like FT3,4 (equivalent to D7,8) and FC5,6 (equivalent to D5,6) may also provide additional informations, for example; for differentiating temporal from frontal origin. In some cases supraorbital electrodes provide additional information on activity of the fronto-orbital cortex. The electrode positions are shown in Figure 5-1A in relation to the brain structures; additional electrode positions are shown in Figure 5-1B.

Sphenoidal Electrodes

In several respects sphenoidal electrodes are used to pick up activity of the mesial temporal lobe. They are superior to nasopharyngeal electrodes and the so-called mini-sphenoidals [2] that are inserted under

the skin because of (a) the vicinity to the mesiobasal structures, (b) the lower risk of confusing left and right hemispheres, (c) fewer artifacts, and (d) the facility to remain implanted for a prolonged period without discomfort to the patient. They consist of insulated (Teflon) wires (silver, steel, or platinum) inserted extracranially from lateral by means of a lumbar puncture needle under the zygomatic arch toward the foramen ovale. The implantation does not require anesthesia. Some authors recommend controlling the final location by x-ray investigations. However, although in some cases small migrations over several days have been observed, in our experience there is no need to be too cautious because the information provided by sphenoidal derivations appears rather stable against moderate variations of their depth location [3].

Electrode Montage and Choice of Reference

From a theoretical point of view, if modern storage facilities are used that allow off-line reformatting with a free choice of reference, the problem of montage and reference choice can be postponed to the phase of analysis. The only required condition is to store signals derived with a common reference (either of a single electrode or arbitrarily averaged). However, for the purpose of on-line visualization or preanalysis of the tracings, the reference problem is crucial because it may either disclose or sometimes even blur the electroencephalographer's vision. Several major solutions to the problem have been applied. (a) Biasing by the reference can be avoided completely by using bipolar montages. Here, the preferred tool of evaluation is the phase reversal between adjacent channels. A drawback to this solution is that focal abnormalities, spreading over several electrodes, are difficult to identify and that low-amplitude signals may lead to critical interference with noise. (b) Theoretically the ideal method (providing an absolute potential scale) would be to measure with respect to a common reference distant from any source of epileptiform activity. For physical reasons, however, this would imply a reduced signal-to-noise ratio; therefore, one might select a scalp area where the impact of epileptic activity can be widely excluded, for example, on the contralateral hemisphere, as soon as the existence of a unilateral focus has been established. Unfortunately, this method is obviously less appropriate for the problem of focus localization (i.e., when the exact position of one focus or even the absence of multiple foci has not yet been proven. (c) Alternatively one might use an artificial common reference by calculating the average potential over all (or a number of selected) electrodes as a function of time. This approach, however, holds only as long as the majority of the electrode locations are not affected by epileptic activity. In contrast to the "simple" common reference method, the *a priori* knowledge of the location of the focus is not necessary. (d) From a theoretical point of view, a favorable solution would be the so-called source derivation, which tries to solve the "inverse problem," that is, concluding from the measured potential differences to the underlying sources. This method is based on rather simple assumptions concerning the potential generators; postulating nearly equidistant electrode positions, the significance decreases toward the boundary regions and finally it is not adequate for sphenoidal recordings. Thus, despite some of its theoretical advantages, its usefulness in focus localization, primarily in the temporal lobe, is somewhat questionable. In our hands, for everyday practice, the montage as used in the Montreal Neurologic Institute [4] proved to be extremely useful; it is shown in the schematic drawing in Figure 5-2A.

Recording and Storing Data

Technical instruments for amplification, transmission, storage, and display of the signals must meet the standards set for clinical EEG monitoring. Currently only preamplifiers with high impedance that are located close to the patient are recommended for am-

plification. Once EEG signals have been picked up and preamplified, they can be led to the remote storage or display unit in different ways, either using conventional hard wire connectors (for long-distance so-called cable telemetry) or wireless radio (or infrared) telemetry; in the most recent generation of instruments digitized and multiplexed signals are transmitted via glass fibers. The problem of data storage is crucial: to achieve a truly representative collection of all types of a patient's habitual epileptic features, both the number of channels and the length of the recordings must be as large as possible. Consequently, an extremely high storage capacity is needed. Moreover, facilities should be available that allow the comparison between electrographic events and clinical or behavioral phenomena stored on video storage device. Different approaches are used for this purpose. (a) If video and EEG recordings are stored on separate media, a time code signal must be on both of them. During the analysis it serves as a synchronizing signal. This method has to be used when 24-hour cassette recorders are the storage media for the EEG (sometimes they are used because they allow very long recording periods even when patients are allowed unrestricted mobility). (b) A modified version (with enhanced accuracy) is used in the recently developed computer-controlled digital EEG storage devices (magnetic or optical disk), combined with a separate video recorder that receives the same master time code. (c) The most common method, however, to record bioelectrical and clinical signals simultaneously is to store both on the same medium after having passed either a splitter-inserter or EEG-video processor; up to now, and if high video quality is required, the medium has been magnetic tape, but in the future it will be replaced by others.

Generally, for each patient under investigation a representative and significant collection of signal epochs must be stored. How the selection should be done is the topic of the following section. We would like to end this section on technical considerations by emphasizing the importance of adequate display devices. These comprise high-quality multichannel cathode ray tube (CRT) monitors (primarily for the purpose of on-line control and off-line screening) and high-resolution hard-copy devices (conventional EEG writer, laser printer, or cam writer).

Monitoring Conditions

One of the problems when recording seizure activity by means of noninvasive electrodes is the amount of

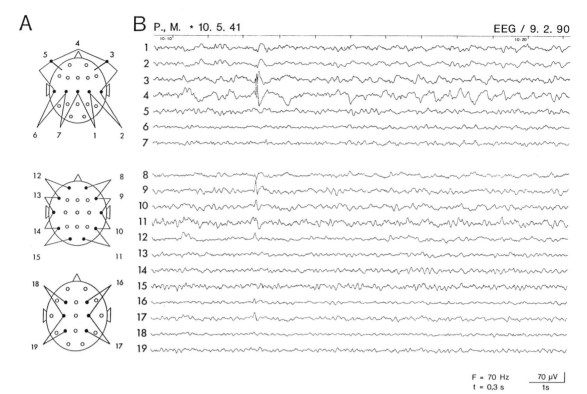

Figure 5-2. Discharge in a montage with sphenoidal electrodes. (*A*) Schematic drawing of the montage. (*B*) EEG tracings. Numbers are related to the numbers in *A*. From Gotman J, Ives JR, Gloor P, et al. Monitoring at the Montreal Neurological Institute. In: Gotman J, Ives JR, Gloor P, eds. Long-term monitoring in epilepsy. *Electroencephalogr Clin Neurophysiol Suppl* 1985;37:327–340, with permission.

artifacts caused by electromyographic activity and body movements. Therefore, in the presurgical evaluation it is very important to record more seizures that stay restricted for a longer period of time. For this purpose, we do not withdraw the anticonvulsant medication immediately and completely, since thereby secondary generalized seizures may predominate and the evaluation with surface EEG is spoiled by artifacts. Rather, we try to taper the drug dosage carefully and to spend more time with the recordings. The provocation of seizures and of interictal activity by means of pharmacologic and physical methods is described in Chapter 4.

In cases where the risk of inducing seizures by reduced medication must be kept low and the seizures are to be short lasting, this state is usually preserved for the (second-level) intracranial investigations. The noninvasive technique, on the other hand, can take advantage of the possibility of prolonging the registration periods and thus also enhancing the chance to register epileptic events. The time to be spent on recording a patient's seizures varies considerably (de-

pending on the frequency and consistency of findings); in our department the average is about 72 hours, including all-night sleep.

Methods of Analysis

The value of long-term EEG monitoring is only as high as appropriate analytical methods are applied to establish the diagnostical conclusions. As mentioned earlier, data reduction is a task that requires the use of analytical considerations in so far as selecting electrode montage and type of reference, and epochs of interest depend on the anamnestic background and/or intended points of interest.

Selecting Epochs of Interest

Apart from the so-called nonspecific EEG alterations, most epileptiform phenomena are more or less transient. This means that only a relatively small part of the registered time is assumed to be diagnostically relevant and therefore has to enter the final storage medium. Selection criteria concern either the symptoms (behavioral, clinical, and/or vegetative) or the electrographic events. For instance, in order to distinguish between pseudoseizures and epileptic seizures, selection of epochs will be done primarily according to behavioral and clinical abnormalities. Epochs must be marked either on-line by the technical staff, by the patient, or by care persons (cassette recorders have been equipped with special push buttons) or off-line by visually reviewing the whole recording. Even using fast-speed playback, this is a time-consuming process and requires a lot of experience in recognizing physiologic and pathologic behavior and motor phenomena, both during daytime and sleep. Under certain conditions it may be easier to go the other way, that is, to apply EEG criteria in order to detect seizures. Finally, to select interictal events, the EEG is the only relevant criterion by definition. Both interictal and ictal EEG patterns can be assessed by visual inspection on the display media or by means of technical supporting devices. As a rather simple tool, some replay instruments are capable of making the EEG signals audible. Since the human auditory system does not work in the frequency range of EEG signals, this can be done only with enhanced replay speed, which means that it works only off-line. By these means, spike-wave complexes, spikes, and especially spike (or sharp-wave) series or even bursts of abnormal theta waves often are better recognized and discerned from artifacts than by visual inspection alone. In particular, the often waxing and waning frequency within ictal patterns can be efficiently and fairly simply recognized.

There are other, more sophisticated kinds of technical support in first-line computer-based pattern-recognition methods. For detection of both ictal and interictal patterns, the most common and widely tested algorithms have been developed by the Montreal group [5]. Their basic idea is to mimic the process of visual analysis as far as possible (hence it is called *mimetic* analysis concept). Elementary steps are decomposition of the EEG traces into half-waves, calculating certain characteristics (such as amplitude, duration, slope, and sharpness), and comparing the actual values at any point in time with an adapted combination of criterion parameters (resembling the nonepileptiform background activity). Since this method is well documented in a series of publications, details may be omitted here. Several alternative methods have been proposed [6,7,8]. Based on the concept of Gotman [5], we have developed a modified version of spike analysis that allows automatic screening,

epoch selection, and classification under visual control, and quantitative-statistical analysis. Details of this method will be given below (see Computer-Assisted Evaluation, below) together with examples of application.

Evaluating Signals

Visual Evaluation

Visual evaluation of recordings comprises different levels of consideration: *Nonspecific* activity (slowing of background) concerns topology. *Interictal-specific* activity (see Fig. 5-2) is described with regard to topology (lateralization, localization), morphology (spikes, sharp-wave, spike-wave, isolated, grouped, or burst-like), and conformity. With respect to *ictal* events (Fig. 5-3) topologic indicators for the very onset of seizure activity are most important; spreading and generalization phenomena in correlation with clinical symptoms should be carefully denoted also in order to get reliable information about the conformity (or variability) of the attacks.

Computer-Assisted Evaluation

The major goals of computer-supported analysis of the EEG are (a) to save time, effort, and storage capacities by means of data reduction; (b) to increase the level of significance by removing artifacts and nonepileptic EEG components, as well as by providing quantitative rather than qualitative parameters; and (c) to reveal regularities and relationships invisible to the naked eye.

For documentation and quantification of *nonspecific* abnormalities (normally in lower-frequency bands) and also of postictal focal signs, power spectral analysis is an appropriate tool; however, it is not used yet for clinical decisions.

Concerning *interictal* epileptiform signs, these have already been pointed out in a previous section; the automatic selection of the epochs of interest must be based on quantitative analytical processes.

A further step in this direction is the use of quantitative parameters not only as markers (for the subsequent visual analysis) but in themselves as the subject of an evaluation procedure. As an example we shall briefly outline the computer-based analysis of epileptiform discharges that we have implemented for this purpose. It comprises several program modules: the first, as a step in data reduction, the detection and storage of suspected spike-containing epochs; the second, editing of the selected epochs and classifying

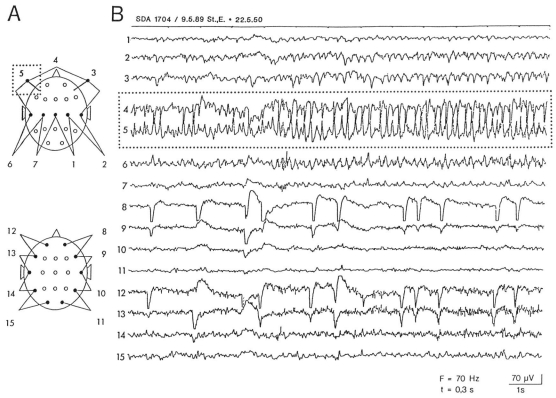

Figure 5-3. Seizure in a sphenoidal recording. (*A*) Schematic drawing of the montage. (*B*) EEG tracings. Numbers are related to the numbers in *A*. From Gotman J, Ives JR, Gloor P, et al. Monitoring at the Montreal Neurological Institute. In: Gotman J, Ives JR, Gloor P, eds. Long-term monitoring in epilepsy. *Electroencephalogr Clin Neurophysiol Suppl* 1985;37:327–340, with permission.

them under visual control; the third, computing the single-spike parameters (frequency, amplitude, duration, and time delay against a reference channel) and averaging these according to the predefined criteria; and finally, display of the results. Spike recognition and parameterization have been based on a special stepwise approximation of the EEG curves by straight lines and segments. Here, the peculiarity lies in the application of linear regression fits modified by means of weighting the resulting correlation coefficient with a factor proportional to the logarithms of the number of data points. This is to counteract the well-known fact that correlation coefficients increase with decreasing number of sample points included (and become 1.0 in the case of two points). Since interchannel amplitude comparison is intended, only common (or average) reference derivations are considered. The representation of the EEG by means of segments of straight lines provides the basis (a) to define elementary wave-form parameters; (b) to compare them with predefined thresholds (here maximum spike/sharp-wave duration, minimum duration and/or slope as discriminator of EMG and movement artifacts, and

minimum relative amplitude) as a tool to differentiate epileptiform, nonepileptic EEG and artifact patterns; and (c) to perform statistical calculations (means and standard deviations). The results are displayed in a simple form of topographic representation of the averaged parameters, registered in different locations (Fig. 5-4). Computerized methods have been developed not only to recognize and describe interictal activity, but also to analyze the *ictal* EEG. One approach is by means of spectral analysis (FFT), for example, in order to describe states as well as dynamic processes in the development of seizures such as the spread of epileptic seizure activity. Power spectra can well illustrate the variation of frequency components (amplitudes) over the electrode locations. Moreover, coherence analysis (based on the cross-spectrum between the signals of two locations) indicates phenomena of enhanced (or even pathologic) synchronization, and the phase spectrum provides a direct measure for the time lag between both signals [9,10,11]. From the theoretical as well as the practical point of view, a problem in the application of spectral methods to seizure lies in the assumption of linearity

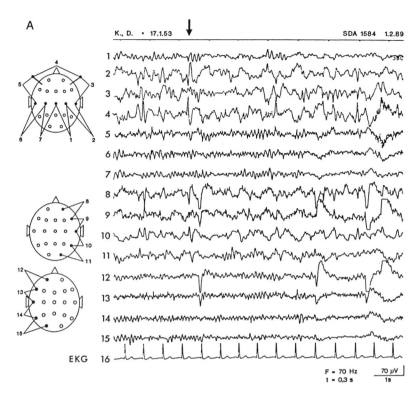

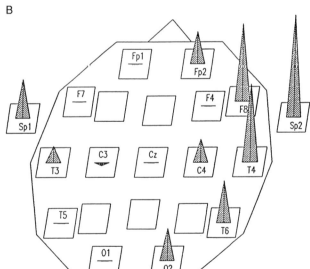

Figure 5-4. Bilateral interictal discharges in sphenoidal recordings. (*A*) Original tracings and montage. (*B*) Spike-topogram of 20 interictal discharges similar to the one marked in *A*.

and stationarity of the process, which obviously is not strictly fulfilled. Therefore, alternatives have been proposed to compute time lags in nonlinear systems, estimating the average amount of mutual information [12,13]. So far, however, these have not been implemented for routine work in presurgical epilepsy diagnostic centers.

Interpretation

As mentioned earlier, long-term EEG recordings in presurgical evaluation are done to determine the presence of epileptogenic areas and, if possible, to provide reliable information about their number, location, and respective contribution to the clinical manifestation of the seizures. In principle, one is faced with the so-called inverse problem of the electromagnetic field theory, that is, the need to draw conclusions about the topographic distribution of generators from the distribution of potential differences measured between distant locations outside the brain [14]. Even assuming homogeneous dipole layers as sources, the problem does not have one unequivocal answer because, for example, several separate dipoles by superimposition may show the same effect as one single dipole. Nevertheless, in many cases the interpretation applying the "solid angle theorem" [15,16] works reasonably well. This concept makes use of the fact that (at a distant point) the potential caused by a dipole is proportional to the solid angle under which the dipole is "visible" from that point. In this context, it is well understood, for example, that dipoles in the surface of a gyrus are easily detectable since the solid angle is large for an electrode immediately above it (and decreases with increasing distance on the surface), so that a dipole in one wall of a sulcus contributes only little, and, finally, a dipole distribution comprising both banks of a sulcus is nearly undetectable by surface electrodes because the difference between the two solid angles (subtended by negative and positive charges, respectively) is approximately zero. Although complex mathematical approaches have been proposed to solve the "inverse problem," the most promising method is to follow the shape of the brain lobes as closely as possible, for example, by means of anterior frontal or sphenoidal electrodes or, on a more invasive level of investigation, by subdural electrodes. The physical properties of the brain and the overlying tissue result in a low-pass filtering of electrical brain signals. Consequently, the epileptiform patterns with highest localizing value are maximally reduced in amplitude, whereas sharp waves (which arise from larger aggregates and therefore have higher amplitudes *per se*) reach the scalp electrodes reduced by only distance factors. Hence the physical properties of the brain and adjacent tissue result in a rather poorly defined localization, which allows lateralization and a coarse regional determination within one lobe.

Significance of Findings

Essentially three types of information are obtained from EEG monitoring: nonspecific (focal), epileptiform interictal, and ictal activity. To describe their respective significance is ambiguous and, to a certain degree, biased by the investigator's individual experience. Objective factors, however, such as stability

and consistency, and the diagnostic task under consideration must also be taken into consideration.

Differential Diagnosis

The differential diagnosis as to whether epileptic seizures (or seizures in addition to other malfunctions) exist in a patient is seldom a problem. Unequivocally epileptiform EEG findings at the time of an attack usually suffice to prove the diagnosis of epilepsy. Exceptionally, however, in some patients only interictal discharges can be recorded, and their occurrence strongly suggests the (presumed) diagnosis of epilepsy. On the other hand, lack of epileptiform patterns in the interictal or even ictal surface EEG does not disprove the existence of an epileptic disorder, particularly if other signs such as clinical symptoms or vegetative parameters (e.g., sudden heart rate alterations during nondisrupted sleep states) are present. If a nocturnal attack occurs without specific EEG alterations during clearly defined (ongoing) sleep activity, a seizure of frontal origin is likely.

Differential Typology

Once *generalized* (e.g., 3-s spike-wave) patterns have been registrated in a patient interictally or ictally, the predominantly focal nature of underlying disease is difficult to prove. There are, in principle, patients in whom both generalized and complex-partial seizures coexist. Here, the importance of a final diagnostic decision is limited because in these cases a surgical intervention will be indicated only exceptionally. However, a number of patients with focal lesions in frontal, parietal, or occipital brain areas exhibit a so-called secondary bilateral synchrony with more or less generalized spike-wave activity.

More often we are concerned with lateralized or focal epileptiform EEG abnormalities and are thus faced with the question of whether a unifocal or multifocal process is involved; in the latter case, there is a question of which focus is the primary or predominant one (i.e., the problem of localization).

Localizing of Epileptic Areas

Observing *nonspecific* focal EEG abnormalities is a helpful supplementary tool for the identification of the primary focus in so far as an interictal epileptiform pattern over the primary focus is rarely associated with a completely normal background. However, no clear data exist concerning the prognostic value of nonspecific focal activity in epilepsy surgery. Therefore, the clinical value is still under discussion.

Interictal epileptiform activity is frequently observed in the region where the primary focus is located. At the convexity, the amplitude distributions of a focus correspond (within limits) approximately to its actual extent [17]. Mesially or basally located foci show characteristic amplitude distributions mainly in sphenoidal, nasopharyngeal, or specially located scalp electrodes [20]. Hence, interictal activity is of confirmatory value as long as it is consistent with the other location indicators, that is, morphologic lesions and neuropsychological deficit [19]. Since interictal activity is not always reliable, however, it alone normally does not suffice to identify the site or even the side of the focus. False lateralization (when restricting oneself to the interictal activity) has been estimated to range between 5% and 33%. On the other hand, it is important to carefully take into consideration whether or not the findings are inconsistent either with each other or with supplementary (ictal electrographic, clinical, neuropsychological, morphologic, and functional neuroimaging) signs. Although interictal activity is usually predominant in the vicinity of the primary focus, those inconsistencies sometimes are substantial indicators of the involvement of bifocal or multifocal processes. Reviewing the reported data, it is generally assumed that interictal signs (under favorable conditions) may miss the very primary focus (in particular when it is concealed in an area distant from the surface), but on the other hand they are helpful in disclosing more widespread abnormalities. Problems frequently arise from the occurrence of temporal interictal epileptiform abnormalities in both hemispheres. Even for bitemporal independent spiking, seizures mostly start from the side of predominant epileptic activity. Statistical data concerning the value of time-lag analysis (resembling neuronal propagation) are not yet available. In this context it should be emphasized that sleep recording may provide additional information. Sammaritano et al. [20] have pointed out that the value of interictal activity during rapid eye movement (REM) sleep is highly localizing, whereas discharge patterns of non-REM sleep are of lower localizing value than those registrated during the waking state. This must be taken into account when sleep recordings are used, because of the long artifact-free periods of recording of scalp EEG.

Ictal epileptiform patterns localized in circumscribed areas of the brain are most informative [21]. Many authors attribute an even higher relative degree of significance to those recorded during spontaneous seizures than to those that are provoked. When the topographic distribution varies over time, the place of first onset of epileptiform patterns is regarded as the primary focus, even if in a later phase the amplitudes over other (often contralateral) areas exceed those observed in the primary focus. A major problem is to define the very first onset of ictal activity, because it is well known that a part of seizure (particularly mesiotemporal) attacks do not project to extracranial (even sphenoidal) electrodes. In two studies at the Montreal Institute [19], the validity of extracranial ictal registrations was estimated to provide clear localization of seizure onsets in 22–40%. The predictive accuracy of scalp and sphenoidal recordings was 82% in a study of patients with focal ictal recordings [22] and 94% in patients with uniformly focal signs. The same study yielded no significant difference in reliability when distinguishing between initial and delayed focal patterns (with respect to the first electrographic feature other than diffuse background suppression). On the other hand, if the first *clinical* symptom precedes the focal EEG onset, the localizing value of the EEG is questionable [19]. The risk of false lateralization is particularly high in patients with gross focal lesions [23].

Recording from scalp and sphenoidal electrodes suffices as long as interictal and ictal findings are congruent with those of clinical, psychometric, and neuroimaging investigations. Even then, however, these recordings must be supplemented by more invasive intracranial (e.g., subdural) derivations, especially in the presence of one of the following conditions: (a) surface recordings speak in favor of bilateral independent foci; (b) the exact location of the focus cannot be differentiated between mesiotemporal and fronto-orbital by characteristics of semiology; (c) temporal and frontal lobe origins are not well enough differentiated; or (d) a primarily occipital and/or parietal focus is rapidly spreading to temporal regions.

Contribution of Scalp and Sphenoidal Recordings

The anterior temporal regions (T1,2; FT3,4; F7,8) turn out to be most frequently concerned when comparing the amount of information provided by various scalp electrodes with respect to how often they were maximally involved [24,25]. These figures reflect the incidence of epileptic focal abnormalities in the various brain areas rather than a quantitative guideline as to how to distribute the electrodes.

It was suggested in earlier studies that sphenoidal electrodes are superior to nasopharyngeal electrodes [26] and able to detect spikes not found in scalp registrations [27]. Sharbrough [28], however, pointed out that this may be due to the fact that the lateral scalp electrodes are often compared in a longitudinal bipolar array, whereas sphenoidal electrodes are linked in transverse montage (hence with longer distances). Examples with direct comparisons have shown that sphenoidal electrodes are not superior to lateral scalp electrodes in every case; their respective amplitudes may sometimes be higher and sometimes lower. Thus, sphenoidal electrodes provide improved information rather than completely new information. In another study comparing sphenoidal and anterior temporal electrodes [29], the latter turned out to be only slightly inferior. In a prospective study [30], sphenoidal recording during wakefulness was less efficient in detecting epileptic discharges than scalp recordings during sleep. Binnie et al. [31] report that sphenoidal recording offers no advantage over suitably placed scalp contacts for detecting interictal discharges, although the latter may help to differentiate between mesial and lateral temporal foci. It is our own experience that sphenoidal electrodes are simple to apply and without any risk, but do cause slight discomfort when placed. Therefore, they provide an easy and practical way to explore the temporal region; in principle, this might also be done by means of other electrodes, which, however, must be attached in the exact positions (see Fig. 5-1).

Conclusion: The Role of Extracranial Recordings within the Presurgical Evaluation Scheme

As mentioned earlier, the main indication for the use of scalp and sphenoidal recordings in patients prior to epilepsy surgery is to establish a reliable hypothesis regarding the type and the location of the intracranial electrodes that must be implanted. Extracranial measuring may help to avoid further invasive procedures under four special conditions: (a) if by EEG methods the psychogenic origin of a patient's attacks can consistently be demonstrated; or (b) if the EEG abnormalities prove that a primary generalized epileptic process is at least coexistent. In both of these cases further steps toward epilepsy surgery are superseded. (c) Similarly, EEG methods together with the clinical history usually are adequate to prove the severe multifocal nature of an epileptic disorder, in which case only a callosotomy rather than focal resection or lobectomy will be indicated. (d) On the other hand, there are circumstances that allow a positive decision on epilepsy surgery, even avoiding additional electrode implantation; this is when ictal and interictal abnormalities from scalp and sphenoidal EEG recordings constantly show a single unilateral temporal focus and, moreover, this focus is consistent with clin-

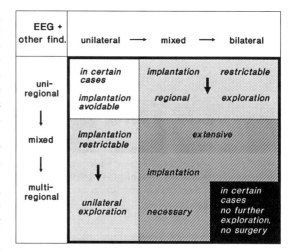

Figure 5-5. Scheme of the decision process in the presurgical work-up using extracranial EEG.

ical, neuropsychological, and neuroimaging signs (Fig. 5-5). In most cases, the findings, even if less unequivocal, serve as the basis for the decision whether to implant intracranial electrodes (subdural strips and grids and depth electrodes). If EEG signs (in agreement with the findings by other examinations) are consistently unilateral (or uniregional, respectively), implantations of subdural electrodes can be limited in their dimension. In any case, the findings of extracranial recordings can be primarily used as indicators where not to place the intracranial contacts, thus minimizing the implantation risk and also the costs for the patient.

Acknowledgment

This work was supported by the Minister of Social Affairs of the Federal Republic of Germany. The authors wish to thank Mrs. M. Schruff, Mrs. A. Kipp, Mrs. K. Schmidt, and Mrs. H. Storma for their technical assistance and Mrs. L. Sarvan for support in preparing the manuscript.

References

1. Cooper A, Winter AL, Crow JH, Walter WG. Comparison of subcortical, cortical and scalp activity using chronically indwelling electrodes in man. *Electroencephalogr Clin. Neurophysiol* 1965;18:217–28.
2. Laxer KD. Mini-sphenoidal electrodes in the investigation of seizures. *Electroencephalogr Clin Neurophysiol* 1984;58:127–9.

3. Wilkus RJ, Thompson PM. Sphenoidal electrode positions and basal EEG during long term monitoring. *Epilepsia* 1985;26:137–42.

4. Gotman J, Ives JR, Gloor P, Quesney LF, Bergsma P. Monitoring at the Montreal Neurological Institute. In: Gotman J, Ives JR, Gloor P, eds. Long-term monitoring in epilepsy. *Electroencephalogr Clin Neurophysiol Suppl* 1985;37:327–40.

5. Gotman J. Automatic recognition of interictal spikes. In: Gotman J, Ives JR, Gloor P, eds. Long-term monitoring in epilepsy. *Electroencephalogr Clin Neurophysiol Suppl.* 1985;37:93–114.

6. Guedes de Oliveira P, Queiroz C, Lopes da Silva FH. Spike detection based on a pattern recognition approach using a micro computer. *Electroencephalogr Clin Neurophysiol* 1983;56:97–103.

7. Ktonas PY. Automated spike and sharp wave (SSW) detection. In: Gevins AS, Rémond A, eds. *Methods of analysis of brain electrical and magnetic signals.* EEG Handbook (rev. series, Vol I). Amsterdam: Elsevier 1987:211–41.

8. Principe JC, Smith JR. Automatic recognition of spike and wave bursts. In: Gotman J, Ives JR, Gloor P, eds. Long-term monitoring in epilepsy. *Electroencephalogr Clin. Neurophysiol Suppl* 1985;37:115–32.

9. Gotman J. Measurement of small time differences between EEG channels: method and application to epileptic seizure propagation. *Electroencephalogr Clin Neurophysiol* 1983;56:501–14.

10. Gotman J. Interhemispheric interactions in seizures of focal onset: data from human intracranial recordings. *Electroencephalogr Clin Neurophysiol* 1987;67:120–33.

11. Lieb JP, Hoque K, Skomer CE, Son XW. Interhemispheric propagation of human mesial temporal lobe seizures: a coherence/phase analysis. *Electroencephalogr Clin Neurophysiol* 1987;67:101–19.

12. Mars NJI, Lopes da Silva FH. Propagation of seizure activity in kindled dogs. *Electroencephalogr Clin Neurophysiol* 1983;56:194–209.

13. Pijn JPM, Vijn PCM, Lopes da Silva FH, van Emde Boas W, Blanes W. The use of signal-analysis for the localization of an epileptogenic focus: a new approach. In: Manelis J, Bental E, Loeber JN, Dreifuss FE, eds. *Advances in epileptology.* XVIIth epilepsy international symposium. New York: Raven Press, 1989;67–71.

14. Ebersole JS. Equivalent dipole modeling: a new EEG method for epileptogenic focus localization. In: Pedley TA, Meldrum BS, eds. *Recent advances in epilepsy 5.* Edinburgh: Churchill Livingstone, 1991;51–71.

15. Gloor P. Neuronal generators, the problem of localization and volume conductor theory in electroencephalography. *J Clin Neurophysiol* 1985;2:327–54.

16. Woodbury JW. Potentials in a volume conductor. In: Ruch TC, Fulton JF, eds. *Medical physiology and biophysics.* Philadelphia: Saunders, 1960;83–91.

17. Lüders H, Hahn J, Lesser RP, Dinner DS, Rothner D, Erenberg G. Localization of epileptogenic spike foci: comparative study of closely spaced scalp electrodes, nasopharyngeal, sphenoidal, subdural and depth electrode. In: Akimoto H, Kazamatsuri H, Seino M, Ward AA eds. *Advances in epileptology.* XIIIth epilepsy international symposium. New York: Raven Press, 1982; 185–9.

18. Ebersole JS, Wade PB. Spike voltage topography identifies two types of frontotemporal epileptic foci. *Neurology* 1991;41:1425–33.

19. Quesney LF, Gloor P. Localization of epileptic foci. In: Gotman J, Ives JR, Gloor P, eds. Long-term monitoring in epilepsy. *Electroencephalogr Clin Neurophysiol Suppl* 1985;37:165–99.

20. Sammaritano M, Gigli GL, Gotman J. Interictal spiking during wakefulness and sleep and the localization of foci in temporal lobe epilepsy. *Neurology* 1991; 41:290–7.

21. Swartz BE, Walsh GO, Delgado-Escueta AV, Zolo P. Surface ictal electroencephalographic pattern in frontal vs temporal lobe epilepsy. *Can J Neurol Sci* 1991; 18:649–62.

22. Risinger MW, Engel J, Van Ness PC, Henry TR, Crandall PH. Ictal localization of temporal lobe seizures with scalp/sphenoidal recordings. *Neurology* 1989;39:1288–93.

23. Sammaritano M, de Lotbiniere A, Andermann F, Olivier A, Gloor P, Quesney LF. False lateralization by surface EEG of seizure onset in patients with temporal lobe epilepsy and gross focal cerebral lesions. *Ann Neurol* 1987;21:361–9.

24. Morris HH, Lüders H. Electrodes. In: Gotman J, Ives JR, Gloor P, eds. Long-term monitoring in epilepsy. *Electroencephalogr Clin Neurophysiol Suppl* 1985; 39:3–26.

25. Quesney LF, Gloor P. Special extracranial electrodes. In: Wieser HG, Elger CE, eds. *Presurgical evaluation of epileptics.* Berlin-Heidelberg: Springer-Verlag, 1987; 162–76.

26. Sperling MR, Mendius JR, Engel J Jr. Mesial temporal spikes: a simultaneous comparison of sphenoidal, nasopharyngeal and ear electrodes. *Epilepsia* 1986; 27:81–6.

27. King DW, So EL, Marcus R, Gallagher BB. Techniques and application of sphenoidal recording. *J Clin Neurophysiol* 1986;3:51–65.

28. Sharbrough FW. Commentary: extracranial EEG evaluation. In: Engel J, ed. *Surgical treatment of the epilepsies.* New York: Raven Press, 1987:167–71.

29. Homan RW, Jones MC, Rawatt S. *Electroencephalogr Clin Neurophysiol* 1988;70:105–9.

30. Neufeld MY, Cohn DF, Korczyn AD. Sphenoidal EEG recording in complex partial seizures. *Clin Electroencephalogr* 1986;17:139–41.

31. Binnie CD, Marston D, Polkey CE, Amin D. Distribution of temporal spikes in relation to the sphenoidal electrode. *Electroencephalogr Clin Neurophysiol* 1989; 73:403–9.

Chapter 6

Chronic Intracranial Monitoring Techniques

ALLEN R. WYLER

The outcome of epilepsy surgery depends primarily on the identification of appropriate surgical candidates and secondarily on completeness of the surgical procedure. As is evident from other chapters in this book, patient selection is usually based on agreement among a variety of data, which include the structural, functional, metabolic, and electrical integrity of the brain. Of these data, the electroencephalogram (EEG) provides the criterion that has most reliably localized the epileptogenic focus. However, there are several points of controversy surrounding the EEG evaluation of surgical candidates and these are reviewed below.

Ictal Versus Interictal Recordings

Historically, epilepsy surgery was first done on only the most easily localized cases, and therefore, as practiced by Foerster and Penfield [1], it usually involved the removal of structural lesions such as chronic depressed skull fractures or atrophic lesions seen by pneumoencephalography. With the advent of EEG, neurologists and neurosurgeons were able to find electrical abnormalities that correlated with the location of the focus in many of the cases, and surgical decisions were then changed to rest on the correlation between structural lesions and EEG data. Because this approach continued to yield fair results, the extrapolation was finally made in 1947 by Dr. Percival Bailey (with the contributions of Frederic and Erna Gibbs) to remove a temporal lobe for the treatment of psychomotor epilepsy based solely on interictal EEG findings [2]. In Bailey's day, long-term ictal monitoring was not available and so obviously only interictal scalp recordings were used. Shortly afterward, Penfield and colleagues began to use interictal recordings

to select patients for surgery, and surgeons began to bring the EEG machine into surgery with the hopes that the intraoperative electrocorticography (ECoG) would further improve their ability to localize the epileptogenic focus. Because the surgeries based on these concepts have had some excellent results, we have developed an almost superstitious acceptance of the localizing value of interictal EEG and ECoG. However, what were the actual results from the early surgical series? According to the psychomotor seizure outcome from the University of Illinois series only 30% of patients were greatly improved, 38% improved, and 32% unimproved [2]. Early results from the Montreal Neurological Institute were not much different [3]. It is interesting to speculate what the outcome might be if patients were submitted to anterior temporal lobectomy at random. For example, given 100 patients without structural lesions who have complex partial seizures, 90% have those seizures coming from the temporal lobes. If all 100 patients are subjected to a right anterior temporal lobectomy, approximately 45 will have undergone the correct operation. If we assume that the interictal EEG has at least some localizing value, it is reasonable to assume that the data it generates could improve patient selection and localization of epileptogenic foci. And, in fact, after the EEG was introduced into epilepsy surgery, the postoperative results from centers such as the Montreal Neurological Institute did improve. However, interictal recordings have several serious drawbacks, which will be listed below. Although many centers that provide epilepsy surgery make decisions based primarily on interictal EEG findings, they deny many potential candidates an opportunity for successful surgery and inappropriately operate on other patients.

There is increasing evidence that long-term EEG/video ictal monitoring is superior to interictal EEG monitoring for lateralizing and localizing epileptogenic foci. Some of the reasons for this superiority are that interictal recordings do not allow the physician to determine seizure type or phenomenology, both important variables for establishing surgical candidacy. (For example, patients who have only tonic seizures do not do well with temporal lobectomy even if there is a preponderance of interictal discharges within a temporal region.) Interictal recordings may appear to be nonfocal or bilateral when in fact the seizure focus is unilateral and the patient may be a good candidate for unilateral anterior temporal lobectomy. In a more recent study from the Montreal Neurological Institute [4], 57 patients with bitemporal independent epileptiform abnormalities and no localized epileptogenic focus by extracranial EEG were subsequently investigated by depth electrode recordings. The majority of patients (77%) were found to have a unilateral focus and subsequently did well after anterior temporal lobectomy [5]. These patients would not have been selected for surgery if invasive monitoring had not been done. Finally, interictal epileptiform discharges may be falsely localizing. For example, Wieser et al. [6] demonstrated that the side of onset of spontaneously occurring seizures agreed with the lateralization of interictal spike activity (recorded from depth electrodes) in only two thirds of cases. Spencer et al. [7] compared ictal scalp recordings to depth recordings and found that the accuracy of scalp ictal EEG readings ranged from 21% to 38% for lobe and 46% to 49% for side of seizure onset. Wyler et al. [8] compared relative localizing values of scalp interictal, scalp ictal, and subdural ictal recordings in a group of 52 patients who became seizure-free after surgery (thereby verifying the location of the epileptogenic focus) with similar results.

Thus, the data indicate that although there is some localizing and lateralizing value to interictal scalp-recorded EEGs, they are insufficient when used by themselves for the selection of surgical patients.

Intracranial Recordings Versus Scalp Recordings

A second area of controversy has been over the relative accuracy of scalp versus intracranial recordings. Data from various sources indicate that invasive ictal recordings provide more accurate lateralization and localization than do scalp interictal or ictal EEG recordings [6–11]. Not only do invasive ictal recordings provide the best localization of epileptogenic foci, they also provide data (not obtainable from scalp recordings) that can determine who should not undergo surgery. For example, the interhemispheric propagation time provides an excellent measurement for predicting surgical outcome. Patients whose seizures spread from one temporal lobe to the other within 5 s or less do not do well following unilateral anterior temporal lobectomy [12].

Thus, there is considerable evidence from various surgical centers that invasive ictal monitoring provides the most accurate data for selecting surgical candidates. The purpose of this chapter is to review techniques and methods for chronic intracranial recordings, pointing out the advantages and disadvantages of each.

Instruments for Chronic Intracranial Monitoring

The most common techniques for chronic intracranial recordings are (a) depth electrodes; (b) epidural or subdural grid electrodes; and (c) subdural strip electrodes. The indications for each technique are slightly different and dependent on the specific information needed. To fully appreciate the differences among these techniques, it is best to begin by discussing how each is implemented.

Depth Electrodes

Depth electrodes are typically made as long thin shafts with small recording surfaces near the tip (Fig. 6-1). The electrode's shaft is usually made of flexible material so that, once embedded in the brain, the electrode can move slightly to accommodate any brain movement. Depth electrodes are inserted intracranially through small holes and then stereotaxically directed through the brain to the target area. In most cases, only the distal portion of the electrode is actually within the gray matter and thus only a small portion of the electrode shaft can have contacts used for recordings. One exception to this rule is the occipital trajectory that Spencer uses to record from hippocampus [13,14]. He inserts depth electrodes through the occipital lobe anteriorly so that the electrode shaft traverses the long axis of the hippocampus. In doing so, multiple contacts at various lengths along the electrode shaft can be used to record mesial temporal ECoG activity.

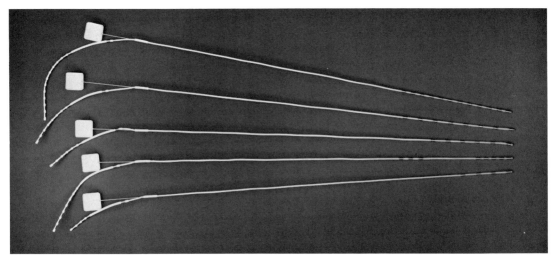

Figure 6-1. Examples of 8-, 12-, and 12-contact (different interelectrode contact spacing) depth electrodes with introducers inserted down the shaft of each electrode. After inserting the electrode to its final target, the introducer is removed, allowing for greater electrode flexibility.

Advantages

Depth electrodes can be placed to record from structures not reached by cortical surface electrodes (e.g., hippocampus or amygdala); they can usually be withdrawn without general anesthesia either in the patient's room or in a minor surgery room, thus decreasing total hospital costs; the definitive surgery can then be scheduled at a later time and the electrodes are easily placed bilaterally.

Disadvantages

Stereotaxic equipment and expertise are needed for proper placement of depth electrodes, and operating room time is greater so that fewer patients can be treated within any one center.

Complications

Because the depth electrode traverses the brain parenchyma, it can tear a vessel during insertion and cause hemorrhage. This complication, although infrequently reported, can be disastrous when it does occur.

Grid Electrode Arrays

Large grids or arrays of electrodes can be purchased commercially or manufactured individually by a laboratory technician trained in working with the proper materials. The electrode contacts in the grid are commonly arranged in rows of 6 to 10 disk contacts, but the grid can be made to any configuration (Fig. 6-2). Some centers use grids with up to 64 electrode contacts. The interelectrode distance is usually 1 cm, but it too can be adapted to the needs of the investigator.

Implanting a grid array requires a large craniotomy to expose the desired portion of the brain. The electrode array is laid either on the cortical surface (subdural) or over the intact dura (epidural). When the electrodes are inserted subdurally, additional strip electrodes can be placed under the temporal lobes or within the interhemispheric fissure to expand the total recording area. The array of cables are brought through the skin either at separate stab wounds or along the craniotomy wound margin (which is less preferable because of increased chances for wound infection). Epidural grid arrays can cover only the brain's convexity and obviously cannot record from locations such as interhemispheric cortex of the frontal lobes. Because of this major limitation, the only good indication for epidural electrode grid insertion is when one needs to investigate a patient from a previous craniotomy whose subdural space is obliterated by adhesions.

Advantage

The advantage of the grid array is that it allows cortical stimulation through the same electrodes used for seizure monitoring. If the suspected seizure focus is near eloquent cortex, the location of cerebral function can be mapped in relation to the location of seizure onset. This strategy is beneficial when dealing with frontal lobe foci within the dominant hemisphere.

Disadvantages

Most disadvantages of the grid array are related to the surgery required for placement and removal. The grid array is not suitable for bilateral implantation. Consequently, one must have excellent evidence that the correct side of seizure onset has been chosen before a large grid electrode array is implanted. The most common indication for intracranial monitoring is to verify the *side* and *site* containing the epileptogenic focus, which cannot be done with a unilateral electrode montage. Because the grid array requires a large craniotomy for placement, the infection rate associated with its use is considerably greater than for either depth or subdural strip electrodes. A second craniotomy under general anesthesia is needed to remove the grid array. In some cases, the definitive epilepsy surgery is done at the time of grid removal so that the correlation between mapped cortical function and the site of seizure onset can be accurately extrapolated to the underlying cortex. When resective surgery is coupled with grid removal, the infection rate for the focal resection is higher than expected.

In a few cases the grid electrode acted as a mass lesion, much the same as an epidural or subdural hematoma, and had to be removed before sufficient information could be obtained. This situation has occurred only when the grid was manufactured at a moderate thickness.

Subdural Strip Electrodes

Subdural strip electrodes are commercially available or can be fabricated [15] (Fig. 6-3). They consist of thin strips made of Silastic or a similar material. Each strip contains from 4 to 12 electrodes in a single row with an interelectrode distance of 1–1.5 cm. The most common strip size is 6 cm and has four electrode contacts. One or more strips can be implanted

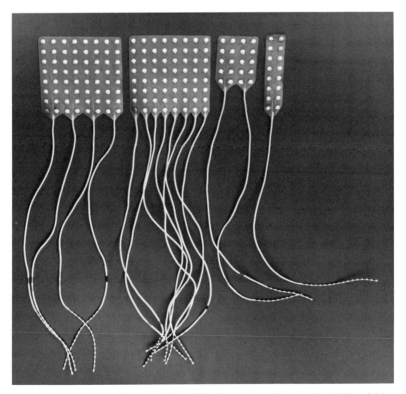

Figure 6-2. Examples of 8 × 8, 4 × 5, and 2 × 8 contact grid electrodes. Grids of this size are implanted through a large craniotomy opening and can be placed either epidurally or subdurally. Often combinations of grids and strips are used together. For example, an 8 × 8 grid can be placed over the lateral frontal lobe and two smaller strip electrodes placed down the interhemispheric fissure, providing coverage of any extent of cortex desired. Because these grids require implantation through a craniotomy flap, they are most often implanted only unilaterally.

through a standard-sized burr hole rather than through the large craniotomy flap needed to implant grid electrode arrays. Because of the flexibility of most commercially available strips (i.e., AD-Tech Co., Racine, Wisconsin), they can be slid over the surface of the brain to deeper regions such as the basal surfaces of the temporal lobe and the interhemispheric fissure. Double, parallel-row strips are also available and can be treated as minigrid arrays and inserted through burr holes.

Advantages

Subdural strip electrodes can also allow cortical stimulation through their electrode contacts; however, the exact correlation with underlying cortex is not as easily reconstructed as with a grid array. They are simple to insert and require no special expertise in stereotaxic surgery. They can be placed in most neurosurgical centers with minimal operating time, therefore allowing for a high volume of cases within any surgical center. At our center a full set of eight electrodes can be inserted within 1 hour. Like depth electrodes, subdural strip electrodes can be placed easily bilaterally. Most thin strip electrodes can be removed percutaneously without the use of an operating room, thus limiting surgical costs. Finally, subdural strip electrodes can cover large expanses of cortex through a single burr hole.

Disadvantages

Subdural strip electrodes cannot be used to record directly from amygdala or hippocampus. Thus, some researchers believe them to be less accurate than depth electrodes in diagnosing temporal lobe foci [16].

Complications

The major risk from subdural strip electrodes is infection. This risk appears to be equal to or less than that with depth electrodes, and both subdural strip electrodes and depth electrodes have an infection rate considerably lower than the infection rate associated with grid arrays.

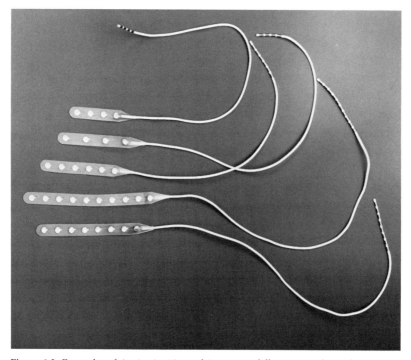

Figure 6-3. Examples of 4-, 4-, 6-, 10-, and 8-contact (different interelectrode spacing) strip electrodes with either multistrand or unistrand attachment wires. Strip electrodes with multistrand wires are often used for acute ECoG during epilepsy surgery, whereas unistrand strip electrodes are best suited for chronic implantation.

Risks and Benefits of Invasive Monitoring

The primary indication for invasive monitoring is to increase the accuracy of patient selection and therefore improve the outcome of epilepsy surgery. Improved patient selection involves the proper identification of the site of seizure onset as well as recognition of patients who are not candidates for focal resection because of multifocal epilepsy. In a review of the literature up to 1980, Spencer [13] noted that monitoring with depth electrodes enabled selection of 36% more patients for surgery by defining otherwise unidentifiable single epileptogenic foci. In addition, depth EEG monitoring could have prevented surgery in another 18% of patients by demonstrating different or additional epileptogenic foci in patients otherwise thought to have a single discharging focus amenable to resection. Spencer concluded that depth electrode monitoring had the potential to alter the surgical decision in more than 50% of patients reported.

In contrast to this view, Ojemann [17] has written:

The outcome of the patients identified by noninvasive criteria is as good as that in most of the cases where selection was based on the depth electrode localization of ictal onset. Because of this, it seems clear that there is little justification for implanting intracranial electrodes in patients who meet these noninvasive criteria. The use of intracranial electrodes clearly introduces some element of additional risk and, although the risk is quite small with modern approaches, it is almost as great as the small risk of resective surgery. Thus, the use of intracranial electrodes almost doubles the risk to the patient who is selected for resection and exposes those patients not selected for resection to some risk without direct therapeutic benefit. Placement of intracranial electrodes also adds substantial cost to the preoperative evaluation, especially when compared to approaches using noninvasive criteria based on interictal EEG recordings.

Ojemann's cost argument is the most easily dealt with. Admittedly, there is cost to implanting electrodes; however, if doing so can shorten the time needed for noninvasive monitoring, then the only additional cost is that of the surgical procedure. At our center, for example, if a patient does not have a structural lesion we monitor the patient only long enough to clearly document that he or she suffers from complex partial seizures. When that is documented, we terminate monitoring and arrange for definitive localizing monitoring using subdural strip electrodes. Thus, the expense of lengthy scalp monitoring is minimized whereas the ultimate confidence for having localized the focus is maximized. Invasive monitoring saves other additional costs during a surgical evaluation such as the cost of a positron emission tomography (PET) scan, intraoperative ECoG, and so on. Thus, an accurate comparison of the total costs of an efficient work-up that utilizes invasive monitoring to one that does not, has not been done. Secondly, what is the cost of a failed operation? There is increasing evidence that substantial psychological, psychiatric, and vocational gains only follow surgery that renders the patient seizure-free [18]. Data indicate that patients whose surgery followed invasive monitoring have a higher probability of being seizure-free than those operated on the basis of noninvasive data [8]. Moreover, reoperation of patients whose resective surgery has failed to eliminate seizures is most likely to result in seizure-free outcome if the patient was initially evaluated with invasive monitoring [19]. Finally, invasive monitoring identifies patients with resectable unilateral seizure foci (with seizure-free outcomes) who would never be considered for surgery because their scalp-recorded EEG demonstrated bilateral discharges or bilateral foci [4,7,8,14]. If one wishes to consider the total cost to society, the most cost-effective result from surgery is the patient who is completely seizure-free because that person is most likely to be rehabilitated socially and vocationally and will most likely become a financially productive person. Patients who are improved and who yet continue to have seizures almost never become financially self-supporting and remain dependent on social services. The patient who has seizures following surgery continues to assume the risk of accidental injury inherent in the seizures themselves and the increased financial cost of continued medical care in comparison to the person who is rendered seizure-free. Finally, the person who has a focal region of brain removed that is not the epileptogenic focus becomes a postoperative disaster: not only do the seizures persist, but the person will show considerable cognitive loss as a surgical result. The probability of a seizure-free outcome is greater when a person has been evaluated before surgery with either depth or strip electrodes.

The second argument against invasive monitoring is that some patients will ultimately be found to not be surgical candidates, yet will have been subjected to the risk of invasive monitoring. This argument is equally weak because if such monitoring had not been done, then the patient may well have had surgery with a poor result. In that case, the patient will have undergone a needless resective surgery with its inherent risk, will still be having seizures, and will probably have a substantial neuropsychological deficit. I would much rather submit a patient to the small risk of invasive monitoring than to the risk of failed surgery.

Finally, the argument that the outcomes of patients operated on based on noninvasive criteria are as good as those operated on following invasive monitoring is fallacious because the data are simply not available. Surgical series based solely on noninvasive data are highly selective and do not necessarily represent the same group of patients operated on at centers that rely on invasively obtained information.

Given the above discussion, who should be monitored invasively and who should not? At our center we have devised the following protocol:

1. All patients have a magnetic resonance imaging (MRI) brain scan prior to initial scalp monitoring.
2. Patients then undergo EEG/video monitoring with scalp electrodes to document spontaneous, typical seizures. Unless the patient regularly has nocturnal seizures, all attempts are made to analyze seizures that have occurred during wakefulness.
3. Patients who have a structural lesion and complex partial seizures are then considered for surgery to remove the structural lesion without further invasive monitoring.
4. Patients who have obvious tonic, atonic, tonic-clonic, or myoclonic seizures without a structural lesion are considered for anterior corpus callosotomy without additional invasive monitoring.
5. Patients who have obvious complex partial seizures are subjected to additional invasive monitoring before considering focal resection.

Choice of Invasive Monitoring Techniques

The most common reason to implant electrodes is to determine the site of seizure onset. Because interictal and ictal scalp recordings have a significant rate of false lateralization, exploratory recordings should be done bilaterally in most cases. Unless there is compelling evidence that the side of seizure onset has been determined unequivocally, bilateral recordings are always preferred. For this reason, large grid electrode arrays have limited indications. The most common indication for a grid electrode is to map functional cortex around the periphery of a known structural lesion prior to planning removal of that lesion. A further discussion of grid electrodes is the subject of Chapter 7.

Some investigators have advocated use of grid arrays when planning resection of speech-dominant temporal lobes. However, most data indicate that the site of seizure onset for idiopathic temporal lobe epilepsy is most commonly within the mesial temporal regions, and a standardized resection can provide excellent results without complicated cortical mapping [20,21].

For determining the lobe, laterality, and discreteness of an epileptogenic focus (i.e., whether the focus is singular or multifocal), the choice is primarily between depth and subdural strip electrodes. The advantages and disadvantages of both have been discussed without clear resolution. The argument in favor of depth electrodes hinges around the fact that they can be inserted into deep structures not reached by subdural strip electrodes (i.e., hippocampus and amygdala). However, the question is whether one always needs to record from hippocampus in order to obtain enough data with which to make an accurate surgical decision. Our experience is that subdural strip electrodes can provide sufficient data to render appropriate surgical decisions.

Summary

No consensus exists as to the indications for invasive EEG monitoring in an evaluation for epilepsy surgery. Yet there are numerous data from various surgical centers to indicate that long-term intracranial ictal EEG monitoring is superior to long-term scalp EEG recordings in lateralizing and localizing epileptogenic foci. Invasive monitoring can provide additional data, such as the presence of bilateral foci, interhemispheric propagation time, and regional versus lateral versus medial temporal ictal onset that cannot be provided with scalp recordings, and these data are crucial in the proper selection of patients who are or not likely to benefit from surgery. Because of an increasing awareness of the value of invasive monitoring, more surgical epileptologists are requiring such recordings as an integral portion of most presurgical evaluations. At our center, we require invasive recordings from any patient considered for focal cortical resection who has complex partial seizures without a causal structural lesion demonstrated on MRI.

Invasive recordings may be accomplished with depth electrodes, subdural strip electrodes, and subdural grid electrode arrays. The indications, advantages, and disadvantages of each method are listed in this chapter. The individual surgical techniques for implanting these recording devices are varied; they are best obtained from individual publications and are not the subject of this chapter.

Acknowledgment

Examples of depth, grid, and strip electrodes were supplied by AD-Tech Medical Instrument Corporation, Racine, Wisconsin.

References

1. Foerster O, Penfield W. *Brain* 1930;53:99–119.
2. Hermann BP, Stone JL. A historical review of the epilepsy surgery program at the University of Illinois Medical Center: the contributions of Bailey, Gibbs, and collaborators to the refinement of anterior temporal lobectomy. *J Epilepsy* 1989;2:155–63.
3. Penfield W, Jasper H. *Epilepsy and the functional anatomy of the human brain.* Boston: Little, Brown, 1954.
4. So N, Gloor P, Quesney LF, Jones-Gotman M, Olivier A, Andermann F. Depth electrode investigations in patients with bitemporal epileptiform abnormalities. *Ann Neurol* 1989;25:423–31.
5. So N, Olivier A, Andermann F, Gloor P, Quesney LF. Results of surgical treatment in patients with bitemporal epileptiform abnormalities. *Ann Neurol* 1989;25:432–9.
6. Wieser HG, Bancaud J, Tacairach J, Bomis A, Szika G. Comparative value of spontaneous and chemically and electrically induced seizures in establishing the lateralization of temporal lobe seizures. *Epilepsia* 1979;20:47–59.
7. Spencer SS, Williamson PD, Bridgers SL, Mattson RH, Cicchetti DV, Spencer DD. Reliability and accuracy of localization by scalp ictal EEG. *Neurology* 1985;35:1567–75.
8. Wyler AR, Richey ET, Hermann BP. Comparison of scalp to subdural recordings for localizing epileptogenic foci. *J Epilepsy* 1989;2:91–6.
9. Lieb JP, Engel J Jr, Gevins A, Crandal PH. Surface and deep EEG correlates of surgical outcome in temporal lobe epilepsy. *Epilepsia* 1981;22:515–38.
10. Engel J Jr, Rausch R, Lieb JP, Kuhl DE, Crandall PH. Correlation of criteria used for localizing epileptic foci in patients considered for surgical therapy of epilepsy. *Ann Neurol* 1981;9:215–24.
11. Engel J Jr, Rausch R, Lieb JP, Kuhl DE, Crandall PH. Correlation of criteria used for localizing epileptic foci in patients considered for surgical therapy of epilepsy. *Ann Neurol* 1981;9:215–24.
12. Lieb JP, Engel J Jr, Babb TL. Interhemispheric propagation time of human hippocampal seizures. I. Relationship to surgical outcome. *Epilepsia* 1986;27:286–93.
13. Spencer SS. Depth electroencephalography in selection of refractory epilepsy for surgery. *Ann Neurol* 1981;9:207–14.
14. Spencer SS, Spencer DD, Williamson PD, Mattson RH. The localizing value of depth electroencephalography in 32 patients with refractory epilepsy. *Ann Neurol* 1982;12:248–53.
15. Wyler AR, Ojemann GA, Lettich E, Ward AA Jr. Subdural strip electrodes for localizing epileptogenic foci. *J Neurosurg* 1984;60:1195–1200.
16. Spencer SS. Depth versus subdural electrode studies for unlocalized epilepsy. *J Epilepsy* 1989;2:123–7.
17. Ojemann GA. Surgical therapy for medically intractable epilepsy. *J Neurosurg* 1987;66:489–99.
18. Hermann BP, Wyler AR, Ackermann B, Rosenthal T. Short-term psychological outcome of anterior temporal lobectomy. *J Neurosurg* 1989;71:327–34.
19. Wyler AR, Hermann BP, Richey ET. Results of reoperation for failed epilepsy surgery. *J Neurosurg* 1989;71:815–9.
20. Spencer DD, Spencer SS, Mattson RH, Novelly RA, Williamson PD. Access to the posterior temporal lobe structures in the surgical treatment of temporal lobe epilepsy. *Neurosurgery* 1984;15:667–71.
21. Crandall PH. Cortical resections. In: Engel J Jr, ed. *Surgical treatment of the epilepsies.* New York: Raven Press, 1987:377–404.

Chapter 7

Functional Mapping of Language Abilities with Subdural Electrode Grids

HANS O. LÜDERS
ISSAM AWAD
ELAINE WYLLIE
LEONARD SCHÄFFLER

Electrical stimulation can be used effectively to investigate the cortical organization of language. This methodology has been applied most extensively in patients who are candidates for surgery of epilepsy [1–6]. In these patients subdural electrodes can be implanted subacutely to record interictal and ictal electroencephalographic (EEG) abnormalities, which permits relatively precise delineation of the epileptogenic zone that has to be removed as completely as possible to achieve good surgical results. In addition, the implementation of electrodes allows electrical stimulation, which represents the most powerful method to define the eloquent cortex surrounding the epileptogenic focus [7]. This information is essential to permit safe removal of the epileptogenic zone without producing neurologic deficits.

Methodology

It is essential to follow some of the basic methodologic rules outlined below to investigate with precision the language function of the human cortex by electrical stimulation. To uncover cortical language areas, it is best to use as high a stimulus intensity as possible, avoiding, however, the eliciting of afterdischarges. *Afterdischarges* represent epileptiform discharges elicited by electrical stimulation and occurring at one or more electrodes, and very frequently are associated with spread of the activation over more or less extensive cortical areas in addition to the stimulated electrode. The presence of afterdischarges

makes interpretation of the results difficult because it is impossible to determine whether the effect is due to the electrode stimulated or to the activation related to the afterdischarges, which, as mentioned above, frequently spreads to involve a more extensive cortical area. It is interesting to mention, however, that not infrequently afterdischarges, even when involving numerous electrodes, may be clinically silent. This is also the case when they involve electrodes that when stimulated produce clear neurologic symptoms or neurologic deficits. A typical example would be when a patient has speech arrest during the stimulation but continuous reading as soon as the stimulus is over, even when the EEG shows a prominent afterdischarge involving many electrodes, including the one that, when stimulated, produced the speech arrest. This finding indicates that the stimulation may produce a more intense disruption of neuronal function or may affect a larger number of neurons than the afterdischarges. Certainly, there are also other cases in which the speech arrest may continue as long as the afterdischarge persists, long after the stimulation has been discontinued. The graded effect of afterdischarges in the production of clinical symptomatology explains the observation that patients with exquisitely focal motor ictal symptomatology (e.g., twitching of one finger) may have an extensive epileptic discharge involving the whole motor strip and adjacent cortex. In these cases, a jacksonian march of a clonic motor seizure may just be determined by a change in the relative intensity of a widespread ictal discharge involving the whole motor cortex simultaneously. The "intensity" of an epileptiform discharge cannot be assessed solely by visual inspection of the waveform or amplitude of the ictal epileptiform discharge.

Ideally we would like to stimulate at the highest stimulus intensity we consider to be safe (50 Hz, 0.3 ms, 15 mA for electrodes of 3 mm or more in diameter). However, very frequently the occurrence of afterdischarges at very low stimulus intensities precludes testing at appropriate intensities at some electrodes. This may leave eloquent areas of cortex uncovered. To avoid this problem the following techniques can be used. In patients who had low afterdischarge thresholds and relatively low blood levels of anticonvulsants, the testing can be repeated after loading with phenytoin or other major anticonvulsants. This procedure is frequently associated with a significant increase of the afterdischarge threshold. We have also observed that no afterdischarges may be elicited when stimulating again shortly after producing an afterdischarge, even when the repeat stimulus was at a higher intensity. With this technique, it is frequently possible to stimulate some electrodes at considerably higher stimulus intensities than the initial "afterdischarge threshold." These special techniques are not always effective and not infrequently may limit our maximum stimulus intensity to relatively low values. In those cases, it is essential to remember that no signs or symptoms when stimulating at 15 mA for 5 s or longer is a fairly reliable sign that the cortex is actually "silent," but that this cannot be said when the cortex underlying an electrode was never tested at more than 2–3 mA because of afterdischarges. This is particularly true for "language electrodes" in the temporal lobe, which usually do not give positive results at intensities below 5–10 mA.

Another extremely important aspect when testing for language function is the reproducibility of the results. To ensure a cause-effect relationship between the stimulation and the observed language deficit, we have to make sure that (a) the patient has no difficulty in executing the language task when no stimulation occurs and (b) that the same effect can be elicited repeatedly when stimulating the same electrode even when the patient is unaware that stimulation was being performed. This is particularly true when testing for more complex language tasks that test the limits of each patient's verbal skills. So, for example, we may ask a patient to list the months of the year backward. If the patient makes some error while being stimulated, we should ask the patient to perform the same task a few times while no stimulation is going on. If the patient makes similar errors under this condition, it is almost impossible to define the effect of stimulation. If he or she makes no error, we

would repeat the same task once or twice while again stimulating the same electrode. Another useful test is to ask the patient to perform a given task *at different stimulus intensities*. The deficit can reliably be attributed to a stimulus effect if it consistently occurs at high stimulus intensities, occurs only occasionally or in incomplete fashion at intermediate stimulus intensities, and disappears completely at low stimulus intensities. For example, this would be the case with a patient who when stimulating a given electrode stops reading at high stimulus intensities, slows down at intermediate stimulus intensities, but has no reading difficulties at low stimulus intensities.

The test results should not only indicate at which electrodes a certain symptom or sign was elicited but also the *maximum stimulus intensity* at which an electrode was tested when no symptoms or signs were elicited. There are many reasons that can prevent the examiner from testing the effect of high stimulus intensities. The most frequent reason, as mentioned earlier, is a too low threshold for afterdischarges and auras or seizures. In other cases, no testing is possible because higher stimulus intensities elicit pain either due to (a) stimulation of nerve fibers included in the dura mater or in cortical blood vessels [8], or (b) to direct stimulation of cranial nerves, particularly the trigeminal nerve when stimulating in the medial temporal region. Stimulation in the medial temporal region may also produce ipsilateral motor twitching of the facial musculature due to excitation of the motor branch of the trigeminal nerve. This may also limit the intensity at which the cortex can be stimulated. Cortex should only be considered as "silent" and therefore safe to resect without producing any neurologic deficit if it was stimulated at or close to 15 mA and no symptoms or signs occurred. When cortical stimulation produces no symptoms or signs at low stimulus intensities, we certainly cannot exclude the possibility of eloquent cortex if testing at high stimulus intensities would have been possible.

It is also important to remember that in many cortical areas stimulation includes only "negative" signs. In other words, stimulation of the cortex elicits no spontaneous signs or symptoms such as muscle twitching or subjective symptoms ("positive" signs). Actually the patient is totally unaware that the stimulation occurred. However, when asked to perform a certain function, the patient is unable to do so. Thus, for example, stimulation of the temporal lobe language areas produces exclusively negative signs. It has been speculated that in these cases the stimulation produces an inactivation of centers that are important for the organization of the task the patient was unable to perform during the stimulation [7]. The exact function of cortical areas is extremely difficult to define by the electrical stimulation method because most higher cortical functions consist of "negative" signs. In other words, they are only detectable by asking the patient to perform a certain task and then watching for interference in the patient's performance of the task. Even in extraoperative settings it is only possible to test at each electrode for a limited number of functions.

How does the investigator decide which functions are going to be tested for? In our laboratory we have used essentially three techniques to decide the testing methodology.

1. After having determined the maximum stimulus intensity that does not produce discharges, the patient is asked to read aloud while stimulating again at an intensity that is immediately subthreshold for afterdischarges. Electrodes at which there is speech interference are then tested for other higher cortical functions.

2. Previous research using different procedures (e.g., the effects of cortical infarcts) is taken into consideration to predict the possible function of the cortex underlying any given electrode. The testing procedure is then adapted to detect "negative signs" related to the predicted cortical function, for example, testing for symptoms of Gerstmann's syndrome in the dominant temporoparietal region [9].

3. Finally, in selected cases we have screened for a particular higher cortical function with all or most of the implanted subdural electrodes, for example, screening all electrodes for short-term memory deficits elicited by electrical stimulation. This procedure is evidently very time consuming and can only be done for very selected functions and using highly simplified testing methods.

The results of electrical stimulation of language areas is best exemplified by the following case report.

CASE REPORT

C.O. is a 20-year-old white female with psychomotor seizures since the age of 15 years. The seizures consisted of a motionless stare, unresponsiveness, and oral and hand automatisms. The seizures lasted from 40 to 130 s. Postically, she was confused and aphasic for up to 5 min. Secondary generalized tonic-clonic seizures never occurred. Neurologic examination was normal. Scalp EEG revealed interictal sharp wave activity arising independently from the left and right temporal lobes. Magnetic resonance imaging (MRI) showed increased signal intensity on T2-weighted images in the lateral aspect of the left temporal lobe, thought to represent a cyst or tumor mass. Despite adequate treatment with phenytoin, carbamazepine, valproate, phenobarbital, and various combinations of these drugs, the patient continued to experience five to six seizures per day. Invasive EEG monitoring with bitemporal depth electrodes showed frequent interictal sharp waves in the left temporal mesial and lateral (85%) and right mesial temporal regions (15%). Psychomotor seizures originated from the left temporal region (anterior and posterior hippocampus). The intracarotid sodium amobarbital (Wada) test showed that the left hemisphere was dominant for language, and both hemispheres could support memory function.

Neuropsychologic testing revealed low-average functioning with a full-scale Wechsler Adult Intelligence Scale (WAIS) intelligence quotient (IQ) of 83 and a Wechsler Memory Scale IQ of 86. The WAIS verbal IQ was 81. She obtained a standard score of 77 on immediate verbal recall but a standard score of 112 for immediate visual memory. Her delayed retention for both verbal and nonverbal material was in the low-average range. The patient manifested significant dysnomia and calculation difficulties despite having normal visuoconstructional and visual-organizational abilities.

The patient had a left frontotemporal craniotomy for placement of a subdural electrode array in the left basal temporal region and in the left temporal convexity. For the next 17 days, the patient was studied by cortical stimulation and interictal and ictal EEG/video monitoring. The seizures originated from the left temporal convexity immediately anterior to the structural lesion. Electrical stimulation revealed a cortical language area (Wernicke's area) immediately posterior and superior to the structural lesion. She underwent a second craniotomy with removal of the posterior temporal lesion (modified temporal lobectomy, which included 2.5 cm of the superior temporal gyrus and 9 cm of the inferior temporal gyrus). Electrocorticography revealed no ictal discharges at the resection margin. Neuropathologic examination of the removed specimen revealed that the removed structural lesion was a ganglioglioma. A mild to moderate anomic aphasia was noticed for 1–2 weeks postsurgically. She has had no seizures or auras since surgery and is on phenytoin monotherapy.

Figure 7-1 shows a diagram with the location of the plate of subdural electrodes and the nomenclature used to identify the electrodes. Figure 7-2 shows the results of electrical stimulation. The location of the lesion is also shown as underlying electrodes A25 and A26. All the electrical stimulation was performed using electrode A64 as the reference electrode. In Figure 7-2 we can identify three language areas: the

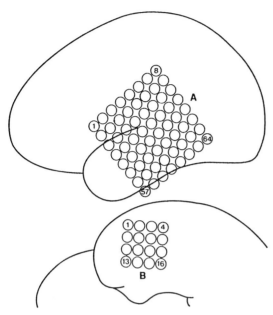

Figure 7-1. Nomenclature used for identifying subdural electrodes. The plate over the convexity was called the *A* plate and the plate over the basal temporal region was labeled the *B* plate. Numbers run left to right, top to bottom (sample numbers shown).

anterior language area ("Broca's area") at electrodes A47 and A39; the posterior language area ("Wernicke's area") at electrodes A21, A28, A20, A12, and A19; and the basal temporal language area at A57,

In addition, we were able to identify the motor area of the jaw (A24); the sensory area of the face and contralateral hand (A6, A7, A15, A14, A23, A30, A31); and negative motor areas (A16, A31, A22) (Table 7-1). At the motor area (A24) the stimulation pulled the tongue to the inside of the mouth and the jaw to the right side. The patient showed speech arrest (most probably due to the positive motor effects described above) but was able to see the words and read them silently ("I can see the words but cannot say them"). Stimulation of the sensory electrodes produced paresthesias in the area indicated in Table 7-1. No negative motor response was recorded at any of these electrodes except at electrode A31. At electrode A38 the patient complained consistently of excessive salivation during the stimulation. At electrode A7 low stimulus intensity (8 mA) elicited paresthesias only, whereas higher stimulation intensity (11–12 mA) also produced motor twitches at the right mouth. Stimulation of A16 elicited a negative motor response of the tongue (unable to wiggle tongue from side to side) and of the right hand (unable to perform rapid alternating movements of the fingers of the right hand) but not of eyes, right foot, or ipsilateral left extremities. At A22 there was a negative motor response of the tongue with speech arrest. The patient, however, was able to write on dictation and read silently with good understanding of the material she had been asked to read. At electrode A31 stimulation at 7 mA produced a mixture of a negative motor response of the tongue, prominent

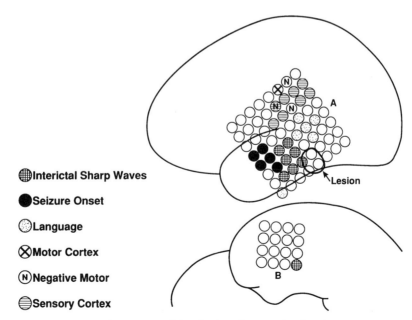

Figure 7-2. Functional mapping and distribution of interictal and ictal activity.

Table 7-1. Results of Electrical Stimulation (Motor and Sensory Effects)

Electrode	Intensity (mA)	Electrode	Sensory Symptoms	Motor Signs	Conclusion
A16	9	A64	—	Arrest of rapid alternating movements of tongue	Negative motor tongue area
A31	7	A64	—	Arrest of rapid alternating movements of tongue	Negative motor tongue area
A22	8	A64	—	Arrest of rapid alternating movements of tongue	Negative motor tongue area
A24	7	A64	—	Pulling of lower jaw to the right; pulling of tongue to the inside of the mouth	Positive motor jaw area
A7	8	A64	"Tingling": right mouth corner	—	Sensory mouth area
A15	4	A64	"Tingling": right lower lips and tip of tongue	—	Sensory mouth and tongue area
A23	5.5; 6.5	A64	"Tingling": right side of tongue	—	Sensory tongue area
A6	9	A64	"Tingling": right thumb	—	Sensory right thumb area
A14	9.5	A64	Numbness: right lower lip and tip of tongue	—	Sensory mouth and tongue
A30	9	A64	"Tingling": right side of lower and upper lips	—	Sensory mouth area
A31	7	A64	"Tingling": tip of tongue; increasing salivation	—	Sensory tongue area

salivation, and paresthesias at the tip of the tongue. Stimulation of the two electrodes in the anterior language area (A47 and A39) produced similar results. The patient was unable to read aloud (speech arrest) or name objects even when testing for a negative motor response of tongue and hand was negative (Table 7-2). Repetition of a single sentence was also impossible but the patient had no comprehension deficit of oral or written material. Interestingly, at both electrodes we were able to demonstrate a mild agraphia. So, for example, the patient wrote "the pencil *off* blue" when asked to write "the pencil is blue." The relatively smaller interference with writing was also clearly demonstrated by the observation that the patient was totally unable to read aloud the sentence she had just written. In summary, we conclude that electrical stimulation of the anterior language area in this patient produced a clinical expressive aphasia with a mild agraphia with clear *dissociation* of input functions comprehension, which was relatively intact.

The results at the posterior language area were significantly more variable (Table 7-3). At four electrodes (A12, A19, A20, and A21) the patient was unable to read aloud ("speech arrest") and also had other expressive difficulties when tested for them (agraphia at three electrodes, anomia at two electrodes, inability to count aloud and inability to repeat a single sentence at one electrode). At two electrodes (A19, A12) this was associated with inability to follow oral or written commands and inability to read silently, indicating that at these two locations the expressive deficit was matched by an equally severe comprehension deficit. At two other electrodes, however, severe expression deficit was not associated with a clear comprehension deficit; at electrode A21 the patient was able to read silently (even if slightly more slowly) and could follow two-step oral commands, and at electrode A20 the patient was even able to follow three-step oral commands. Also of interest is the observation that the patient made paraphasic errors during naming when stimulating electrode A20.

Table 7-2. Results of Stimulation Testing in Anterior Speech Area

	Electrode	
	A47	A39
Reading aloud	+ + +	+ + +
Confrontation naming	+ + +	+ + +
Repetition of sentences	+ + +	+ + +
Writing sentences to dictation	+	+
Commands, oral: Two-step	−	−
Silent reading of questions and understanding	−	−
RAMs of tongue	−	−
RAM of fingers: L and R hand	−	−

Abbreviations: L, left; R, right; RAM, rapid alternating movements; + + + = total speech arrest or total inability to perform the task; + = slight impairment to perform the task; − = no abnormality produced by electrical stimulation.

Finally, at electrode A28 we were able to elicit a predominant comprehension deficit by electrical stimulation. In other words, the patient was able to continue reading aloud with only slight slowing down when she was totally unable to follow two-step written or oral commands. At all five electrodes we tested for a negative motor response of the tongue or hand with negative results. From these observations we can conclude that electrical stimulation of the posterior language area can produce a variety of language deficits including global aphasias, predominantly expressive aphasias, and predominantly receptive aphasias. In this case, it appears that electrodes that produced predominantly comprehension deficit were located most anteriorly (A28), those that produced predominantly expressive deficit were located more superiorly (A20, A21), and those that produced mixed expression/comprehension deficits were located most inferiorly and posteriorly (A12, A19) within the posterior language areas. Systematic studies in our laboratory are currently underway to define if within the posterior language area we can identify areas of subspecialization that occupy different anatomic loci.

In this case we were able to identify only one electrode, A57, that was localized approximately in the region we have identified as the basal temporal language area. Stimulation of that electrode produced inability to read aloud or to write, but no further systematic testing was performed.

Figure 7-2 also shows the distribution of interictal sharp waves and of ictal activity at the onset of the seizures.

Results and Conclusion

The effects of stimulation of language areas using the technique detailed above have been reported in numerous publications [8,10–18]. In all these studies we required the following test results to define a cortical area as a language area by electrical stimulation:

1. Speech arrest, significant slowing of speech, or other language interference at a stimulus intensity that does not produce any positive signs or symptoms and also elicits no afterdischarges

Table 7-3. Results of Stimulation Testing in Posterior Speech Area

	Electrode				
	A20	A21	A28	A12	A19
Reading aloud	+ + +	+ + +			
Confrontation naming	+ + +	+ + +	+	+ + +	+ + +
Repetition of sentences	+ + +	NT	NT	+ + +	NT
Counting forward	NT	NT	NT	+ + +	NT
Repetition of sentences	NT	NT	NT	+ + +	NT
Writing sentences to dictation	+ + +	+ + +	NT	+ + +	NT
Commands, oral					
One-step	−	NT	NT	NT	NT
Two-step	−	−	+ + +	+ + +	+ + +
Three-step	−	NT	NT	NT	NT
Comprehension of written questions/commands (silent reading)	−	−	+ + +	+ + +	+ + +
RAMs of tongue	−	−	−	−	−

Abbreviations: NT, function not tested during electrical stimulation; + + + = total speech arrest or total inability to perform the task; + = slight impairment to perform the task; − = no abnormality produced by electrical stimulation; other abbreviations as in Table 7-2.

2. Clear proof from additional testing that the apparent language interference is not due to a negative motor effect. This is only necessary when the testing for language function included a motor component (e.g., reading aloud).

According to this definition, we have been able to define language areas in the following three regions:

1. Anterior language area (in the inferior and intermediate frontal gyrus immediately in front of the face motor strip) corresponding approximately to what has been labeled as Broca's area
2. Posterior language area (in the parietoposterior temporal region) corresponding to what approximately has been labeled Wernicke's area
3. Basal temporal language, which is located in the base of the temporal lobe

In the supplementary motor area, which has been considered the "superior language area" by Penfield and Roberts [1], we have been unable to elicit a pure language deficit by electrical stimulation. Speech arrest occurs frequently but in our experience has consistently been due to a negative motor effect. However, our experience with stimulation of the supplementary motor cortex is still relatively limited (nine cases) and conclusive evidence will require additional testing in more patients. Negative motor responses can also be elicited frequently from the anterior language area [19,20], but, in addition, pure language disturbances are also common in the anterior language area. Negative motor responses occur only very infrequently from the postrolandic area and are always immediately adjacent to the rolandic fissure at a distance from the classic Wernicke's area.

The effect of electrical stimulation is relatively similar in all three language areas. Total speech arrest can be seen when stimulating electrodes in the posterior or basal temporal language area, and comprehension deficits have been described when stimulating Broca's area [21]. This is illustrated well by the case presented earlier. Quantitative comparative analyses are now underway to compare the effect of electrical stimulation on different input or output language functions in these three areas.

The results of exact cortical mapping of language areas, like those of other aspects of eloquent cortical cases, have been used effectively by surgeons to plan a safer surgical procedure, and in many cases exact knowledge of the boundaries of eloquent cortical areas has allowed significantly more complete resection of the epileptogenic zone. There is evidence indicating that a more complete resection of the epileptogenic focus is associated with a better outcome [22], making cortical mapping techniques essential for epilepsy surgery centers treating more complicated cases, particularly patients with extramesiotemporal epileptogenic loci.

References

1. Penfield W, Roberts L. *Speech and brain mechanisms.* Princeton, NJ: Princeton University Press, 1959.
2. Rasmussen T, Milner B. Clinical and surgical studies of the cerebral speech areas in man. In: Zülch KJ, Creutzfeldt O, Galbraith GC, eds. *Otfried Foerster symposium on cerebral localization.* New York: Springer-Verlag, 1975:238–57.
3. VanBuren J, Fedio P, Frederick G. Mechanism and localization of speech in the parieto-temporal cortex. *Neurosurgery* 1978;2:233–9.
4. Ojemann GA. Individual variability in cortical localization of language. *J Neurosurg* 1979;50:164–9.
5. Rapport R, Tan C, Whitaker H. Language function and dysfunction among Chinese and English-speaking polyglots: cortical stimulation, Wada testing and clinical studies. *Brain Lang* 1983;18:42–66.
6. Lesser RP, Lüders H, Morris HH, et al. Comprehension deficits produced by stimulation of Wernicke's area in candidates for temporal lobectomy. *Ann Neurol* 1985;18:118–9.
7. Lüders H, Lesser RP, Dinner DS, et al. Commentary: chronic intracranial recording and stimulation with subdural electrodes. In: Engel J Jr, ed. *Surgical treatment of the epilepsies.* New York: Raven Press, 1987:297–321.
8. Lesser RP, Lüders H, Klem G, Dinner DS, Morris HH III, Hahn J. Ipsilateral trigeminal sensory responses to cortical stimulation by subdural electrodes. *Neurology* 1985;35:1760–3.
9. Morris HH, Lüders H, Lesser RP, Dinner DS, Hahn J. Transient neuropsychological abnormalities (including Gerstmann's syndrome) during cortical stimulation. *Neurology* 1984;34:877–83.
10. Lesser RP, Lueders H, Hahn J, et al. Location of the speech area in candidates for temporal lobectomy: results of extraoperative studies. *Neurology* 1982;32:1.
11. Lesser RP, Lueders H, Dinner DS, Hahn J. The anatomical relationship of the frontal speech area to the inferior motor strip: results of extraoperative cortical stimulation. *Neurology* 1983;33:9.
12. Lesser LP, Lüders H, Dinner DS, Hahn J, Cohen L. The location of speech and writing functions in the frontal language area: results of extraoperative cortical stimulation. *Brain* 1984;106:275–91.
13. Lüders H, Lesser RP, Hahn JF, et al. Basal temporal speech area demonstrated by electrical stimulation. *Neurology* 1985;35:220.
14. Lesser RP, Lüders H, Morris HH, et al. Electrical stimulation of Wernicke's area interferes with comprehension. *Neurology* 1986;36:658–63.

15. Lüders H, Lesser RP, Dinner DS, Morris HH, Wyllie E, Klem G. Comprehension deficits elicited by electrical stimulation of Broca's area. *Epilepsia* 1986;27:598–9.

16. Lüders H, Lesser RP, Dinner DS, Morris HH, Wyllie E. Language deficits elicited by electrical stimulation of the fusiform gyrus. In: Engel J Jr, Ojemann GA, Lüders HO, Williamson PD, eds. *Fundamental mechanisms of human brain function.* New York: Raven Press, 1987: 83–9.

17. Wyllie E, Lüders H, Dinner DS, Morris HH, Hahn J, Lesser RP. Cortical electrical stimulation of frontal and temporal speech areas in the evaluation of epilepsy surgery in children and adolescents. *Epilepsia* 1987; 28:622.

18. Lüders H, Lesser RP, Dinner DS, Morris HH, Wyllie E, Godoy J. Localization of cortical function: new information from extraoperative monitoring of patients with epilepsy. *Epilepsia* 1988;29:556–65.

19. Lüders H, Lesser LP, Dinner DS, Morris HH, Hahn J. Inhibition of motor activity elicited by electrical stimulation of the human cortex. *Epilepsia* 1983;24:519.

20. Lüders H, Lesser LP, Dinner DS, et al. Negative motor response elicited by electrical stimulation of the human frontal cortex. In: Delgado-Escueta A, Chauvel P, Hargren E, Bancad J eds. *Frontal lobe seizures.* New York: Raven Press, 1992;149–57.

21. Lüders H, Lesser RP, Hahn J, et al. Basal temporal language area demonstrated by electrical stimulation. *Neurology* 1986;36:505–10.

22. Wyllie E, Lüders H, Morris HH, et al. Clinical outcome after complete or partial cortical resection for intractable epilepsy. *Neurology* 1987;37:1634–41.

Chapter 8

The Role of Neuropsychological Assessment in the Presurgical Evaluation of the Epilepsy Surgery Candidate

GORDON J. CHELUNE

Since the pioneering efforts of Horsley in 1886 [1], surgical resection of epileptogenic brain tissue has become an increasingly accepted treatment option for patients with focal seizure disorders that are refractory to conventional therapies [2–5]. With advanced preoperative methods of evaluation, it is now estimated that about 80% of individuals with intractable complex-seizure disorders, especially those of temporal lobe origin, could become seizure-free or experience significant reductions in seizure frequency following epilepsy surgery [5–9]. In his review of the incidence and prevalence rates of focal seizures in the United States, Dreifuss [6] estimates that perhaps as many as 75,000 persons in this country have intractable disorders and could be eligible for such surgical intervention given current surgical criteria.

The purpose of this chapter is to examine the potential contributions of neuropsychological assessment in the preoperative evaluation of these epilepsy surgery candidates. We begin first with an examination of the nature and content of neuropsychological assessment and then review the major applications of these procedures within an epilepsy surgery program. Although clinical examination of memory and language functions during intracarotid injection of Amytal Sodium (i.e., the Wada test [10]) is an important form of preoperative neuropsychological assessment among surgery candidates at many centers [11], we limit our discussion here to the potential utility of standardized psychometric assessment procedures.

The Neuropsychological Evaluation

Clinical Neuropsychology

Clinical neuropsychology can be broadly defined as the study of brain-behavior relationships and the application of this knowledge to clinical problems arising from disturbances of cognitive and behavioral ability associated with brain dysfunction. Over the course of the past 60 years a myriad of standardized test procedures have been developed to assess the wide variety of human abilities dependent on the cortical integrity of the brain [12]. The sensitivity of these neuropsychological procedures to the presence and location of both focal and diffuse cortical lesions is well documented in the literature and compares favorably with surgical information and other neurodiagnostic procedures [13–21].

Because seizures arise from paroxysmal disturbances of the normal electrical activity of the brain, considerable attention has been given to studying the neuropsychological correlates of various seizure characteristics and electroencephalographic (EEG) parameters among epilepsy patients, especially those with complex-partial disorders [22–29]. Recent research has also shown a strong association between indicators of focal functional deficit on neuropsychological testing and changes in regional cerebral blood flow among patients with focal seizure disorders [30]. It is therefore not surprising that formal neuropsychological assessment has become an integral part of the comprehensive evaluation of seizure surgery patients.

In surveying epilepsy surgery centers about their typical evaluation approaches, Engel [5] found that "a standard psychometric assessment is routinely performed on all patients in 86% of responding centers" and "occasionally" in another 11% of centers. While the nature of these "standard psychometric" evaluations is not delineated by Engel, they are typically neuropsychological in orientation. That is, these evaluative processes involve the use of standardized psychometric procedures to gather data that are then interpreted within the broader nomothetic framework of neuropsychological research and theory to identify and delineate the cognitive and behavioral deficits associated with a patient's seizure disorder. The tests employed generally sample a broad range of ability domains, including such areas as intelligence, problem solving, attention, learning and memory, language, visuospatial functions, motor skills, and sensory-perceptual ability. It is not necessarily the tests that make the evaluations *neuropsychological* in nature, but the conceptual framework within which the data are interpreted [31]. The specific test procedures may vary from program to program, but the purpose of the neuropsychological examination is always to generate empirical referents from which neuropsychological inferences can be made about the patient.

Nature of the Evaluation

The typical neuropsychological evaluation employs a comprehensive battery of tests in which the patient must demonstrate specific skills or abilities. The tests are designed to sample a broad range of cognitive and behavioral abilities within a multitrait-multimethod paradigm [32] that allows for both convergent and discriminant validation on several inferential levels. Because multiple procedures are used, the neuropsychological evaluation is time-intensive and may require several hours to a full day to complete. In addition, the nature of the tasks presented requires the active participation of the patient; that is, without adequate levels of patient cooperation and effort, it is not possible to conduct a reliable and valid neuropsychological evaluation.

Multitrait-Multimethod Paradigms. Although use of multiple-ability measures is labor-intensive, it is critical to the efficacy of the neuropsychological evaluation. Given our developing knowledge of the functional organization of the brain and the multifaceted effects of brain dysfunction on cognitive activity, it is clear that a multivariate (multitrait) assessment approach is necessary if the neuropsychologist is to attempt to delineate the nature and scope of cognitive dysfunction associated with a central nervous system (CNS) disturbance. It is through the examination of the patterning of a patient's strengths and deficits that inferences concerning specificity arise. Multiple sampling of a given ability domain is also important to establish the reliability of a deficit and to distinguish it from transient lapses of effort or attention [27].

Since performance on any given behavioral task is an end point that can be adversely affected at different levels by complex biologic processes located in disparate neural substrates, multiple methods of sampling a cognitive domain are important to delineate the manner in which a cognitive skill breaks down [33]. A qualitative analysis of performance deficits can provide further clues as to possible localization of a focal disturbance within the functional system [34]. For example, neuropsychologists will often employ material-specific (verbal versus visual) measures of free recall, cued recall, recognition memory, and rate of acquisition when examining a patient's "memory," a cognitive domain of particular interest among individuals with complex-partial seizure disorders of temporal or frontal origin [7,11,26,27,35–38]. Careful examination of potential differences arising from these multimethod modes of sampling an ability such as "memory" provides useful information for the possible lateralization and localization of the seizure focus.

Inferential Approaches. To evaluate and derive neuropsychological implications from the large data set that is produced by a multifactorial test battery, the clinician uses several inferential methods of analysis [39]. These methods include an examination of the patient's *level of performance* with respect to appropriate population norms and standards. With knowledge of a patient's level of ability on individual tests, one can perform a *profile analysis* of the data to determine if there are differential patterns or dissociations between related tests that suggest a specific ability deficit. *Intraindividual comparisons* between the right and left sides of the body can be made for tests of motor function and sensory-perceptual capacity. By extension, intraindividual comparisons are also made between abilities that are typically assumed to be mediated by the left (e.g., language) versus right (e.g., complex visuospatial recognition) hemispheres. Finally, individual responses are qualitatively examined for *pathognomonic indications* of subtle deficit that may affect the interpretation of the data as a whole (e.g., a subtle dysnomia could adversely affect performance on a task of primary visual-organizational ability if the test requires a verbal answer for a response) or reflect a subtle deficit that might otherwise not be suspected.

Although the content of neuropsychological test batteries varies widely from one epilepsy center to another, there is a great deal of overlap in the ability areas assessed, if not in the actual procedures used. It is beyond the scope and intent of this chapter to detail the most commonly used tests in the presurgical evaluation of seizure patients, but the interested reader is referred to the excellent paper by Rausch [40] for a survey of such procedures. For our purposes it is sufficient to appreciate the nature and process of the neuropsychological examination as it is used in the presurgical evaluation of epilepsy patients.

Let us now turn our attention to how neuropsychological assessment can contribute to the work-up of the surgical candidate.

Role of the Neuropsychological Evaluation

Neuropsychologists are generally not directly involved in the ongoing care of the epileptic patient. Rather, they are asked to evaluate the patient in the role of a consultant whose task it is to provide specialized input that addresses the concerns of the professionals who are managing the clinical care of the patient. The value of the report generated on the basis of the neuropsychological evaluation in this context can be measured in terms of "how it influences subsequent decisions about the patient and how beneficial those decisions are for the patient" [41]. Within an epilepsy surgery program, the ultimate decision that must always be addressed is whether a given patient is a suitable candidate who will benefit from surgical intervention. Understanding the desired outcome of epilepsy surgery and the fundamental criteria for patient selection defines the range of questions that the preoperative neuropsychological evaluation attempts to address.

Selection Criteria and Goals of Epilepsy Surgery

The ultimate goal of epilepsy surgery is to eliminate or substantially reduce a patient's seizures by excising "the epileptogenic tissue in its entirety but without resection of normal tissue, particularly brain tissue essential for full functional capacity" [42]. To achieve this goal, careful attention must be given to the se-

lection of appropriate surgical candidates. McNaughton and Rasmussen [43] have noted that "without doubt, the proper evaluation and selection of patients for surgical management of the symptom, epilepsy, is the most important single factor in determining the success or failure of this form of treatment in reducing the seizure tendency."

Over the course of the past 10–15 years, a general consensus has emerged concerning the fundamental criteria for selecting those patients who are most apt to benefit from surgical management of their epilepsy [2–4,6,43,44]. First, the ideal candidate for epilepsy surgery should be intractable to conventional therapies, having failed one or more adequate trials of anticonvulsant medications despite evidence of good compliance and blood levels high within the therapeutic range. Next, the patient's seizures should be of sufficient severity and frequency, occurring over an extended period of time, to disrupt normal patterns of daily living. It is also felt that the seizures should arise from a relatively focal brain region that is amenable to resective surgery without undue risk of significant neurologic or cognitive deficit. Finally, patients "should be sufficiently intellectually intact and free from disabling psychotic disturbances as to be able to benefit from rehabilitation" [6].

Issues to Be Addressed by the Neuropsychological Examination

Given the selection criteria and desired outcome described above, the neuropsychologist reformulates these into a set of questions that neuropsychological assessment procedures might appropriately address. For the purpose of our discussion, these are grouped under four general headings: baseline assessment, localization and lateralization, seizure control, and neuropsychological outcome.

Baseline Assessment

Perhaps the single most common purpose for obtaining a comprehensive neuropsychological evaluation prior to surgical intervention for epilepsy is to provide an objective description of the patient's presurgical cognitive status that can serve as a baseline against which future comparisons can be made. Although neuropsychological assessments are generally not obtained within epilepsy surgery centers until a patient's seizure disorder is considered intractable, their inclusion early among other clinical, EEG, and imaging studies can help provide a "clear, informed interpretation of the problem to the patient, the family, and the physician" [2]. They also provide a basis for monitoring the effects of intractable seizures on the individual's cognitive capabilities over time.

Although not without controversy, the literature suggests that cognitive deterioration can occur in epilepsy and is associated with a variety of factors. Seizure frequency [45–48], age of seizure onset [45, 49–53], seizure type [54,55], etiology [6,56], duration of condition [45,50,57], and use of anticonvulsant medication [58–61] have all been implicated in the occurrence of cognitive deterioration among individuals with intractable seizure disorders. Generally, those with more frequent seizures beginning at an earlier age and lasting for a longer period of time are more likely to show signs of mental deterioration than those with infrequent seizures and having recent onsets beginning later in life. Patients with major motor seizures often have a more deleterious course than those with complex-partial seizures, as do those with progressive neurologic conditions compared to those with static etiologies. Long-term use of high doses of anticonvulsant medications can also lead to cognitive deterioration, although this is not independent of seizure frequency, duration, or etiology. In the context of such variables, test-retest neuropsychological testing can provide "useful guidance in evaluating whether or not a seizure problem is malignant from a cognitive point of view" [2]. Objective evidence of mental decline speaks to the criteria of severity and disruption of normal living patterns and should accelerate the clinician's consideration of the patient as a potential surgery candidate.

Since the benefits of increased seizure control must be weighed against possible decrements in cognitive ability [2,6,62], it is also essential to have a comprehensive presurgical neuropsychological baseline against which postsurgical performances can be compared. These presurgical-to-postsurgical comparisons allow the neuropsychologist to determine what, if any, cognitive losses have resulted from surgery. Using data from such comparisons, research by Milner [37,63] and others [7,8,64–69] has documented a number of potential deficits that can result from epilepsy surgery. In doing so, these researchers have greatly enhanced our understanding of the nature and manner in which the temporal and frontal lobes contribute to the functional organization of cognition and memory.

Although there is a relative paucity of published research on the topic, the preoperative neuropsychological baseline evaluation has also been used to predict various outcome parameters such as likelihood of seizure control [70] and the potential effects of surgery on subsequent neuropsychological functioning

[71]. The emphasis is on finding signs or predictors within the baseline neuropsychological data set that can be used to identify patients at possible risk for negative outcomes. Because of their potential importance, these uses of neuropsychological assessment will be discussed separately in subsequent sections.

Localization and Lateralization

The correct lateralization and localization of the epileptogenic focus prior to surgical intervention are critical to the potential success of epilepsy surgery. Given the documented sensitivity of neuropsychological procedures to other types of focal neurologic lesions and their correlation with various seizure characteristics and EEG parameters noted earlier, it is not surprising that neuropsychologists frequently attempt to draw inferences concerning the potential location of the epileptic focus on the basis, when present, of a circumscribed functional deficit manifested in the data accrued during the preoperative neuropsychological evaluation. Although such inferences are rarely definitive, they "can often help to identify a focal functional deficit that has localizing value, particularly when attempting to differentiate between dominant and nondominant, and temporal and extratemporal lesions" [5]. As might be expected, the concurrence of a focal pattern of neuropsychological deficit implicating a specific cortical region and evidence of discrete electrophysiologic excitability of an epileptiform nature arising from the same area suggests that the correct localization of the seizure focus has been made [72].

Although there is often concordance between focal neuropsychological findings and electrophysiologic data [37], it is not infrequent to find the neuropsychological data at some variance with the EEG findings. In such instances, the utility of neuropsychological data is open to question and depends on why the two sources of data are discrepant. As noted by Engel [5], "focal functional deficit alone, when epileptogenicity has not been well localized by EEG, is never a sufficient basis for performing surgery," although "the absence of a functional deficit contralateral to an EEG-identified epileptic focus is often considered sufficient to recommend surgical resection."

Perhaps the most frequent reason that discrepancies occur derives from the inherent differences in the intent of the two data sources. Whereas electrophysiologic measures are designed to reflect neural patterns of electrical activity, data derived from neuropsychological assessment of cognitive and behavioral abilities reflect the behavioral output of the brain.

These data are not "specific" to seizure activity but to the conditions producing the epileptogenic activity. For example, diffuse neurologic disorders such as encephalitis or closed head trauma are often associated with diffuse patterns of neuropsychological deficit, yet have focal regions of epileptogenicity that may be amenable to surgical resection. We have seen cases in our center where the neuropsychological results correlated very closely with the presence of focal encephalomalacia secondary to a depressed skull fracture in one hemisphere only to find, via intensive scalp and invasive EEG studies, that the seizure focus was localized to a discrete region in the contralateral hemisphere.

Other variables also influence the degree of concordance between electrophysiologic data and the nature and patterning of cognitive performance on neuropsychological batteries. Generally, the earlier the age at seizure onset, the lower and more generalized the pattern of cognitive deficit, presumably because intractable disorders from an early age disrupt the normal acquisition of a wide range of cognitive ability regardless of the locus of the seizure focus [33, 50–53]. Early insults to the brain have also been associated with atypical patterns of functional organization. Among the most dramatic of these is the behavioral reorganization of language abilities to the right hemisphere that occasionally occurs after early left hemisphere injuries [73,74]. In such cases, language functions may be relatively well preserved and may even appear somewhat superior to visuospatial functions [53,75–77].

It should be clear that use of neuropsychological assessment for lateralization and localization among intractable seizure patients is a complex and difficult task. At best, when neuropsychological signs of focal functional deficit coincide with similar focal findings from electrophysiologic and neuroimaging sources, one's confidence that the correct localization of the seizure focus has been made is enhanced. However, when the neuropsychological data are at variance with other data sources, one must ask how and why the data are discrepant. In some instances, the neuropsychological data may reflect more widespread cortical impairment, involving extratemporal regions or possibly even the contralateral hemisphere. In other cases, discrepancies may signal the presence of pathologic patterns of functional organization that should be further explored via other procedures such as the Amytal Sodium technique [11,70,78–80]. While such discrepant signs of functional deficit do not negate the presence of focal EEG findings, they should give rise to caution and careful consideration of their possible implications for seizure control and neuropsychological outcome following surgery.

Prediction of Seizure Control

The primary goal of epilepsy surgery is the elimination or substantial reduction of a patient's seizure tendency. To achieve this goal, careful attention must be given to selecting patients who are most apt to benefit from surgical intervention. The decision to proceed with surgery rests heavily on the prognostic value of a wide variety of preoperative variables. Based on their review of the literature concerned with predicting seizure control, Dodrill et al. [70] suggest that the relevant presurgical variables can be grouped into five general areas: demographic variables, seizure history, electrophysiologic characteristics, radiologic and surgical parameters, and neuropsychological and personality findings. By far the most common groups of variables examined for their prognostic value were seizure history variables and EEG characteristics. However, the handful of studies that examined the utility of neuropsychological and personality factors for predicting extent of seizure control generally reported positive results [51,65,69,81–83]. In fact, neuropsychological and personality factors were able to predict postsurgical seizure relief as often as the other classes of variables, including EEG characteristics [70].

The pioneering study by Bengzon et al. [81] in 1968 at the Montreal Neurological Institute represents the first systematic attempt to link preoperative neuropsychological characteristics to seizure control after surgery. Of 650 patients who had undergone temporal lobectomies, 104 were chosen whose pathologic lesion was neither a tumor nor an arteriovenous malformation and for whom there was at least 5 years of follow-up data. Fifty patients were essentially seizure-free, whereas 54 showed little or no improvement following surgery. Patients who were improved but not seizure-free were not included. Using chi-square analyses, two findings of prognostic value emerged. First, those patients with poor seizure control demonstrated more frequent neuropsychological evidence of bilateral cerebral dysfunction than those who experienced a good surgical outcome. Second, those patients whose neuropsychological data suggests restricted temporal lobe dysfunction were more apt to have a positive response to surgery than those with test findings suggestive of extratemporal dysfunction, with or without temporal lobe involvement. These findings were in good agreement with EEG data, which also suggested that patients with bilateral abnormalities or widespread disturbances extending beyond the temporal region have a less favorable prognosis than those with more circumscribed, unilateral temporal lobe dysfunction.

Consistent with the findings of Bengzon et al. [81], Wannamaker and Matthews [51] also reported a relationship between degree of preoperative neuropsychological impairment and subsequent seizure control after surgery among a small group of patients with mixed seizure disorders. Using the Halstead-Reitan Battery, these investigators found that those patients with evidence of widespread neuropsychological deficits had a worse prognosis for seizure control than those with less impairment. Age at onset was also correlated with both seizure control and presurgical level of neuropsychological functioning. Patients with early seizure onsets had a poor prognosis for seizure control and demonstrated the greatest degree of cognitive impairment prior to surgery.

While Bengzon et al. [81] failed to find a relationship between preoperative intelligence quotient (IQ) levels and subsequent seizure control, several studies from the group at the University of California at Los Angeles (UCLA) have found that patients with higher preoperative IQ levels were more likely to have good seizure control following focal temporal lobe resections than those with lower IQ scores [65,69,83]. Rausch [28] interprets this relationship to be a manifestation of the IQ measure's sensitivity to "brain integrity." Patients with lower IQ scores are thought to have "more diffuse brain involvement" and, hence, are at greater risk for poor seizure control than those with higher preoperative IQ levels. While such a relationship would be consistent with data derived from other sources (i.e., EEG), Rausch [28] suggests that inferences drawn from the presurgical neuropsychological evaluation are complementary, but not necessarily redundant, to those from other medical diagnostic procedures.

Although neuropsychological status appears to be of some prognostic value in predicting potential reduction in seizure tendency following surgery, little attention has been given to using neuropsychological data in combination with other preoperative variables to enhance prognostic predictions. The study by Dodrill et al. [82] and its extension [70] are notable exceptions. In a multivariate, multidisciplinary study of extent of seizure relief among 100 patients during their second postoperative year, Dodrill et al. [82] examined 71 variables from several data sources (e.g., demographic, EEG, neuropsychological). These variables were considered individually and then in multivariate combination. Eight variables discriminated between patients who were significantly improved following surgery from those who were not. Four of these were EEG variables, two were neuropsychological scores, and two were personality-test variables. Correct classification rates for individual variables ranged from 57–73%, with the neuropsychological and personality variables yielding 71–73% correct classifications. When multiple cutoff scores and multiple regression techniques were applied to these eight scores, the classification rates increased to 80% and 76%, respectively.

In an extension of their original study, Dodrill, Wilkus, and Ojemann [70] followed 30 patients from their original sample over longer periods of time (4 to 5-year and 9 to 10-year intervals) and examined a new sample of 22 patients followed at similar intervals. Prediction rates using their original multiple cutoff procedure were considerably less for the two groups (63% and 67%, respectively), suggesting some loss of predictive accuracy over time. Nonetheless, Dodrill and his colleagues find their multivariate, multidisciplinary approach to prognostic prediction useful and "use this system in counseling patients prior to their making decisions about surgery" [70].

In summary, preoperative neuropsychological data appear to have some prognostic value for predicting potential relief of seizures following surgery. Although the research is quite limited, the data suggest that patients with evidence of diffuse neuropsychological impairment may be less likely to become seizure-free after surgical intervention than those who are cognitively more intact. To what degree this information is independent of age at onset, etiology, EEG findings, and other preoperative data is not clear. Clearly, additional research is needed to explore the potential prognostic value of neuropsychological baseline data for predicting seizure control, especially within a multivariate, multidisciplinary framework.

Prediction of Neuropsychological Outcome

Patients considering surgical options for relief of intractable seizure disorders must be advised of their chances of experiencing decrements in functional ability that might arise as a result of surgery, as well as of the likelihood of obtaining improved seizure control. To provide such risk-to-benefit information concerning cognitive abilities, it is essential to know the typical patterns of cognitive change associated with epilepsy surgery, in addition to possible preoperative variables that might moderate such modal patterns of change for the individual patient. The preoperative neuropsychological evaluation provides the baseline against which postoperative performances can be evaluated to establish such patterns of "expected" change. In addition, it also represents a rich source of preoperative data that may yield information concerning individual risk factors for potential cognitive impairment. Since the vast majority of epilepsy surgery cases involve cortical resections of the temporal lobes [11], we will limit our discussion to the findings associated with temporal lobectomy (TL).

The test-retest paradigm has been widely used to evaluate the general effects of surgical treatment of epilepsy on cognitive capacity. Reports of selective improvements and impairments have been noted in the literature, and they appear to be moderated by such factors as side of surgery, nature and extent of resection, degree of seizure control, length of recovery, and age at seizure onset. Those cognitive abilities most extensively examined have been intelligence, memory functions, and language ability. The literature concerning the cognitive changes in each of these domains has been extensively reviewed elsewhere [40,71,84–86] and will be only briefly reviewed here.

Intelligence. Postoperative measures of general intelligence typically demonstrate some initial decrement from baseline immediately following TL of either hemisphere [37,66]. These decrements generally are reported to resolve over time, and some investigators note mild improvements at extended follow-up intervals [7,8,37], especially among right TL patients [7,66,68,69]. Selective changes in verbal and performance IQ scores on the Wechsler Intelligence Scales [87,88] have also been reported to interact with side of surgery [7,69,89]. Verbal intellectual abilities tend to be mildly diminished after dominant TL but modestly improved after TL of the nondominant hemisphere. Performance IQ scores generally improve or remain unchanged regardless of the side of surgery. Whether an individual patient demonstrates a decrement or improvement on repeat intelligence testing appears to be related to his or her degree of seizure control. Those obtaining good seizure relief are more apt to show improvements on formal intelligence testing than those who failed to benefit substantially from surgery [65,69]. Whether improvements on postoperative intelligence testing reflect actual increases in intellectual capacity or simply differential practice effects has recently been questioned by Chelune et al. [90]. These investigators found no differences in observed improvements in IQ among left and

right TL patients and among a matched sample of nonoperated, intractable-seizure controls who were retested over a 7-month interval.

Memory Functions. Alterations in learning and memory have long been attributed to temporal lobe dysfunction and have been extensively studied in relation to epilepsy surgery. It is well recognized that bilateral damage or surgical resection of the anterior temporal lobes and their mesial structures can produce a severe and lasting anterograde amnesia [91–93]. Although unilateral TL generally does not produce such global amnestic syndromes [11], milder, material-specific deficits are frequently observed [7,11,37,66–68, 94]. Typically, dominant-hemisphere TL results in decrements in the acquisition and retention of semantic material, whereas nondominant-hemisphere TL can produce decrements of learning and memory for complex visuospatial material [37,67,94], although the latter has not been universally observed [7,35,66]. Similar to the effects on measures of intelligence, material-specific decrements are more pronounced within the first month after surgery than at 1-year or longer follow-up intervals [37,66,68]. However, significant deficits are still apparent after these longer follow-up periods, such that some investigators feel that "verbal memory deficits remain a major complication of anterior temporal lobectomy of the dominant hemisphere" [68].

Degree of seizure relief has been found to moderate the severity of verbal memory deficits following dominant TL [66,68], although not completely, with verbal memory deficits still evident among seizure-free patients [68,69]. Several authors have also reported "release of memory function" or improvement in material-specific memory functions in the hemisphere contralateral to the side of surgery [7,66–69]. That is, patients with dominant TL have experienced improvements in memory for visuospatial material despite decrements in learning and retention of verbal information. Conversely, memory for verbal material has been found to increase after nondominant TL despite diminished or unchanged performances on nonverbal memory tasks. The generality of these findings has recently been called into question by Saykin et al. [53], who found age at seizure onset to be a major moderating variable. Although sample sizes were small, patients with seizure onsets at or before the age of 5 years who underwent dominant TL were found to show no change in verbal memory but had marked decrements in figural memory. In contrast, patients with late seizure onsets showed decrements in verbal memory but had improved scores on figural memory tasks. Those patients who underwent nondominant TL manifested increases in both semantic and figural memory regardless of age at seizure onset. The authors concluded that "age of onset affects not only the level, but the pattern of memory changes produced by temporal lobectomy, and that the effects depend on the side of focus" [53].

Given the important role of the temporal lobes for the acquisition and retention of new information, it is not surprising that the location and extent of surgical resection incurred during epilepsy surgery affects the nature and severity of memory difficulties observed afterward. Milner [95] first observed that decrements in short-term recall of prose passages and verbal paired associates were more related to resection of the lateral cortex of the dominant temporal lobe than its mesial structures. Similar relationships between short-term, material-specific memory deficits and extent of lateral resection have been found following both dominant [68] and nondominant [94] TL. However, it is difficult to separate extent of lateral versus mesial resection since the two resection parameters covary closely. Recent attempts [96,97] using a magnetic resonance imaging (MRI)-based compartmental model [98] to independently assess extent of lateral, basal, and mesial resection have found that the efficiency of material-specific delayed retention was correlated with extent of mesial and basal resection, but not with lateral resection, following both dominant and nondominant TLs. Clearly, more research is necessary to tease out the relative effects of various resection parameters on memory functions following temporal lobe epilepsy surgery.

Language. The preoperative neuropsychological evaluation typically assesses a number of basic language skills and can provide a means of evaluating the adequacy of the lanaguage-dominant hemisphere. Although in most cases this is the left hemisphere, it is not always the case [71,72]. It is here that the Wada technique [10,11] is invaluable in determining the actual lateralization of language functions. The value of the neuropsychological evaluation is largely descriptive and serves as a baseline for postsurgical comparisons.

Patients with well-defined dominant-hemisphere seizure foci often manifest more impaired language abilities than either neurologically intact individuals or those with nondominant-hemisphere seizure foci [64,99]. Although surgical resection of the dominant temporal lobe has some morbidity in terms of language functions, only mild decrements in language skills compared with baseline performances are generally noted immediately after surgery [68], and these are typically not apparent at 6-month [64] or at

1-year [68] follow-up. In the most comprehensive prospective study of the effect of TL on language skills, Hermann and Wyler [64] found no significant losses in language functions for either right or left TL patients at 6-month follow-up. In fact, the dominant-hemisphere TL group manifested significant gains in both receptive language comprehension and verbal fluency. However, the authors do note considerable individual variability in language changes that could not be attributed to gender, seizure control, or extent of lateral resection. They described this individual variability as "psychometric noise" [64]. While these investigators were not able to identify predictors of this observed variability in their study, it is precisely the identification of such predictors of individual change that is necessary for advising the individual patient of his or her potential risks.

Prediction of Individual Risks. In the above sections, we have described the modal changes in cognitive ability that are most commonly associated with epilepsy surgery and noted some of the variables that moderate these changes. While such information is useful in identifying some of the potential risks associated with surgery, it is based on group data and does not address the issue of individual risk factors. Ivnik et al. [7] have recognized the need to counsel patients about their individual risks for developing cognitive deficit and have compiled base-rate tables describing the likelihood that "any specific patient may have none, one, or multiple areas of compromised cognition after temporal lobectomy." Although such tables provide useful information about the overall risks of cognitive deficit attendant to surgery, they do not identify specific markers that might identify which patients are most at risk and for what type of deficit.

Although there is a paucity of research at this time, the most reliable preoperative neuropsychological predictor of individual cognitive change is level of performance. Studies by Rausch et al. [100,101] have shown that patients with high preoperative verbal memory scores were more apt to show greater decrements following dominant TL than those with lower presurgical verbal memory scores. Similar trends were observed for nonverbal memory scores following nondominant temporal resections. These findings were recently replicated using the Wechsler Memory Scale-Revised (WMS-R) [102], but only for dominant TL patients [103]. Chelune et al. [35] examined this relationship in further detail using multiple measures of memory, language, and visuospatial skills. Preoperative ability status was consistently associated with the magnitude of postsurgical losses across the memory and language measure, but not the visuospatial tasks, for the dominant TL group. The nondominant TL group failed to demonstrate any consistent relationship between preoperative ability status and changes in any of the three ability domains.

As a further refinement, Chelune et al. [35] calculated base-rate tables for the scores from the WMS-R [103] in a manner that can be directly used to advise individual patients. For example, the data suggest that patients who score in the "average" range or above (≥ 90) on the WMS-R Verbal Memory Index and who were being considered for dominant TL have a 75% chance of experiencing a 10% or greater decrement in verbal memory at 6-month follow-up. While these data are preliminary and it is not known whether observed deficits resolve over longer follow-up intervals, construction of empirically derived base-rate tables is greatly needed to provide a practical guide for counseling prospective epilepsy patients of their attendant cognitive risks should they elect to proceed with surgery.

Summary

The preoperative neuropsychological evaluation of the epilepsy surgery candidate is an important and integral component of the clinical evaluation of these patients. Although time-intensive, presurgical neuropsychological assessment provides useful functional data about a patient's cognitive and behavioral abilities. These data are not only descriptive, but also provide a baseline for evaluating changes in mental status over time—whether after pharmacologic intervention or after surgery. They can also provide useful corroborative information, within limits, concerning seizure lateralization and localization, or they may yield discrepant findings that signal the need for more careful and in-depth investigation. As a predictor of outcome, research suggests that preoperative neuropsychological variables have some bearing on eventual seizure control, although they have not been examined in detail, as noted by Dodrill et al. [70].

Much of the neuropsychological research in the area of epilepsy has used test-retest evaluations to elucidate often subtle changes in cognitive ability that result from resective surgeries, especially of the temporal lobes. Such test-retest investigations have added greatly to our knowledge and understanding of brain-behavior relationships. However, there is a paucity of information concerning potential predictors of individual cognitive change. Since cognitive deficits, especially memory deficits, remain a major complication of epilepsy surgery, clinicians have an obligation to advise their patients of the cognitive risks attendant to surgery. To do so in a meaningful way requires knowledge of the patient's baseline neuropsychological status and the relevant risk factors that affect cognitive outcome. Although growing attention is given to these issues, much more research is needed to identify empirical markers that can be used to counsel individual patients. The preoperative neuropsychological evaluation represents a rich source of potentially useful data and needs to be further explored.

References

1. Horsley, Sir V. Brain surgery. *Br Med J* 1886;2:670–5.
2. Anderman F. Identification of candidates for surgical treatment of epilepsy. In: Engel J Jr, ed. *Surgical treatment of the epilepsies*. New York: Raven Press, 1987:51–69.
3. Delgado-Escueta AV, Treiman DM, Walsh GO. The treatable epilepsies: Part I. *N Engl J Med* 1983; 308:1508–14.
4. Delgado-Escueta AV, Treiman DM, Walsh GO. The treatable epilespies. Part II. *N Engl J Med* 1983; 308:1576–84.
5. Engel J Jr. Approaches to localization of the epileptogenic lesion. In: Engel J Jr, ed. *Surgical treatment of the epilepsies*. New York: Raven Press, 1987:75–95.
6. Dreifuss FE. Goals of surgery for epilepsy. In: Engel J Jr, ed. *Surgical treatment of the epilepsies*. New York: Raven Press, 1987:31–49.
7. Ivnik RJ, Sharbrough FE, Laws ER. Anterior temporal lobectomy for control of partial complex seizures: information for counseling patients. *Mayo Clin Proc* 1988;63:783–91.
8. Olivier A. Risk and benefit in the surgery of epilepsy: complications and positive results on seizure tendency and intellectual function. *Acta Scand* 1988;78 (Suppl 117):114–21.
9. Walczak TS, Radtke RA, McNamara JO, et al. Anterior temporal lobectomy for complex partial seizures: evaluation, results, and long-term follow-up in 100 cases. *Neurology* 1990;40:413–8.
10. Wada J, Rasmussen, T. Intracarotid injection of Sodium Amytal for the lateralization of cerebral speech dominance: experimental and clinical observations. *J Neurosurg* 1960;17:266–82.
11. Jones-Gotman M. Commentary: psychological evaluation—testing hippocampal function. In: Engel J Jr, ed. *Surgical treatment of the epilepsies*. New York: Raven Press, 1987:203–11.
12. Lezak MD. *Neuropsychological assessment* (2nd ed). New York: Oxford, 1983.
13. Anthony WZ, Heaton RK, Lehman RAW. An attempt to cross-validate two actuarial systems for neuropsychological test interpretation. *J Consult Clin Psychol* 1980; 48:317–26.
14. Damasio H, Damasio AR. *Lesion analysis in neuropsychology*. New York: Oxford, 1989.

15. Filskov SB, Goldstein SG. Diagnostic validity of the Halstead-Reitan neuropsychological battery. *J Consult Clin Psychol* 1974;42:382–8.

16. Golden CJ, Kane R, Sweet J, et al. Relationship of the Halstead-Reitan Neuropsychological Battery to the Luria-Nebraska Neuropsychological Battery. *J Consult Clin Psychol* 1981;49:410–7.

17. Kertesz A, ed. *Localization in neuropsychology.* New York: Academic Press, 1983.

18. Reitan RM, Davison LA, eds. *Clinical neuropsychology: current status and applications.* New York: Hemisphere, 1974.

19. Russell EW, Neuringer C, Goldstein G. *Assessment of brain damage: a neuropsychological key approach.* New York: Wiley, 1970.

20. Snow WG. A comparison of frequency of abnormal results in neuropsychological vs neurodiagnostic procedures. *J Clin Psychol* 1981;37:22–8.

21. Swiercinsky DP, Leigh G. Comparison of neuropsychological data in the diagnosis of brain impairment with computerized tomography and other neurological procedures. *J Clin Psychol* 1979;35:242–6.

22. Aarts HP, Binnie CD, Smit AM, Wilkins AJ. Selective cognitive impairment during focal and generalized epileptiform EEG activity. *Brain* 1984;107:293–308.

23. Bornstein RA, Pakalnis A, Drake ME, Suga LJ. Effects of seizure type and waveform abnormality on memory and attention. *Arch Neurol* 1988;45:884–7.

24. Delaney RC, Rosen AJ, Mattson RH, Novelly RA. Memory function in focal epilepsy: a comparison of nonsurgical, unilateral temporal lobe and frontal samples. *Cortex* 1980;16:103–17.

25. Dodrill CB, Wilkus RJ. Neuropsychological correlates of the encephalogram in epileptics: III. Generalized nonepileptiform abnormalities. *Epilepsia* 1978,19:453–62.

26. Hermann BP, Wyler AR, Richey ET, Rea JM. Memory function and verbal learning ability in patients with complex partial seizures of temporal lobe origin. *Epilepsia* 1987;28:547–54.

27. Loring DW, Lee GP, Martin RC, Meador KJ. Material specific learning in patients with partial complex seizures of temporal origin: convergent validation of memory constructs. *J Epilepsy* 1988;1:53–9.

28. Rausch R. Differences in cognitive function with left and right temporal lobe dysfunction. In: Benson DF, Zaidel E, eds. *The dual brain.* New York: Guilford, 1985:247–61.

29. Wilkus RJ, Dodrill CB. Neuropsychological correlates of the electroencephalogram in epileptics: I. Topographic distribution and average rate epileptiform activity. *Epilepsia* 1976;17:89–100.

30. Homan RW, Paulman RG, Devous MD, Walker P, Jennings LW, Bonte FJ. Cognitive function and regional blood flow in partial seizures. *Arch Neurol* 1989;46:964–70.

31. Chelune GJ, Ferguson W, Moehle K. The role of standard cognitive and personality tests in neuropsychological assessment. In: Incagnoli T, Goldstein G, Golden CJ, eds. *Clinical application of neuropsychological test batteries.* New York: Plenum, 1986:75–119.

32. Campbell DT, Fiske DW. Convergent and discriminant validation by the multitrait-multimethod matrix. *Psychol Bull* 1959;56:81–105.

33. Tarter RE, Edwards KL. Neuropsychological batteries. In: Incagnoli T, Goldstein G, Golden CJ, eds. *Clinical application of neuropsychological test batteries.* New York: Plenum, 1986:135–53.

34. Luria AR. *The working brain.* New York: Basic Books, 1973.

35. Chelune GJ, Naugle RI, Lüders H, Awad IA. Prediction of cognitive change as a function of ability status among temporal lobectomy patients seen at 6-month follow-up. *Neurology* 1991;41:399–404.

36. Lee GP, Loring DW, Thompson JL. Construct validity of material-specific memory measures following unilateral temporal lobe ablations. *J Consult Clin Psychol* 1989;3:192–7.

37. Milner B. Psychological aspects of focal epilepsy and its neurosurgical management. In: Purpura D, Penry J, Walter R, eds. *Advances in neurology,* Vol 8. New York: Raven Press, 1975:299–321.

38. Mungas D, Ehlers C, Walton N, McCutchen CB. Verbal learning differences in epileptic patients with left and right temporal lobe foci. *Epilepsia* 1985;26:340–5.

39. Reitan RM. Methodological problems in clinical neuropsychology. In: Reitan RM, Davison LA, eds. *Clinical neuropsychology: current status and applications.* New York: Hemisphere, 1974:19–46.

40. Rausch, R. Psychological evaluation. In: Engel J Jr, ed. *Surgical treatment of the epilepsies.* New York: Raven Press, 1987:181–95.

41. Cleeland CS. Inferences in clinical psychology and clinical neuropsychology: similarities and differences. *Clin Psychologist* 1976;29:8–10.

42. Lüders H, Lesser RP, Dinner DS, et al. Commentary: chronic intracranial recording and stimulation with subdural electrodes. In: Engel J Jr, ed. *Surgical treatment of the epilepsies.* New York: Raven Press, 1987:297–321.

43. McNaughton FL, Rasmussen T. Criteria for selection of patients for neurosurgical treatment. In: Purpura DP, Penry J, Walter R, eds. *Advances in neurology,* Vol 8. New York: Raven Press, 1975:37–48.

44. Ward AA. Perspectives for surgical therapy of epilepsy. In: Ward AA, Penry J, Purpura DP, eds. *Epilepsy.* New York: Raven Press, 1983:371–90.

45. Dikmen S, Matthews CG. Effect of major motor seizure frequency upon cognitive intellectual function in adults. *Epilepsia* 1977;18:21–30.

46. Dodrill CB, Troupin AS. Seizures and adaptive abilities: a case of identical twins. *Arch Neurol* 1976;33:604–7.

47. Lennox WG, Lennox MA. *Epilepsy and related disorders.* Boston: Little, Brown, 1960.

48. Seidenberg M, Beck N, Geisser M, et al. Academic achievement of children with epilepsy. *Epilepsia* 1986;27:753–9.

49. Bourgeois B, Prensky A, Palkes H, Talent B, Busch S. Intelligence in epilepsy: a prospective study in children. *Ann Neurol* 1983;14:438–44.

50. Dikmen S, Matthews CG, Harley JP. The effect of early versus late onset of major motor epilepsy upon cognitive intellectual function. *Epilepsia* 1975;16:73–81.

51. Wannamaker BB, Matthews CG. Prognostic implications of neuropsychological test performance for surgical treatment of epilepsy. *J Nerv Ment Dis* 1976; 163:29–34.

52. O'Leary DS, Seidenberg M, Berent S, Boll TJ. The effects of age of onset of tonic-clonic seizures on neuropsychological performance in children. *Epilepsia* 1981;22:197–203.

53. Saykin AJ, Gur RC, Sussman NM, O'Connor MJ, Gur RE. Memory deficits before and after temporal lobectomy: effect of laterality and age of onset. *Brain Cogn* 1989;9:191–200.

54. Matthews CG, Klove H. Differential psychological performances in major motor, psychomotor, and mixed seizure classifications of known and unknown etiology. *Epilepsia* 1967;8:117–28.

55. Tarter RE. Intellectual and adaptive functioning in epilepsy: a review of fifty years of research. *Dis Nerv Sys* 1972;33:763–70.

56. Lesser RP, Lüders H, Wyllie E, Dinner DS, Morris HH. Mental deterioration in epilepsy. *Epilepsia* 1986; 27(Suppl 2):S105–23.

57. Mirsky AF, Primac DW, Ajmone MC, Rosvold HE, Stevens JR. A comparison of the psychological test performances of patients with focal and nonfocal epilepsy. *Exp Neurol* 1960;2:75–89.

58. Dodrill CB. Diphenylhydantoin serum levels, toxicity, and neuropsychological performance in patients with epilepsy. *Epilepsia* 1975;16:593–600.

59. Dodrill CB, Troupin AS. Psychotrophic effects of carbamazepine in epilepsy: a double blind comparison with phenytoin. *Neurology* 1977;27:1023–8.

60. Thompson PJ, Trimble MR. Anticonvulsant drugs and cognitive functions. *Epilepsia* 1982;23:531–44.

61. Trimble MR, Thompson PJ. Neuropsychological aspects of epilepsy. In: Grant I, Adams K, eds. *Neuropsychological assessment of neuropsychiatric disorders*. New York: Oxford, 1986:321–46.

62. Dasheiff RM. Epilepsy surgery: is it an effective treatment? *Ann Neurol* 1989;25:506–9.

63. Milner B. Disorders of learning and memory after temporal lobe lesions in man. *Clin Neurosurg* 1972; 19:421–6.

64. Hermann BP, Wyler AR. Effects of anterior temporal lobectomy on language function: a controlled study. *Ann Neurol* 1988;23:585–8.

65. Lieb JP, Rausch R, Engel J Jr, Brown WJ, Crandall PH. Changes in intelligence following temporal lobectomy: relationship to EEG activity, seizure relief, and pathology. *Epilepsia* 1982;23:1–13.

66. Novelly RA, Augustine EA, Mattson RH, et al. Selective memory improvement and impairment in temporal lobectomy for epilepsy. *Ann Neurol* 1984;15:64–7.

67. Nilsson LG, Christianson SA, Silfvenius H, Blom S. Preoperative and postoperative memory testing of epileptic patients. *Acta Neurol Scand* 1984;99:43–56.

68. Ojemann GA, Dodrill CB. Verbal memory deficits after left temporal lobectomy for epilepsy. *J Neurosurg* 1985; 62:101–7.

69. Rausch R, Crandall PH. Psychological status related to surgical control of temporal lobe seizures. *Epilepsia* 1982;23:191–202.

70. Dodrill CB, Wilkus RJ, Ojemann LM. Use of psychological and neuropsychological variables in selection of patients for epilepsy surgery. *Epilepsy Res* 1992;5(supplement):71–75.

71. Chelune GJ. Using neuropsychological data to forecast postsurgical cognitive outcome. In: Lüders H, ed. *Epilepsy surgery*. New York: Raven Press 1991:477–85.

72. Engel J Jr, Crandall PH, Rausch R. The partial epilepsies. In: Rosenberg RN, Grossman RG, Schochet S, Heinz ER, Willis WD, eds. *The clinical neurosciences*, Vol 2. New York: Churchill Livingstone, 1983:1349–80.

73. Rasmussen T, Milner B. The role of early left-brain injury in determining lateralization of cerebral speech functions. *Ann NY Acad Sci* 1977;299:355–69.

74. Rausch R, Walsh GO. Right hemispheric language dominance in right handed epileptic patients. *Ann Neurol* 1984;14:1077–80.

75. Dennis M, Whitaker H. Language acquisition following hemidecortication: linguistic superiority of the left over the right hemisphere. *Brain Lang* 1976;3:404–33.

76. Levy J. Possible basis for the evolution of lateralized specialization of the human brain. *Nature* 1969; 224:614–5.

77. Smith A. Speech and other functions after left (dominant) hemispherectomy. *J Neurol Neurosurg Psychiatry* 1966;29:467–71.

78. Loring DW, Lee GP, Meador KJ, et al. The intracarotid amobarbital procedure as a predictor of memory failure following unilateral temporal lobectomy. *Neurology* 1990;40:605–10.

79. Strauss E, Wada J. Lateral preferences and cerebral speech dominance. *Cortex* 1983;19:165–77.

80. Wyllie E, Lüders H, Murphy D, et al. Intracarotid amobarbital (Wada) test for language dominance: correlation with results of cortical stimulation. *Epilepsia* 1990;31:156–61.

81. Bengzon AR, Rasmussen T, Gloor P, Dassault J, Stephens M. Prognostic factors in the surgical treatment of temporal lobe epileptics. *Neurology* 1968;18:717–31.

82. Dodrill CB, Wilkus RJ, Ojemann GA, et al. Multidisciplinary prediction of seizure relief from cortical resection surgery. *Ann Neurol* 1986;20:2–12.

83. Lieb JP, Rausch R, Engel J Jr, Crandall PH. Complementary prognostic value of EEG and IQ data with respect to surgical outcome in temporal lobe epilepsy. *Soc Neurosci Proc* 1980;6:850.

84. Awad IA, Chelune GJ. Temporal lobectomy: outcome and complications. In: Wyllie E, ed. *The treatment of*

the epilepsies: principles and practice. Philadelphia, Lea & Febiger, 1993:1084–1091.

85. Naugle RI. Neuropsychological effects of epilepsy. In: Lüders H, ed. *Epilepsy surgery.* New York: Raven Press, 1991:637–45.

86. Saykin AJ, Robinson LJ, Stafiniak P, Kester DB, Gur RC, O'Connor MJ, Sperling MR. Neuropsychological changes after anterior temporal lobectomy: acute effects on memory, language, and music. In: Bennett T, ed. *The neuropsychology of epilepsy.* New York: Plenum Press, 1992:263–90.

87. Wechsler D. *Wechsler Adult Intelligence Scale: manual.* New York: Psychological Corporation, 1955.

88. Wechsler D. *Wechsler Adult Intelligence Scale-Revised: manual.* New York: Psychological Corporation, 1981.

89. Mullen J, Chelune, GJ, Plesec T. Utility of the Speech Sounds Perception and Seashore Rhythm tests as measures of lateralized function in temporal lobectomy patients. Paper presented at the annual meeting of the National Academy of Neuropsychologists, Chicago, 1987.

90. Chelune GJ, Naugle RI, Lüders H, Awad IA. Individual change following epilepsy surgery: practice effects and base-rate information. *Neuropsychology* in press.

91. Butters N, Miliotis P, Albert MS, Sax DS. Memory assessment: evidence of the heterogeneity of amnesic symptoms. In: Goldstein G, ed. *Advances in clinical neuropsychology*, Vol. 1. New York: Plenum Press, 1984:127–59.

92. Mayes AR. Learning and memory disorders and their assessment. *Neuropsychologia* 1986;24:25–39.

93. Scoville WB, Milner B. Loss of recent memory after bilateral hippocampal lesions. *J Neurol Neurosurg Psychiatry* 1957;20:11–21.

94. Jones-Gotman M. Right hippocampal excision impairs learning and recall of a list of abstract designs. *Neuropsychologia* 1986;24:659–70.

95. Milner B. Brain mechanisms suggested by studies of the temporal lobes. In: Darley F, ed. *Brain mechanisms underlying speech and language.* New York: Grune & Stratton, 1967:122–45.

96. Chelune GJ, Katz A, Awad IA, Naugle RI, Lüders H, Kong A. Relationship of memory changes to resection parameters in temporal lobectomy patients. *J Clin Exp Neuropsychol* 1989;11:23.

97. Katz A, Awad IA, Kong AK, et al. Extent of resection in temporal lobectomy for epilepsy. II. Memory changes and neurologic complications. *Epilepsia* 1989;30:763–71.

98. Awad IA, Katz A, Hahn JF, Kong AK, Ahl J, Lüders H. Extent of resection in temporal lobectomy for epilepsy. I. Interobserver analysis and correlation with seizure outcome. *Epilepsia* 1989;30:756–62.

99. Mayeux R, Brandt, J, Rosen J, Benson DF. Interictal memory and language impairment in temporal lobe epilepsy. *Neurology* 1980;30:120–5.

100. Kosaka B, Rausch R, Ary C. Predictors of psychological change following left temporal surgery. *J Clin Exp Neuropsychol* 1985;7:639.

101. Rausch R, Babb TL, Ary C, Crandall PH. Memory changes following unilateral temporal lobectomy reflect preoperative integrity of the temporal lobe. Paper presented at the annual meeting of the International Neuropsychological Society, Houston, 1984.

102. Wechsler D. *Wechsler Memory Scale-Revised: manual.* New York: Psychological Corporation, 1987.

103. Naugle RI, Chelune GJ, Lüders H. The relationship between presurgical memory function and memory changes following temporal lobectomy. *Epilepsia* 1988;29:669.

Chapter 9

Psychiatric Evaluation of Patients with Unilateral Temporal Lobectomy for Epilepsy

DIETRICH BLUMER

The surgical treatment of seizure disorders is largely directed at temporal lobe epilepsy and has sparked a sizable literature on the associated psychiatric complications. Temporal lobe epilepsy (TLE) is in most cases primarily a disorder of the limbic (mesial-temporal) system, and the candidates for surgical treatment tend to suffer from the more severe and chronic forms of the disorder. These patients therefore appear to be particularly vulnerable to experience psychiatric complications of their seizure disorder, and their study brings in focus most of the questions that have been raised about the psychiatric aspects of epilepsy.

We argue that specific major and minor emotional and behavioral changes may develop in many patients with chronic TLE as a result of the activity of a temporal-limbic epileptogenic focus. Since it is evident that surgical removal of a localized epileptogenic focus may eliminate the seizure disorder, the study of the psychiatric effects of a successful operation is of exceptional interest. Such a study, carried out with patients in whom the preoperative role of the epileptogenic focus has been carefully assessed, can be carried out with a properly selected control group of patients with only partial surgical success and can provide a better understanding of the psychiatric indication or contraindication for the surgical treatment of epilepsy.

In Chapter 20 of this volume, Peter Fenwich reviews the literature on the psychiatric aspects of temporal lobectomy. We discuss here our recent findings of the nature of the psychiatric disorders of chronic epilepsy, as well as our own experience with patients

who underwent surgical treatment of their epilepsy, and propose an appropriate method of evaluating the patients prior to and after surgical treatment.

The confusing wealth of psychopathology reported in association with epilepsy has led many observers to doubt the existence of emotional and behavioral changes that could be specifically related to seizure disorders. Furthermore, it appears impossible to sort out the respective roles of psychosocial factors, brain damage, medication, and the seizure condition *per se*. An individual's support system and his or her social and occupational opportunities are unquestionably of great importance for well-being and may be decisive pathogenetic factors. However, it is generally recognized in modern psychiatric thinking that biologic factors of either genetic or neural origin represent the crucial etiologic factors determining not necessarily the manifestation but the characteristics of mental phenomena in a given individual, from psychosis to subtle personality traits [1]. Patients who undergo surgery for epilepsy will have a comprehensive assessment of the extent and type of both brain damage and seizure disorder, and their relative impact can be differentiated. Their medication remains largely the same after surgery, at least for a prolonged time. This population of patients, studied before and after the attempt at surgical elimination of a seizure focus, indeed represents a prime group for the investigation of the psychiatric complications of epilepsy.

We first review the evidence for the existence of a complex yet specific syndrome of emotional, behavioral, and personality changes associated with TLE of some severity and duration. For practical purposes one can differentiate between minor personality and behavioral changes on the one hand, and major changes of evident clinical significance on the other.

Characteristics of the Minor and Major Mental Changes Associated with Temporal Lobe Epilepsy

Upon the advent of a modern classification of the epilepsies, Henri Gastaut has been a proponent of the rhinencephalic (temporal-limbic) origin of the psychiatric changes that had been previously associated with "genuine epilepsy." He pointed out that dating back to the 19th century neuropathologists had found Ammon's horn sclerosis in 30–70% of institutionalized patients with epilepsy then termed genuine, that is, epilepsy without gross evidence of brain damage [2]. Subtle lesions of the temporal-limbic zones appear to be responsible for the mental changes. Patients with primary generalized epilepsy tend to show no psychiatric disorders, and patients with partial epilepsies in the absence of limbic involvement are likewise mentally intact. Gastaut's views were based on a series of controlled studies carried out in the early 1950s [3,4]. These studies were published in French at a time when the link of any psychopathology to epilepsy was deemphasized, and they were virtually ignored by the English-speaking investigators. We have summarized Gastaut's studies elsewhere [5] and will relate here only the essential findings.

In a major study based on the large population of his epilepsy clinic, Gastaut documented that only the patients with TLE and the much smaller number of patients with secondary generalized epilepsy showed the characteristic findings of mental slowness (viscosity) and impulsive behavior (irritability). In a related study, Gastaut and coworkers documented that viscosity and significant irritability were present in over two thirds of 60 outpatients with TLE. Between the interictal outbursts of anger the patients tended to be unusually calm, or even depressed, and hypersocial. In a separate investigation, Gastaut and Collomb showed for the first time that a majority of patients with TLE suffered from a global hyposexuality, a trait absent among patients with primary generalized epilepsy [6]. Gastaut emphasized that the behavioral and personality changes in TLE tended to develop only about 2 years after the onset of clinical seizures.

Gastaut then compared his behavioral findings in TLE with those of bilateral temporal lobe resections in animal experiments [7]. The interictal behavior traits of patients with TLE (heightened emotionality, viscosity, and hyposexuality) represent the very opposite of the placidity, flighty attention span (hypermetamorphosis), and hypersexuality observed as characteristic traits of the Klüver-Bucy syndrome. Gastaut notes that this is not a surprising finding if one considers that interictally, owing to the effect of the irritative lesions, the TLE patient tends to present a state of excitation, instead of a state of depression, of the temporolimbic system. Thus one can distinguish two opposite forms of the temporal lobe syndrome: the experimental form of temporal disconnection and the clinical form of temporal hyperconnection in TLE.

Gaustaut's findings correlate well with the views of Geschwind [8], Bear [9], and Szondi [10]. The latter authors have elaborated on the positive "hypersocial" aspects of the interictal personality and behavior traits. Indeed, the frequent finding of a tendency toward episodic build-up of anger, with at times paroxysmal explosive outbursts, contrasts characteristically with a usually more predominant good-natured, ethical, and religious-spiritual attitude that may be at times enhanced to a marked degree. The general intensity of emotions tends to be associated with a significant lability of moods.

Two major points have to be made. First, the tendency toward a slow–detail-bound–circumstantial (viscous) behavior and the moodiness and irritability tend to be expressed in individual cases to exceedingly variable degrees and may be just faintly expressed [11]. Kraepelin had correctly noted: "On superficial observation, the more permanent epileptic changes are recognized only in more severe cases," and one can understand why the existence of these peculiar interictal personality and behavior traits has remained controversial. Second, it is correct that some patients are significantly handicapped in their relationships with others by their intense, slow, and detailed manner of communication, but the explosive anger in only some patients may reach clinical significance and require psychiatric intervention. The global hyposexuality in many patients with TLE tends to result in celibacy, particularly among males, but is generally a subtle trait. We have thus far dealt only with the relatively subtle aspects of emotional and behavioral changes related to the presence of a temporal-limbic focus. The major, clinically significant psychiatric disorders associated with epilepsy have become well recognized.

Depressive episodes are the predominant disorder requiring psychiatric treatment among patients with epilepsy [12–15]. The suicide rate among patients with epilepsy tends to be five times higher than in the general population [16,17]. Furthermore, anxiety has been cited as a problem perhaps as frequently as depression among patients with epilepsy [18–20]. Surveys have indicated that about 7% of patients with epilepsy may suffer at one time or another from a psychosis [21]. Postictal psychoses occur after a brief lucid interval following a flurry of seizures, remit spontaneously after several days, and are confusional in nature. Interictal psychoses with paranoid, delusional, and/or hallucinatory symptoms have been described as the schizophrenia-like episodes of epilepsy [22].

It is correct to list depressive moods, schizophrenia-like psychotic episodes, explosive irritability (often mislabeled "aggressivity"), and perhaps anxiety as major clinical mental changes associated with epilepsy. We have shown, by the careful study of a series, that patients with epilepsy and psychiatric complications usually present with a highly complex psychopathology [12]. Most prominent were rapid shifts in moods with predominant depression. Episodic irritability that occasionally became explosive and schizophrenia-like episodes with paranoia, hallucinations, and/or delusions were frequently present. Recurrent attacks of anxiety, symptoms of somatization disorder, and episodes of amnesia and/or confusion occurred. In fact, the experience with a large number of patients with chronic epilepsy shows that perhaps most of the phenomena described as characterizing psychiatric disorders can be present in the epileptic patient. It is standard practice in epilepsy to separate recognized neurologic seizure manifestations from the psychiatric symptomatology, with the latter being cataloged according to the psychiatric disorders of nonepileptic patients. Closer scrutiny, however, suggests significant differences between the mental abnormalities of epileptic patients and those present in the nonepileptic psychiatric patients.

Thus, the mood changes associated with epilepsy differ from those of manic-depressive illness by their rapid shifts (rapid cycling). Schizophrenia-like symptoms occur in patients with epilepsy, who tend to be very emotional and not schizoid, and are able to relate warmly to others. Overall the mental changes of epilepsy tend to be atypical for the psychiatric disorder they resemble; they tend to occur in highly intermittent form, often with sudden onset and termination; and they tend to be pleomorphic in a given patient, with a variety of different symptoms presenting simultaneously or in succession. A precise traditional diagnostic classification is usually not possible. In addition, the patients with epilepsy and significant psychiatric complications tend to manifest, on close scrutiny, a range of the more subtle yet relatively

stable personality and behavioral changes (hyperemotionality, viscosity, hyposexuality) that have been called interictal personality traits and that are characteristic for the inverse Klüver-Bucy syndrome.

Our present understanding of the psychopathology associated with epilepsy can then be formulated as follows: With a chronic temporal-limbic epileptogenic focus, more or less subtle personality and behavior changes tend to develop in the form of viscosity, hyposexuality, and an enhanced and labile emotionality, characterized by a good-natured, ethical, and at times very religious and spiritual personality, which often contrasts with a heightened irritable-angry disposition manifesting itself intermittently. These core changes are unique for epilepsy but, with the exception of episodes of explosive anger, tend to be of relatively minor clinical significance. The heightened emotionality, on the other hand, may manifest itself in a wide range of psychiatric syndromes of any type, which are characteristically atypical, intermittent, and pleomorphic. Of major concern are rapid-cycling mood changes with predominant depression and schizophrenia-like psychotic episodes. The finding that the psychiatric complications of epilepsy, although seemingly so diverse, all tend to respond to a relatively simple pharmacologic treatment consisting of monotherapy with psychotropic anticonvulsants (carbamazepine and valproate) combined with an antidepressant drug (or lithium) confirms the specificity of the psychopathology [12]. The major psychopathology associated with epilepsy is of neural origin and is more akin to the mental changes of a delirious state, which we clearly cannot press into the traditional functional psychiatric categories.

If one can view, in fact, the temporal-limbic focus as the primary cause of the emotional disorders, what can one expect from the surgical removal of the focus?

Mental Changes Following Unilateral Temporal Lobectomy for Epilepsy

If it can be assumed that specific emotional and behavioral changes in the direction opposite to the Klüver-Bucy syndrome tend to result from the presence of a chronic temporal-limbic epileptogenic focus, it would follow that removal of the focus might reverse this process. Specifically, patients treated successfully would become more sexually aroused, less viscous, and less hyperemotional, that is, less prone to suffer mood changes, irritability with outbursts of temper, and psychosis.

The follow-up study of 50 patients treated by unilateral temporal lobectomy for epilepsy at the Johns Hopkins Hospital led us to a number of conclusions [23–25]. These patients were carefully studied for their psychiatric condition prior to the operation and in repeat follow-up evaluations for an average of 17 years (range 12–30 years).

Most conspicuous was the prompt postoperative improvement of irritability and temper. Twenty-nine patients had presented a problem to others prior to the operation because of their episodic irritability with outbursts of anger, at times to the point of rage. Twenty-two of these patients showed a significant and at times striking improvement of their disposition after the operation. This improvement could be observed as an immediate effect of the operation and was generally associated with relief of seizures, although it sometimes also occurred to a degree even though seizures persisted.

The global hyposexuality present among 26 patients preoperatively remitted in nine patients beginning with the second postoperative month. All nine patients had become free of any type of seizures; the mere persistence of fleeting auras was associated with persistence of the hyposexuality. The close relationship between presence and absence of a seizure focus and sexual arousal was furthermore clearly demonstrated by three additional patients who had been previously hyposexual, were free of any seizures after the operation, and experienced a period of hypersexuality terminating on recurrence of seizures.

Six patients in our series suffered from schizophrenia-like psychosis, and none of them showed any improvement postoperatively. Two patients were of particular interest because they both had become completely seizure-free after surgery. One of them died of bone cancer only 3 years after the surgical intervention for epilepsy, whereas the other began to again suffer from infrequent complex partial seizures several years after surgery. The latter patient was the only one of the six patients with psychosis who had shown no conspicuous symptoms of a psychotic process prior to surgery.

The slow, detail-bound, circumstantial, and pertinacious personality traits subsumed under the label *viscosity* appeared to be essentially unchanged, although a few patients may have become somewhat more fluid in communicating and relating to others. We employed no psychological measures of this set of traits in our study.

It is regrettable that we did not assess systematically the presence of depressive symptoms in our series. We know of one patient who committed suicide about 2 years after the operation; a second patient was an apparent suicide several years after the operation. Both patients were not seizure-free after surgery. Depressive symptoms were commonly present at the time of last systematic follow-up.

The findings in the Johns Hopkins series are similar to those reported from the Guys-Maudsley series as recently reviewed by Taylor [26]. In this British series the mood changes were likewise not systematically assessed. However, Taylor reports that of 193 patients providing a minimum follow-up of 5 years, nine had died by suicide and six in unclear circumstances, carrying the total suicide risk to 50 times the expected figure for the British population. Half the patients who died by suicide reportedly had no seizures since their operation. The prime importance of the problems of depression in patients surgically treated for chronic TLE is thus clear.

For the understanding of the emotional and behavioral disorders associated with TLE and its surgical treatment, a case-by-case analysis is required of those with depression, marked irritability, viscosity, hyposexuality, and psychosis, by comparing the respective outcomes of both the seizure disorder and the psychiatric status. It has been customary in reports of series of surgically treated patients to list all patients who have become free of any episodes involving a loss of consciousness as a full success, since the persistence of a mere aura seems of little consequence. However, the comparison of patients who have become completely free of any seizure manifestations postoperatively with those who were left merely with occasional auras is of particular interest. It has been shown recently that, as far as depression is concerned, a successful postoperative outcome appears to be associated with complete seizure freedom [27]. Although only occasional cases of TLE and interictal psychosis have benefited psychiatrically from the operation, it is still possible that complete surgical abolishment of a temporal lobe focus, as documented by persistent freedom from any seizure manifestations, may be associated with remission of a psychotic disorder. Follow-up studies of operated patients over several years will be required.

The lack of response to surgical intervention of both interictal psychotic disorders (which are in general late complications of the epilepsy) and of the more subtle personality traits termed *viscosity* requires more careful studies. On the other hand, irritability and hyposexuality (which develop early after onset of TLE) appear to respond particularly well to successful surgical intervention. The postoperative depressive manifestations associated with chronic

TLE are of prime importance and need to be much better understood.

With the advent of an effective pharmacologic treatment of the psychiatric disorders associated with epilepsy [12], a new method is available to aid patients operated on for TLE. The employment of optimal modern anticonvulsant therapy combined with a modest amount of antidepressant medication can bring about remission not only of depressive disorders but also of an overly irascible disposition and even of psychotic disorders. By the same token, psychiatric complications of epilepsy can be looked on with a lessened concern as surgical treatment is considered.

We have discussed the biologic effects of the removal of a temporal-limbic epileptogenic focus and have stressed the need for careful assessment of specific mental changes that may develop following onset of the epilepsy and may or may not remit after surgery. The impact of the psychosocial circumstances needs to be assessed in every patient, and proper intervention needs to be carried out.

The respite of chronically recurrent seizures after a successful surgical procedure should bring about a sense of greater emotional well-being for the patients. Some patients, for whom their illness served as a long-standing "crutch," may experience difficulties adjusting to their new-found health and to an ensuing set of expectations, in particular if a long-extended support from the family may now lag and be missed [28]. For most patients, however, freedom from seizures represents, an obvious psychological benefit.

Method of Evaluation

We describe here our method of evaluating patients psychiatrically before and after surgical treatment for epilepsy. The psychiatric evaluation is carried out at the time of the initial extracranial electroencephalographic (EEG) evaluation. If necessary, the evaluation can be finalized at the time of the subsequent intracranial EEG study with subdural electrodes. Next of kin are available at the time of the preoperative evaluations. A comprehensive neuropsychological evaluation, carried out at the same time, is described elsewhere in this volume.

The psychiatric evaluation is initiated with the completion of a questionnaire and of a neurobehavioral inventory by the patient and next of kin. The questionnaire is completed jointly, whereas the inventory is completed separately by patient and next of kin. Next, the responses to the questionnaire and the inventory are reviewed for accuracy and completeness by interviewer of the patient and next of kin. The findings are then rated, and a global score is arrived at for all critical items.

Questionnaire for Seizure Disorders (Appendixes A and B)

The questionnaire inquires first about the seizure history, anticonvulsant medication, current seizure frequency, precipitating factors, seizure prodrome, the aura, the observable events, and the postictal phase. Other medical problems are to be listed. Next, the educational and occupational histories are explored, as are the present living situation, marital history, sexual interests and activities, and social life and past-times. An inquiry follows about past and present emotional adjustments, in particular about current signs of depression, lability of moods, irritability and outbursts of temper, paranoid trends, anxieties, and fears; and about confusional episodes (in the absence of seizures), prominent personality traits (good naturedness, viscosity), history of substance abuse, and interest in religious issues. Finally, the family history is explored for major illnesses, including disorders that have been shown to be related to epilepsy.

The examining physician then conducts a semistructured interview with patient and next-of-kin in an effort to obtain complete and accurate information on all the areas outlined by the questionnaire. The interview should be initiated in the presence of both parties in order to obtain an impression of their interaction; separate interviews are mandatory in order to obtain the most candid responses.

The examiner investigates the frequency of sexual arousal and response; the polarity, rate, and duration of mood swings; and the nature and frequency of irritability and angry outbursts. Finally, a detailed family tree including first- and second-degree relatives is completed by the examiner.

A postoperative follow-up questionnaire (Appendix B) focuses on the areas where changes may occur. Again, it elicits first a written documentation by the patient and next of kin and is followed by an interview for completeness and accuracy of the data. The postoperative follow-up evaluation is carried out 3 months, 6 months, and 12 months after the operation and at yearly intervals thereafter.

Neurobehavior Inventory for Next-of-Kin (Appendix C)

The 100-item Neurobehavior Inventory is a revision of the inventory developed by Bear and Fedio [29], specifically to sample the interictal personality and behavior traits of patients with TLE. The ten items from the Lie Scale of the Minnesota Multiphasic Personality Inventory (MMPI) were omitted; five new items probing physical well-being were added for scrutiny of common somatic symptoms of a depressed state (insomnia, aches and pains, anergia, hypochondriasis, somatic misperceptions); five new items exploring fearfulness and suspicion were added; and the items pertaining to attitudes about sex were revised to address hyposexuality.

A copy of the Neurobehavior Inventory is included as Appendix C, in the format to be completed by the next of kin. The same 100 items are listed for the patient without subheadings, in a scrambled fashion, and in the appropriate format (e.g., "It makes good sense to keep a detailed diary"; "I write poetry, stories, or biography").

The Neurobehavior Inventory samples states that tend to be episodic and may be of clinical importance (mood, irritability, suspiciousness, and fearfulness), as well as generally more stable and subtle traits (viscosity, emotionality, spirituality, and hyposexuality). The self-report score is compared with the score obtained from the next of kin, and the reason for inconsistencies is clarified by interviewing both the patient and next of kin. Discrepancies between the inventory scores and the impression gained on completion of the questionnaire data are similarly scrutinized.

Comprehensive Scoring Sheet (Appendix D)

The Neurobehavior Inventory is not primarily employed to obtain an independent score. It serves rather to ensure a comprehensive sampling of the characteristic mental states and traits. A comprehensive scoring sheet is completed preoperatively and at each reevaluation. On this sheet the number of items from each five-item category endorsed on the inventory by patient and next of kin are entered. The overall clinical rating of each category is rated as either none (0), mild (1), moderate (3), or marked (5)—"mild" meaning a trait or state is identifiable but presents no problems to the patient or others; "moderate" meaning there is a problem but it is manageable without treatment intervention; and "marked"

meaning treatment intervention is indicated. The global rating for the principal changes is achieved from the combination of patient input, next-of-kin input, and clinical scrutiny by the methods described.

Conclusion

The psychiatric evaluation described here intends to establish the preoperative and postoperative profiles of each patient's mental states and traits. The format of the evaluation is semistructured, permitting broad documentation of individual findings while systematically setting sight on all the significant psychiatric aspects of patients with TLE who undergo surgical treatment. In the preoperative and postoperative study each patient serves as his or her own control. Patients with similar psychiatric findings can then be grouped together and their psychiatric outcome can be compared with the degree of surgical success in eliminating the epileptogenic zone. Patients who remain completely free of seizure activity after surgery presumably demonstrate a markedly better psychiatric outcome than those who still experience minor seizure activity even though the latter may be free of episodes of loss of consciousness.

The role of presence and absence of a seizure focus appears to be best documented for episodes of anger (often mislabeled aggressivity) and for sexual arousal. Why schizophrenia-like disorders may not remit even with full surgical success still needs to be better understood; it is plausible that the brief episodes of schizophrenia-like psychosis may have a better prognosis than the more chronic psychoses. Our method of evaluation permits a comparison of the personality trait labeled *viscosity* before and after operation. Most importantly, the evaluation is designed to clarify the problem of the postoperative persistence or emergence of depressive disorders. The evaluation also focuses on the presence of anxiety states, a generally neglected aspect.

We have discussed in considerable details the evaluation of the interictal mental changes associated with TLE because of their complexity and in view of their importance for the postoperative outcome. The psychosocial and vocational rehabilitation tends to be the concomitant of a surgical procedure that proves successful as far as both the seizure disorder and the emotional adjustment are concerned. However, the roles of the individual's cognitive abilities (documented by the neuropsychological findings), of the quality of the individual support system, of the duration of the epilepsy, and of other factors documented in the preoperative and postoperative assessments must also be considered.

The treatment of patients with epilepsy, by medication or by surgical intervention, must be aimed not solely at seizure control but also at an optimal quality of life. For patients with chronic epilepsy who undergo surgical treatment, expert psychiatric assessment and intervention should be routinely available, both before and after operation.

References

1. Blumer D. Diagnosis and treatment of psychiatric problems associated with epilepsy. In: Smith DB, ed. *Epilepsy: current approaches to diagnosis and treatment.* New York: Raven Press, 1990:193–204.

2. Gastaut H. État actuel des connaissances sur l'anatomie pathologique des épilepsies. *Acta Neurol Belg* 1956;56: 5–20.

3. Gastaut H, Roger J, Lesèvre N. Différenciation psychologique des épileptiques en fonction des formes électrocliniques de leur maladie. *Rev Psychol Appl* 1953;3:237–49.

4. Gastaut H, Morin G, Lesèvre N. Étude du comportement des épileptiques psychomoteurs dans l'intervalle de leurs crises. *Ann Med Psychol* (Paris) 1955;113:1–27.

5. Blumer D. The psychiatric dimension of epilepsy: historical perspective and current significance. In: Blumer D, ed. *Psychiatric aspects of epilepsy.* Washington, DC: APA Press, 1984:37–45.

6. Gastaut H, Collomb M. Étude du comportement sexuel chez les épileptiques psychomoteurs. *Ann Med Psychol* (Paris) 1954;112:657–96.

7. Gastaut H. Interpretation of the symptoms of psychomotor epilepsy in relation to physiological data on rhinencephalic function. *Epilepsia* 1954;3:84–8.

8. Geschwind N. Behavioral changes in temporal lobe epilepsy. *Psychol Med* 1979;9:217–9.

9. Bear D. Temporal lobe epilepsy: a syndrome of sensory–limbic hyperconnection. *Cortex* 1979;15:357–84.

10. Szondi L. *Schicksalanalytische Therapie.* Bern: Huber, 1963.

11. Blumer D. The psychiatric dimension of epilepsy: historical perspective and current significance. In: Blumer D, ed. *Psychiatric aspects of epilepsy.* Washington, DC: APA Press, 1984:36.

12. Blumer D, Zielinski JJ. Pharmacologic treatment of psychiatric disorders associated with epilepsy. *J Epilepsy* 1988;1:135–50.

13. Mendez MF, Cummings JL, Benson DF. Depression in epilepsy. *Arch Neurol* 1986;43:766–70.

14. Betts TA. A follow-up study of a cohort of patients with epilepsy admitted to psychiatric care in an English city. In: Harris P, Maudsley C, eds. *Epilepsy: proceedings of Hans Berger centenary symposium.* Edinburgh: Churchill Livingstone, 1974:326–38.

15. Robertson MM, Trimble MR. Depressive illness in patients with epilepsy: a review. *Epilepsia* 1983;22: 515–24.

16. Zielinski JJ. Epilepsy and mortality rates and causes of death. *Epilepsia* 1974;15:191–201.

17. Matthew WS, Barabas G. Suicide and epilepsy: a review of literature. *Psychosomatics* 1981:22:515–24.

18. Currie S, Heathfield KWG, Henson RA, Scott DF. Clinical course and prognosis of temporal lobe epilepsy: a survey of 666 cases. *Brain* 1972;94:173–90.

19. Betts TA. Depression, anxiety and epilepsy. In: Reynolds EH, Trimble MM, eds. *Epilepsy and psychiatry.* Edinburgh: Churchill Livingstone, 1981:60–71.

20. Trimble MR, Perez MM. Quantification of psychopathology in adult patients with epilepsy. In: Kulig BM, Meinardi H, Stores G, eds. *Epilepsy and behavior '79.* Lisse: Swets and Zeitlinger, 1980:118–26.

21. Gudmundsson G. Epilepsy in Iceland: a clinical and epidemiological investigation. *Acta Neurol Scand* 1966; 25(Suppl 43):1–124.

22. Slater E, Beard AW. The schizophrenia-like psychoses of epilepsy. *Br J Psychiatry* 1963;109:95–150.

23. Blumer D, Walker AE. Sexual behavior in temporal lobe epilepsy. *Arch Neurol* 1967;16:37–43.

24. Walker AE, Blumer D. Long-term effects of temporal lobe lesions on sexual behavior and aggressivity. In: Fields WS, Sweet WH, eds. *Neural bases of violence and aggression.* St. Louis: Green, Inc. 1975:392–400.

25. Walker AE, Blumer D. Behavioral effects of temporal lobectomy for temporal lobe epilepsy. In: Blumer D, ed. *Psychiatric aspects of epilepsy.* Washington, DC: APA Press, 1984:295–323.

26. Taylor DC. Psychiatric and social issues in measuring the input and outcome of epilepsy surgery. In: Engel J Jr, ed. *Surgical treatment of the epilepsies.* New York: Raven Press, 1987:485–503.

27. Hermann BP. Depression before and after temporal lobectomy. Presented at the 143rd Annual Meeting of the APA, New York, May 1990.

28. Ferguson SM, Rayport M. The adjustment to living without epilepsy. *J Nerv Ment Dis* 1965;140:26–37.

29. Bear DM, Fedio P. Quantitative analysis of interictal behavior in temporal lobe epilepsy. *Arch Neurol* 1977;34:454–67.

Chapter 10

Intracarotid Amobarbital (Wada) Assessment

DAVID W. LORING
GREGORY P. LEE
KIMFORD J. MEADOR

Wada testing, or intracarotid amobarbital assessment, is an integral part of the preoperative evaluation of epilepsy surgery. Its primary role is to establish cerebral language dominance and to identify patients at risk for the development of postsurgical anterograde amnesia. Additionally, the Wada test may also be employed as a measure of functional asymmetry and to help confirm seizure-onset laterality. The Wada procedure typically involves injection of 100–200 mg sodium amobarbital into a single internal carotid artery. This pharmacologically inactivates the distribution of the anterior and middle cerebral arteries for several minutes, during which time the patient is presented with multiple cognitive tasks. As with pre operative neuropsychological assessment, the procedure varies from center to center, reflecting the training and theoretical biases of the examiner. This chapter describes the use of amobarbital testing to determine language and memory function and highlights some difficulties and limitations of this technique.

Language Assessment

The first use of local anesthesia to functionally inactivate potential cerebral language areas was described in 1941 by Gardner [1]. Two left-handed patients were being evaluated for surgery, and Gardner was aware that the patients' handedness raised the potential of altered cerebral lateralization. Procaine hydrochloride was injected into the cortex thought to potentially subserve language. No linguistic changes were noted in either patient following the injection,

and both patients underwent surgery without the development of postoperative aphasia.

The first English-language article describing amobarbital administration to determine language representation appeared in 1960 [2]. Twenty patients received amobarbital injections of 150–200 mg via a common carotid artery approach without complication, thereby establishing both the technical and practical applicability of this technique. Surgery was performed in 17 patients, all of whom appeared to be correctly classified based on the presence or absence of immediate postoperative aphasia.

The most commonly cited paper describing cerebral language laterality and its relationship to early neurologic injury and handedness is that of Rasmussen and Milner [3]. They reported that of 92 left-handed patients with early left brain injury, 26 (28%) were left cerebral dominant, 49 (53%) were right cerebral dominant, and 17 (19%) displayed bilateral speech representation. Of 42 right-handed patients with early left hemisphere injury, 34 (81%) were left hemisphere speech dominant, five (12%) displayed right hemisphere speech, and three (7%) were mixed speech dominant. Across the entire series of patients without respect to handedness or age of probable brain injury, approximately twice as many patients displayed right hemisphere language (19.7%) as mixed speech dominance (9.6%). These data suggest that if language is not exclusively represented in the left hemisphere, language is more likely to be under exclusive right hemisphere control than bilateral representation by a 2:1 ratio.

Because Wada testing was developed at the Montreal Neurological Institute, these reports provided the first estimates regarding language laterality. As

Woods et al. [4] noted, the Montreal results are frequently cited without reservation as representative of the general population. However, only nondextral patients, or patients for whom concern for cerebral laterality existed, were tested. Consequently, incidence estimates can be expected to vary from those of other institutions and series based on subject inclusion criteria, techniques of language assessment, criteria of language impairment, and amobarbital dosage administered.

Several of these points are illustrated by the Branch et al. [5] paper on Wada testing at the Montreal Neurological Institute. This is an initial report that was subsequently extended by Rasmussen and Milner [3]. One patient who was determined by Wada testing to be right hemisphere speech dominant suffered a mild but definite aphasia following left hemisphere resection involving Broca's area. Apparently the language assessment failed to indicate left hemisphere language representation. Wyllie et al. [6] observed a similar pattern in two patients determined to be right hemisphere speech dominant by amobarbital testing but who also displayed left hemisphere language representation with cortical mapping using subdural electrode arrays. Thus, the sensitivity of amobarbital testing to language representation depends on multiple factors, one of which likely includes how language is assessed during the period of hemispheric anesthesia. In addition, bilateral studies were conducted in only 97 of 119 patients; 22 of these patients, or 18%, underwent unilateral testing only, thereby precluding the possibility of determining the presence of bilateral speech.

Reports from other centers using different techniques of assessment have suggested that mixed cerebral language representation may occur more frequently than purely right cerebral language. Hommes and Panhuysen [7] observed right hemisphere language impairment during Wada testing in nine of 11 depressed patients (10 dextral, 1 nondextral), although the magnitude of impairment was much less than that following left hemisphere injections. Oxbury and Oxbury [8] reported that eight of 23 patients (17 dextral, 6 nondextral) became aphasic following left hemisphere injection only, one patient displayed aphasic errors following right hemisphere injection only, and 14 patients developed aphasic errors including naming and forward/backward series recitation (e.g., days of the week, months of the year, counting) following injection to either cerebral hemisphere. Powell et al. [9] reported on 27 patients (18 dextral, 9 nondextral) and observed mixed cerebral dominance in six patients (22%) and right hemisphere speech in only four patients (15%). Although Rey et al. [10] described greater right than bilateral language representation in their patient sample of 73

(17 [23%] right dominant versus 11 [15%] mixed dominant), 15 patients presented with a right-sided hemiparesis, which would increase the likelihood of exclusive right hemisphere speech representation. Overall, 29 patients were dextral and 44 were nondextral. Zatorre [11] reported in his sample of 61 patients that 35 (57%) were left hemisphere dominant for speech, whereas 22 (36%) were considered bilateral, and four (7%) were right hemisphere speech dominant.

We studied hemispheric language representation using incremental injections (mean dosage = 122.5 mg) in 103 patients undergoing Wada testing with adequate bilateral studies and no evidence of a structural lesion outside the temporal lobes (91 dextral, 12 nondextral) [12]. Seventy-nine patients (77%) had exclusive left hemisphere language representation, two patients (2%) had exclusive right hemisphere language representation, and 22 patients (21%) had language to varying degrees in each hemisphere. Seventeen of 22 bilateral language patients (77%) displayed asymmetric representation (13 left > right, 4 right > left); language was represented equally in the remaining five patients. Thus, the consensus across multiple centers is that in the absence of exclusive left hemisphere language representation, mixed language dominance is much more frequently observed than right hemisphere language dominance unless there is evidence of significant neurologic dysfunction in the left hemisphere.

A significant portion of the discrepancy regarding the frequency of right hemisphere language dominance and mixed cerebral dominance is due to the criteria for inferring the presence of impaired linguistic function following amobarbital injection. Snyder et al. [13] surveyed 55 epilepsy surgery centers and found widely disparate estimates of mixed speech dominance. Of the 47 centers reporting specific percentages, there was a range from 0% speech bilaterality to 60% bilaterality (Table 10-1). In addition, diverse criteria for inferring language representation were reported. Most centers (93%) employed naming as a criterion for establishing speech lateralization for the dominant hemisphere. Other criteria included unspecific dysphasic signs (78%), counting ability (80%), familiar word/phrase repetition (61%), and unfamiliar word/phrase repetition (65%). In contrast, heterogeneous criteria were utilized for inferring the presence of speech in the nondominant hemisphere. These criteria included attempts to mouth appropriate words, groaning sounds, singing ability, object naming, partial phoneme vocalization, serial rote speech, and expression of familiar words.

Snyder et al. [13] then subjected the criteria for inferring language representation to a discriminant

Table 10-1. Percentage of Mixed Speech Dominance Across 47 Epilepsy Surgery Centers*

Percentage Mixed Speech	Centers Reporting	
0	$n =$	11 (20%)
1–2	$n =$	2 (4%)
5–6	$n =$	9 (17%)
10	$n =$	13 (24%)
15	$n =$	4 (7%)
16–29	$n =$	7 (13%)
60	$n =$	1 (2%)
	TOTAL 47	
	(87% of centers responding)	

*Seven additional centers (13%) did not respond to this specific question. (Source: Snyder PJ, Novelly RA, Harris LJ. Mixed speech dominance in the intracarotid sodium Amytal procedure: validity and criteria issues. *J Clin Exp Neuropsychol* 1990;12:629–43.)

function analysis. Nearly 70% of centers responding were classified correctly into one of two groups (0–6% mixed language incidence versus 10–20%, plus an additional center reporting 60% mixed language representation) based on whether vocalization of partial phonemes, serial rote speech, and expression of familiar words were assessed to determine language representation. A lower prevalence of mixed language was associated with procedures employing serial rote speech, expression of familiar words, or production of partial phonemes as evidence of language representation in the hemisphere contralateral to injection. The survey by Snyder et al. [13] also indicated that approximately 15% of the centers do not perform Wada testing on all surgical candidates but rather only on those patients with evidence of bilateral brain disease. Thus, without consecutive patient series, nonbiased estimates cannot be obtained. Further, estimates will vary based on the primary patient population being evaluated (e.g., temporal lobectomy candidates versus hemispherectomy candidates with hemiplegia). Although causality cannot be inferred based on correlational results since the relationship may be due to a different variable (such as whether all patients are included), the Snyder data illustrate the importance of method variance when attempting to interpret the amobarbital literature.

Clinical Application

In the evaluation for epilepsy surgery, assessment of language representation is an important factor that frequently affects the type of procedure performed and extent of surgical resection. The determination of language representation is usually an easy task, since patients typically stop talking following left hemisphere injection and continue to converse following right hemisphere injection. However, cases involving bilateral language may require explicit criteria for language representation, since occasionally patients with bilateral language may be missed [e.g., 5]. In addition, right hemisphere language can be observed in patients with right seizure onset. We reported three patients in whom bilateral language representation was indicated by Wada testing (2 left > right, 1 right > left) who underwent subsequent right temporal lobectomy [14]. Formal language assessment was conducted during the initial week following surgery on one patient, and significant paraphasic responses were present during assessment of core linguistic functions [15]. Similarly, Rosenbaum et al. [16] reported a patient with a right seizure onset in which right hemisphere language was present. In both reports, functional cortical mapping of language regions disclosed a combination of either posterior frontal or perisylvian regions that, when stimulated, produced speech arrest or paraphasic substitution. In addition, right hemisphere language may be observed in right-handed patients with seizures originating from the left temporal lobe [17]. These reports illustrate the necessity of establishing language functioning in all epilepsy surgery candidates, since language can be represented in the right hemisphere regardless of whether seizures are originating from the left temporal lobe in a right-handed patient. Consequently, we believe that all patients should receive bilateral evaluation for language representation, not just those suspected of atypical language representation.

Memory Testing

The primary goal of testing memory during hemispheric anesthesia is to identify patients who, without special precautions, would otherwise develop an amnestic syndrome following temporal lobectomy [18]. When hippocampal tissue is dysfunctional, recent memory systems may be assumed by other brain structures, although memory performance may not be at the level expected without temporal lobe pathology. Removal of the hippocampus and surrounding tissue therefore does not necessarily produce a significant loss of memory function. In fact, altered neuronal activity in the hippocampus may result in a greater disruption of certain kinds of learning than that resulting from hippocampal resection [19]. However, significant memory impairment may be present following unilateral temporal lobectomy if occult contralateral mesial temporal dysfunction is present, although the magnitude of memory impairment is not as severe as the amnesia displayed by patient HM following bitemporal lobectomy [20]. Penfield and Mathieson demonstrated extensive atrophy of the right hippocampus at autopsy in one patient who developed significant memory impairment following left temporal lobectomy [21]. The rationale underlying memory testing is that intracarotid amobarbital injection produces a state of temporary dysfunction ipsilateral to the side of proposed surgery that models the potential effects of temporal lobectomy on memory function. If the patient fails to remember a sufficient number of stimuli presented following the injection ipsilateral to the side of seizure onset, the patient is believed to be at risk for a postresection amnesia.

Milner et al. [22] initially described 50 consecutive patients undergoing memory testing following a 200-mg amobarbital injection. However, not all patients were studied bilaterally; 44 received dominant hemisphere injections and 46 received nondominant hemisphere injections. Memory failure occurred following 12 of 90 (13%) injections (dominant = 5, nondominant = 7). In 11 cases (12%), the memory deficit occurred after injection contralateral to the epileptogenic lesion. In the remaining case, the amobarbital was injected rapidly, creating bilateral neurologic impairment, and the assessment was considered invalid.

Of the 20 patients evaluated by Kløve et al. [23] with 180-mg injections ipsilateral to the side of seizure onset, four failed the memory test based on a consensus of raters. The 20% failure rate was contrasted with an *expected* frequency of postresection memory deficits of 10–20% [24]. Blume et al. [25] tested 9 patients for their ability to remember material presented during amobarbital anesthesia (125-mg injection) after the medication had worn off. No patient failed the memory test (at least two of the pictures were recalled following injection ipsilateral to the side of seizure onset or the side of greater seizure activity), and no clinical memory impairment was present in the six patients who subsequently underwent temporal lobectomy.

In the three reports above, no patient who successfully performed the memory portion of the assessment displayed clinically apparent memory deficits after temporal lobectomy. Consequently, inclusion of a memory component during intracarotid amobarbital testing has been widely adopted to screen patients for possible bilateral hippocampal dysfunction before unilateral temporal lobectomy [26]. However, there have been few systematic studies examining memory performance during amobarbital evaluation, and results of Wada memory testing have

been relied on despite limited validation from independent surgery centers.

Assumptions and General Assessment Strategies

Three assumptions are made when employing Wada memory testing to predict anterograde amnesia following temporal lobectomy: (a) Inactivation of a single temporal lobe is not in itself capable of producing a generalized anterograde memory defect, (b) critical memory regions resected with temporal lobectomy will be functionally inactivated by injection into the internal carotid artery, and (c) if temporal lobe structures contralateral to amobarbital injection are severely dysfunctional such that removal of the epileptogenic side will result in an amnestic syndrome, then the injection will produce a transient amnesia due to temporary bilateral temporal lobe inactivation.

There is considerable variability in the approach to memory assessment at various epilepsy surgery centers [20,26]. However, most procedures can be conceptualized as following one of two principal formats. One method employs an ongoing stimulus-distractor-recognition paradigm in which a stimulus is presented and the subject is asked to identify it by either naming, reading, or matching. After a distractor task is performed, recall of the original stimulus is obtained either by free recall or recognition. The time until successful return to baseline memory levels may be used as the index of memory performance, or a recognition test may be administered after the medication effects have worn off. The other approach involves presentation of discrete items during the period of hemispheric anesthesia, testing recall after the amobarbital anesthetization has worn off. Snyder and Novelly [27] reported that of the 55 epilepsy surgery centers surveyed, 19 (29%) employed a stimulus-distractor approach, whereas 39 centers (71%) employed discrete item presentation. However, both the number and type of stimuli vary between and within techniques. Explicit scoring criteria are frequently not presented, making comparisons across centers and studies difficult.

Because of the perceived risk of temporal lobectomy to anterograde memory, Wada memory testing has been used to establish surgery candidacy despite the absence of controlled studies. However, for Wada memory testing to have appropriate statistical predictive validity in identifying risk for postsurgical amnesia, a consecutive series of patients would need to undergo temporal lobectomy independently from Wada memory data. If the Wada memory data are used to establish surgical candidacy, the dependent variable is confounded with the predictor variable requiring validation. When patients who appear to be at risk for postsurgical anterograde memory loss are excluded from temporal lobectomy or undergo limited resection that spares hippocampus on the basis of intracarotid amobarbital results, one cannot determine whether the procedure is truly predictive since those patients believed to be at risk do not receive a standard temporal lobectomy or are never operated on. The number of false-positive identifications cannot be determined. If a significant false-positive error rate exists, many patients who might benefit from surgery could potentially be condemned to a life with intractable seizures. Thus, the frequency of false-positive identifications is not a trivial issue. Greater discussion of the methodologic limitations of Wada memory testing is available elsewhere [20,28].

Because of the above consideration, results of Wada memory testing should be interpreted within the following framework to evaluate indirectly the sensitivity and specificity of the procedure: (a) What is the sensitivity of Wada memory testing to bilateral dysfunction as evidenced by failure with injection contralateral to the side of eventual surgery? (b) What are the effects of language representation on memory results? and (c) What are the effects of surgery if the results of Wada memory testing are discounted?

Continuous Material Recognition Studies. Few studies using a distractor/recognition paradigm have been presented in the literature. Fedio and Weinberg [29] investigated memory in 12 patients with temporal lobe epilepsy (TLE) who were left cerebral language dominant (6 left, 6 right). Photographs of familiar objects were presented alternating with the word "and." The task was to identify "and," to name each object, and then to recall the name of the immediately preceding object. Object naming ($p < .01$) and recall ($p < .001$) were poorer following left hemisphere injection. However, no differential memory performance as a function of seizure onset laterality was observed, suggesting that this procedure was not necessarily sensitive to contralateral temporal lobe dysfunction.

Rausch et al. [30] examined recovery time for different behaviors following unilateral amobarbital injection of 125 mg in 17 TLE patients (6 left, 11 right). A continuous recognition task was used in which common objects, written words, and unfamiliar forms were presented. Different left versus right injection efforts were present for the left TLE and right TLE patient groups, showing a differential effect as a function of seizure focus laterality for short-term

recognition of pictures, words, and forms. However, when examining memory following return to baseline, differential ipsilateral versus contralateral effects as a function of seizure laterality were present only for picture recall.

Although statistical analyses of the simple main effects of injection in left TLE and right TLE groups were not conducted independently, it appears that there was little performance difference in left TLE patients as a function of whether the left or right cerebral hemisphere was injected. In contrast, patients with right TLE performed more poorly following left (contralateral) hemisphere injection. Ipsilateral versus contralateral performance asymmetry using this technique was present for right TLE patients only. Consequently, this approach appears best suited to assess only the functional memory capacity of the left temporal lobe in right TLE patients. However, nondominant temporal lobectomies are generally felt to produce a much smaller risk to recent memory than language-dominant temporal lobe resections [31]. Based on the reports of Fedio and Weinberg [29] and Rausch et al. [30], the stimulus-distractor approach employing the stimuli reported above may have limitations in assessing the memory capacity of the right hemisphere in patients whose seizures originate from the left temporal lobe.

Discrete Item Memory Studies. The majority of Wada memory studies published have employed discrete item presentation. Milner [32] described memory for two line drawings and a nursery rhyme, presented approximately 3 minutes following injection, and observed anterograde amnesia for the postinjection material only 27 times following 226 injections (12%). Failure to remember all items occurred in 25 of 110 injections (23%) contralateral to the side of the lesion, but in only two of 116 injections (2%) ipsilateral to the side of the lesion. When cases with only one error were eliminated (equivocal memory failure), 18 patients failed the amobarbital memory test, all of whom had injection contralateral to the seizure focus. Milner [33] recommended that at least two recognition errors using the above technique be used as the criterion of memory impairment.

The Montreal approach to Wada memory testing evolved with increasing experience with this technique. More recently, when the presentation of two real objects in addition to the line drawings and rhyme was included during the drug effect, patients with a clear unilateral seizure onset had a 41% failure rate following contralateral injection but only a 15% failure rate following ipsilateral injection [18]. In contrast, patients with bilateral seizure onset had a

60% failure rate with injection contralateral to the proposed surgery site and a 50% failure rate with injection on the side of the proposed resection. The number of subjects studied was not specified.

Silfvenius et al. [34,35] examined Wada memory performance in patients with unilateral and bilateral temporal lobe seizures and others with frontal lobe seizures. Of the three left TLE patients, only one had adequate recognition memory for pictures (4 of 6) following left hemisphere injection. The remaining two patients could recognize only a single picture. In contrast, two of these patients displayed better recognition memory following nondominant right hemisphere injection (2 of 6 and 4 of 6 correct, respectively). Although the sample is extremely small, this pattern is opposite that which would be expected since right hemisphere injections contralateral to the epileptogenic left temporal lobes should have created a greater memory deficit.

The five right TLE patients also displayed superior performances following nondominant hemisphere injection. Two patients demonstrated partial recognition of the pictures with scores of at least 3 of 6 after dominant injection. The remaining three right TLE patients were unable to recognize any pictures. Following right hemisphere injection, all five patients recognized at least 2 of 6 pictures, and three patients recognized at least 3 of 6. As with studies employing continuous memory recognition, Silfvenius demonstrated a convincing performance asymmetry in the expected direction for right temporal lobe patients only, the group in whom there is less concern for postoperative amnesia [31].

Additional reports have appeared suggesting that memory testing is less equivocal when the right hemisphere is injected. Badour et al. [36] reported six of six right TLE patients obtained higher memory scores following ipsilateral injection of 125 mg of amobarbital. In contrast, three of six left TLE patients had equal performance following both injections, and three of six had *higher* scores following contralateral (i.e., right) hemisphere injection. Although specific numbers were not presented, Walker and Laxer [37] observed superior recognition memory following ipsilateral injection in greater than 80% of the patients, "particularly if the seizure focus was in the hemisphere nondominant for speech."

This does not indicate that memory cannot be adequately tested if the seizures originate from the left temporal lobe. Lesser et al. [38] examined memory performance for discrete objects presented during the early mute state commonly seen immediately following left hemisphere injection. The left hemisphere confusional period was operationally defined as that period prior to (a) clearing of confusion or clearing of contralateral electroencephalographic (EEG) slowing; (b) resumption of any speech, intelligible or unintelligible; or (c) any return of muscle tone. The number of objects presented varied between 3 and 55. These authors found that 18 of 24 patients with left temporal seizure onset but only 4 of 12 with right temporal seizure onset could correctly recognize at least two thirds of the objects presented following left hemisphere injection. However, six additional left TLE patients did not meet the two-thirds correct recognition criterion. At least three of the patients failing to recognize two thirds of the objects underwent temporal lobectomy without development of an amnestic syndrome. Twenty-one of the 24 left TLE patients had undergone left temporal lobectomy, and no significant memory impairment was reported.

Powell et al. [9] employed discrete item presentation to assess memory in 27 temporal lobectomy candidates (left = 14, right = 13). Although Powell et al. did not employ formal criteria of memory failure, they directly addressed false-positive responses during recognition memory assessment. The authors considered memory performance invalid if false-positive responses were present. Since false-positive response frequency within subjects was not presented, it is difficult to know to what degree false-positives contributed to the rate of memory failure ipsilateral to the side of seizure onset, thereby precluding surgery. In their series of 27 patients, 10 patients (37%) were not operated on due to poor amobarbital memory testing results that were subjectively determined (left $n = 5$, right $n = 5$). However, false-positives cannot be totally ignored, for a patient may correctly "recognize" all material but also "recognize" items never presented. False-positive errors may reflect poor baseline memory function [39].

Rausch et al. [40] described memory performance using discrete items in 30 patients with unilateral temporal lobe seizure onset (left $n = 13$, right $n = 17$). Following administration of 125 mg of amobarbital, discrete memory items were presented during the period of drug-induced unilateral EEG slowing and hemiparesis. The items included stimuli regarded as functionally appropriate for the noninjected hemisphere. Thus, verbal items were not considered critical for assessing the memory ability of the nondominant hemisphere. A passing score was correct recognition of at least 67% of the critical items. All patients recognized at least two thirds of the material following ipsilateral injection. In contrast, 19 of 30 patients failed memory performance following injection to the hemisphere contralateral to the side of seizure onset. These results confirmed the findings of Lesser et al. [38], demonstrating that many left TLE patients can perform recognition assessment following left hemisphere injection. However, these findings are inconsistent with many other studies in which memory performance following left hemisphere injection was poorer than that following right hemisphere injection regardless of seizure-onset laterality. Without greater detail regarding the number of stimuli presented and length of stimulus presentation, it is difficult to determine the potential contribution of method variance to account for the Rausch et al. [40] findings.

We studied early and late memory components of the amobarbital evaluation in 57 TLE patients by employing incremental amobarbital injections [41]. Eight common objects (i.e., "early" items) were presented for approximately 4 s each following demonstration of hemiplegia. After return of minimal language function, "late" items were presented, which included two objects, a nursery rhyme, and two visual discrimination items. Recognition memory for both the early and late objects was tested using appropriate foils. Both early and late item memory components were sensitive to bilateral temporal dysfunction (one side due to injected amobarbital, the other side due to the patient's seizures) by virtue of significantly poorer overall group performance after the injection contralateral to seizure onset.

Despite the statistical sensitivity to bilateral temporal lobe dysfunction, the individual predictive ability of Wada memory testing results appeared poor. We employed conservative criteria for establishing the performance threshold for memory failure (corrected scores of 2 of 8 or less on early objects, corrected scores of 1.5 of 5 or less on late items). Thirteen patients failed either the early or late item recognition memory tests. However, based on performance of other tasks (i.e., electrical hippocampal stimulation with simultaneous memory testing and memory assessment following hippocampal cooling at the time of surgery), 10 patients received standard temporal lobectomies including the anterior hippocampus. None of the 10 patients developed an amnestic syndrome, indicating that the amobarbital memory test may have a high degree of misidentification of patients at risk for a postoperative amnestic syndrome. This high degree of false-positive identifications indicates that some appropriate surgical candidates might either be denied surgery if the amobarbital memory results are used as a strict exclusionary criterion or

undergo a more limited resection with a decreased likelihood of a good seizure outcome.

Data from independent centers similarly demonstrated that memory failure with amobarbital testing does not necessarily indicate risk for postoperative amnesia. Girvin et al. [42] reported three patients who failed Wada memory testing using the Montreal approach but who underwent standard temporal lobectomy. All three patients had bitemporal EEG abnormalities, displayed verbal and nonverbal memory deficits on baseline neuropsychological testing, and had borderline to mildly mentally retarded IQ levels. Magnetic resonance imaging revealed a left temporal structural lesion in two cases. All three patients underwent left temporal lobectomy including anterior hippocampus, and none displayed a postoperative amnestic syndrome.

Both the Montreal Neurological Institute [43] and Yale University [44] described repeat Wada testing in which patients initially failed the memory component but subsequently passed on repeat assessment at the same or lower dose. These centers reported changes in pass/fail clinical performances ranging from 28–84%. The patients who failed the initial Wada test but subsequently passed on repeat assessment underwent temporal lobectomy without the development of a postoperative amnesia. If these patients had simply undergone surgery without repeating the Wada, they would have been equivalent to those reported in our patient series described above.

Methodologic Limitations. The timing of stimulus presentation is potentially an important variable. By presenting items soon after demonstration of contralateral hemiplegia, the maximal anesthetic effects are present. Thus, hippocampal function soon after injection is more similar to the state that will be created following surgery. However, medication effects on other cognitive functions are also maximal. With left hemisphere injection, global aphasia is usually present for several minutes following injection. In addition, since patients are frequently akinetic and abulic, one cannot be certain to what degree the items were attended. As the medication effects recede, cognitive impairments are less severe, but the presumed effects on the hippocampal formation are also less. Thus, the danger is that performance on items presented later is not sufficiently sensitive in certain patients due to less medication effect on temporal lobe function.

In addition to subtotal anesthetization at the time of late item presentation, there is the potential that memory items will be presented at different times following injection of the left and right hemispheres. By waiting to present stimuli until minimal language has returned, items will be presented later following left hemisphere injection than following right hemisphere injection. This problem is not associated with early object presentation. We have also illustrated a lack of correspondence between "early" and "late" memory items when applied on an individual patient basis, despite both measures being sensitive to contralateral dysfunction on the group level [41].

If the presence of amnesia following temporal lobectomy is estimated at 1%, then surgery would be expected to produce a severe anterograde memory impairment in 1% of the patients when no predictive procedures are employed. If Wada memory testing correctly classifies 90% of those individuals at risk for memory impairment (correct identification) but also misidentifies 30% of patients not at risk (false-positive identification), then the correct classification will be 70.2% (correct identification of risk = .9 × .01 = 0.9%, correct identification of risk absence = .7 × .99 = 69.3%), which is actually a reduction in predictive accuracy compared to no attempt at prediction (99%).

Interpretation of Wada memory results may be complicated by inattentiveness, mental confusion, emotional lability, and strong perseverative tendencies [45–47]. Memory performance may be affected by the impairment of other "supportive" cognitive functions that are necessary for the formation of new memories. Testing memory for many types of material is not feasible due to the short duration of drug effect and the medical risk associated with repeated injections. McGlone and MacDonald [48] also reported that although changes in pass/fail memory ratings were obtained in 8 of 18 repeat injections, 7 of 8 changes were associated with identifiable external factors, such as technically unsatisfactory studies, unusual emotional response, or even failing to wear eyeglasses. Thus, for many reasons, patients may fail Wada memory tests due to factors not directly related to the integrity of the contralateral mesial temporal lobe to sustain memory function. Finally, since the anatomic region of interest, the hippocampal formation, obtains its blood supply from both the internal carotid and the posterior cerebral systems, it remains unknown to what degree the hippocampus is affected in each patient tested. Milner [33] stated that filling of the posterior cerebral artery is not a prerequisite for obtaining memory loss. Thus, Wada memory testing may primarily test the competency of the neocortical contribution to recent memory. Others have postu-

lated that perfusion of the septal region of the basal forebrain contributes to the memory impairment following amobarbital injection in certain patients [49].

Although there has been recent acknowledgment of and discussion about the heterogeneity of the procedures employed to assess memory during amobarbital anesthesia, no generally accepted framework exists for evaluating the method variance that may be influencing patient performance. Rausch [50], in a survey presented at the 1992 International Palm Desert Conference on the Surgical Treatment of the Epilepsies, reported that some centers never observe "failure" ipsilateral to the side of surgery, whereas others report that more than 30% of their patients fail the test. Similarly, some centers report that no patients fail contralateral to the side of surgery, whereas others report that between 60% and 80% of their patients fail. Thus, the clinical sensitivity and specificity of Wada memory testing cannot be generalized from center to center. Since the amobarbital dosages administered ranged from 60 mg to 200 mg, dosage is likely one variable that contributes to these discrepant results. We have observed poorer recognition memory performance associated with higher dosages of amobarbital [51].

Posterior Cerebral Artery Injection. Because of the limitations associated with standard intracarotid artery amobarbital injection, a posterior approach through the vertebrobasilar system to anesthetize the medial temporal lobe was developed at the Mayo Clinic by Jack et al. [52]. They reported 17 patients who were candidates for epilepsy surgery and who underwent unilateral injection of the posterior cerebral artery (PCA) ipsilateral to the presumed seizure focus. All patients remained oriented and cooperative throughout the procedure, avoiding the confounding effects of aphasia and attentional impairment on memory function. No language impairments were present, and all patients had satisfactory memory performance.

Jack et al. [52] concluded that given the absence of behavioral confounds, as well as more closely modeling the effects of temporal lobectomy by affecting the hippocampal formation, the PCA Wada technique might develop into a more appropriate method to assess risk for postsurgical amnesia than the conventional carotid technique. However, since the appearance of this report, the PCA Wada is no longer conducted at the Mayo Clinic. One patient from their series of approximately 50–60 patients undergoing the PCA Wada developed a brainstem stroke as a consequence of this procedure. Even if this risk were only 1% and the sample size were sufficient to make this determination, the risk-to-benefit ratio was not felt to be low enough to routinely subject patients to this evaluation, since the risk for postsurgical amnesia is likely less than 1%. The PCA technique offers advantages for cognitive testing and may have a role in the evaluation of a select subset of patients (e.g., those patients who have some evidence of dysfunction contralateral to the proposed surgery), although we would recommend a repeat standard carotid Wada prior to a PCA evaluation. The PCA Wada should be conducted only by radiologists who routinely perform interventional neuroradiologic techniques (e.g., arteriovenous malformation embolization).

Clinical Considerations. At the Medical College of Georgia, we interpret poor results following amobarbital testing as suggesting only a possible risk to recent memory and conclude that additional studies of hippocampal function will be needed. When a strong recognition asymmetry is observed (e.g., 5 of 8 or more early objects with injection ipsilateral to seizure onset and 2 of 8 or fewer contralaterally), we conclude that surgery including the hippocampus will not produce a serious anterograde amnesia, and intraoperative cooling or memory testing is not performed. In this context, the test identifies low-risk patients rather than accurately predicting those with potential postresection memory difficulty. In addition, a comparison of Wada memory performances of each hemisphere helps to lateralize temporal lobe dysfunction in certain places [53,54]. Thus, a marked memory asymmetry may help decrease the necessity for intracranial evaluation in a patient whose seizure onset laterality is otherwise suggestive but not conclusive.

A marked asymmetry, with poorer performance obtained ipsilateral to the side of proposed surgery, may signal risk to recent memory. For example, we observed an asymmetry in early object memory following amobarbital in a patient with right cerebral language dominance, with 8 of 8 objects recalled following left hemisphere injection but 0 of 8 objects recalled following right hemisphere injection. Recall was normal for all items presented later in the procedure (3 of 5 items with no false-positive responses), and no left/right difference was observed. Despite depth-electrode implantation, seizures could not be localized with confidence, and a decision regarding this patient's surgery was deferred. The family, however, pursued surgery at a different center. The pa-

tient was reevaluated with invasive EEG procedures, and his typical spontaneous seizures were found to originate from the right temporal lobe; a right temporal lobectomy was subsequently performed. Following surgery, a significant language deficit was noted. In addition, a profound recent memory deficit was observed, and this has persisted for approximately 1 year (decrease in Wechsler Memory Scale-Revised, General Memory Index, from 84 to 58). Thus, given the large performance asymmetry on early objects, we would have performed hippocampal cooling studies before right hippocampal resection and would have resected only the temporal tip, unless there were strong evidence at the time of surgery to suggest that the hippocampus could be resected safely. This patient illustrates the differential sensitivity discussed above of early- and late-item memory when applied to an individual patient and illustrates that relying solely on late-item performance may fail to indicate risk to memory.

When poor memory is obtained following amobarbital injection ipsilateral to the side of proposed surgery, several options are available depending on the philosophy of the surgical institution in which the patient is being evaluated. The patient may be excluded from surgery. However, this may needlessly exclude candidates who can benefit from the surgery. The patient may also undergo resection of the temporal tip, sparing the hippocampus [18], but this may decrease the surgical efficacy. Some institutions, including our own, will repeat the Wada memory test at the same or lower dose [11,55]. If adequate performance is obtained on repeated assessment, then temporal lobectomy may be performed. Alternatively, special memory testing may be conducted, such as with a specialized posterior amobarbital technique [52].

If despite poor amobarbital memory there is sufficient evidence suggesting temporal lobe pathology (i.e., strict unilateral seizure onset, presence of a structural lesion by computed tomography or magnetic resonance imaging, asymmetrical hippocampal dysfunction by measures of limbic evoked potentials, single photon emission computed tomography, positron-emission tomography, and neuropsychological testing), a temporal lobectomy including hippocampus may be considered in certain cases and the amobarbital memory results discounted [41,42]. We believe that Wada memory results should not be considered absolute but rather should be interpreted within the entire clinical context of preoperative evaluation for epilepsy surgery.

Wada Protocol at the Medical College of Georgia

Wada assessment is performed on all epilepsy surgery candidates. Bilateral studies are performed because we use asymmetrical Wada memory results as a measure of lateralized temporal lobe dysfunction and we have observed right hemisphere language representation in right-handed patients whose seizures originate from the right temporal lobe. The protocol below is the core of our current clinical procedure, although additional tests are frequently included to address specific theoretical issues of brain-behavior relationships. A copy of our protocol form is included (see Appendix E) [20].

Prior to the procedure, the purposes of the test are described to the patient and a practice trial of the procedure without presentation of the memory items is administered. Patients are told that they will be asked to remember most of the material presented during the procedure. They are shown a picture of a cup and a shoe, asked to repeat the sentence "It's a fine day today," and told to remember that material because they will be questioned for those items during the test. The same preinjection pictures and sentence are used for both injections because little weight is given to performance on these tasks, given the general absence of retrograde memory effects of amobarbital.

Wada assessment is conducted with the patient in the supine position immediately following angiography. The procedure is videotaped to allow review of ambiguous findings, thereby minimizing the need for repeat assessment. Administration of test materials is performed by the neuropsychologist, while monitoring of neurologic function, as well as initial behavioral rating, is performed by the behavioral neurologist. Following completion of the test, the neuropsychologist and behavioral neurologist discuss the patient's performance to arrive at rating consensus, and the videotape is reviewed if necessary to resolve disagreements regarding language or other behavioral ratings.

At the onset of testing, patients hold both hands straight up with palms turned rostrally and fingers spread. They then begin counting repeatedly from 1 to 20. An initial injection of 100 mg of amobarbital sodium is administered by hand via catheter over a 4-s interval following a transfemoral approach into the internal carotid artery. Since we have previously demonstrated a relationship between medication dosage administered and Wada memory performance, we presently do not administer additional amobarbital unless a marked hemiplegia does not develop. Left and right amobarbital evaluations and arteriograms are performed on the same day separated by at least 30 minutes, and the order of amobarbital injection is sequentially alternated. Patients are tested prior to the second injection to ensure return to baseline.

The initial expressive language rating is made immediately following demonstration of hemiplegia. Initial expressive language is rated on a 5-point scale based on alterations in counting, with 0 reflecting normal expression and 4 indicating complete speech arrest. If a pause in counting occurs, patients are repeatedly urged to resume counting to ensure that the disruption is not caused by acute medication effects or sedation. If no resumption occurs, patients are asked to start counting again at 1 since the initial portion of the sequence tends to be more overlearned and is more resistant to sedative effects. If counting is resumed within 20 s without paraphasic difficulty, speech is rated as normal. Two types of counting perseveration are noted, both of which are scored as 1. Patients may continue counting beyond the number 20, despite adequate practice, or may fail to stop counting despite repeated urging to do so by the examiner. Sequencing errors, scored 2, include responses such as "12, 15, 16, 17, 15." Occasionally a patient may perseverate on a single number, such as "3-3-3-3-3," and this error is scored as a 3. Finally, complete speech arrest exceeding 20 s is scored as 4.

Subsequent behavior ratings are rated on a 4-point scale (normal, mild, moderate, and severe). Spontaneous eye gaze deviation is rated, as is the ability to cross midline in the hemispace contralateral to the side of injection. The patient is requested to execute a simple command (e.g., "touch your nose"). Eight common objects (i.e., "early" items) are then presented for approximately 4 s each and the name of each object is repeated twice to the patient. Examples include a toy car, a battery, and a clothes pin. The patient's eyes are held open as necessary, and the objects are presented in the visual field ipsilateral to the hemisphere injected. During the period of early object presentation, the patient's level of consciousness is assessed using a modified Glasgow Coma Scale [56].

Multiple language tasks are then administered. Language rating is based on performance on four additional linguistic tasks (namely, comprehension, naming, repetition, and reading). Comprehension is assessed by a modified token test in which four geometric shapes of different colors are presented vertically to the subject's ipsilateral visual field. Commands of decreasing complexity are administered:

1. "Point to the red circle after the green square."
2. "Point to the red circle and then point to the green square."
3. "Point to the red circle."

A score of 0 is awarded for completion of the complex two-stage command with inverted syntax; a score of 1 reflects successful execution of the simple two-stage command; a score of 2 is given for the one-stage commands; and a score of 3 is given if the subject does not perform any commands. Minimal return of language function (e.g., following simple midline commands such as "stick out your tongue," or spontaneous vocalization) is required prior to additional testing and presentation of the "late" memory items. Our decision to wait until some return of language function prior to late-item presentation is to reduce encoding deficits of the "late" memory items secondary to aphasia and to ensure some similarity to the protocol employed at the Montreal Neurological Institute [18]. First, the subject is instructed to name two new objects. If the patient is unable to name the item, its name is repeated twice to the patient. A nursery rhyme phrase is then read to the patient and its repetition requested. If the patient is unable to repeat the rhyme, it is read to the patient again. The presence of dysarthria is rated at this time. A simple sentence is presented for the patient to read. Repetition, dysarthria, and reading are all scored on a 4-point rating scale, with 0 reflecting normal function and 3 being severely impaired. Specific paraphasic errors are recorded. Two visual spatial discrimination items from the Florida Kindergarten Screening Battery Recognition-Discrimination subtest are then presented [57]. The nonverbal discrimination items are presented to provide balance against the primarily verbal aspects of the other late memory stimuli.

Following presentation of the "late" memory items, the patient is asked to recall the two pictures presented earlier in the hospital room (i.e., cup and shoe), as well as the sentence. The two pictures are then presented with four foils, and the patient is requested to name each picture. In addition, recognition memory for the two pictures is assessed in the absence of picture free recall. However, recognition memory of the preinjection material is not used to determine risk for postresection memory impairment.

Language classification is determined by performance on each of four language categories assessed (i.e., counting disruption, comprehension, naming, and repetition). Because considerable differences exist regarding reaction to the medication and duration of the anesthetic effects, we employ a conservative classification for language representation. For language impairment to be inferred, as distinct from confusion or abulia, one of two error configurations must be detected. In the first, impairments (scores > 0) need to be present in at least two categories, with one of the scores greater than 1. In the second pattern, language representation would be inferred if at least three fourths of language categories are only mildly impaired (e.g., scores of 1). Since we have only recently added the reading task to our protocol, we have not yet formally incorporated it into our language criteria.

After the amobarbital effect has worn off, as demonstrated by complete return of 5/5 strength, absence of pronator drift and bradykinesia, normal repetition of the phrase "no ifs, ands, or buts," and ability to execute complex two-stage commands involving inverted syntax, recognition memory of material presented during the procedure is tested. To assess early object memory, the eight target items are presented individually with 16 randomly interspersed foils, and the subject indicates whether the item has been presented previously. To correct for response bias and guessing, we incorporate a correction by subtracting one half of the incorrect (false-positive) responses from the total correct responses. Thus, any average of guessing without recognition would yield an expected value of 0 [e.g., (8 correct) − 0.5 × (16 incorrect) = 0]. Early-item memory performance is our primary recent memory measure.

To assess late-item memory, several tasks are administered. If the patient is unable to recall the two late objects spontaneously, the names of five objects are read and the patient is instructed to identify those objects. The number of objects is not indicated. Similarly, if unable to freely recall the rhyme, four nursery rhymes are read to the patient for recognition assessment. Although we feel more confident if the patient freely recalls the late material, only recognition assessment is analyzed, with free recall scored as evidence of correct recognition. A multiple-choice recognition assessment is obtained for the two visual spatial discrimination designs, with the two targets interspersed on the same recognition sheet with four foils. Again, the number of targets is not indicated, and the subject is asked following each response, either correct or incorrect, if any additional items are recognized. To correct for guessing, one half of the number of false-positive responses is subtracted from the sum of the correctly recognized items. Free recall of the sentence read orally is then requested, and multiple-choice recognition is administered if necessary.

Similarly, free recall of the previously named late line drawings is obtained (which included the cup and shoe), followed by recognition assessment. After completion of the formal memory assessment, the ability to recall weakness and language deficits is assessed. Affect change, response perseveration, paraphasic responses in spontaneous speech, attentional deficits, and ptosis are also noted.

Our primary memory measure is recognition of the eight early objects, although we do not employ fixed pass-fail criteria. We generally consider corrected memory scores from the injection ipsilateral to the side of proposed surgery of 0–1 to be impaired, 1.5–2.5 as borderline, and 3 and above as normal. However, if a patient obtains a corrected score of 2 but performs well on the later items (subjectively defined), there is less concern for postresection memory impairment. Thus, depending on other measures of temporal lobe function, specialized memory procedures during surgery may not be deemed necessary. In conclusion, we employ general guidelines for interpreting memory performance, but these are not fixed and will be altered based on a patient's baseline level of cognitive abilities, pattern of performance on the "late" memory items, behavioral response to medication, and variations in the patient's cerebral vasculature.

Acknowledgments

We thank Patricia A. Downs for her help with manuscript preparation, and Drs. Don W. King and Cheryl A. Gratton for their review of this chapter.

References

1. Gardner WJ. Injection of procaine into the brain to locate speech area in left-handed persons. *Arch Neurol Psychiatry* 1941;46:1035–38.
2. Wada J, Rasmussen T. Intracarotid injection of sodium Amytal for the lateralization of cerebral speech dominance: experimental and clinical observations. *J Neurosurg* 1960;17:266–82.
3. Rasmussen T, Milner B. The role of early left-brain injury in determining lateralization of cerebral speech functions. *Ann NY Acad Sci* 1977;299:355–69.
4. Woods RP, Dodrill CB, Ojemann GA. Brain injury, handedness, and speech lateralization in a series of amobarbital studies. *Ann Neurol* 1988;23:510–18.
5. Branch C, Milner B, Rasmussen T. Intracarotid sodium Amytal for the lateralization of cerebral speech domi-

nance: observations in 123 patients. *J Neurosurg* 1964;21:399–405.
6. Wyllie E, Lüders H, Murphy D, et al. Intracarotid amobarbital (Wada) test for language dominance: correlation with results of cortical stimulation. *Epilepsia* 1990;31:156–61.
7. Hommes OR, Panhuysen LHHM. Bilateral intracarotid Amytal injection: a study of dysphasia, disturbance of consciousness and paresis. *Psychiatr Neurol Neurochir* 1970;73:447–59.
8. Oxbury SM, Oxbury JM. Intracarotid Amytal test in the assessment of language dominance. In: Rose FC, ed. *Progress in aphasiology.* New York: Raven Press, 1984;115–123. (Advances in neurology, vol. 42.)
9. Powell GE, Polkey CE, Canavan AGM. Lateralisation of memory functions in epileptic patients by use of the sodium Amytal (Wada) technique. *J Neurol Neurosurg Psychiatry* 1987;50:665–72.
10. Rey M, Dellatulas G, Bancaud J, et al. Hemispheric lateralization of motor and speech functions after early brain lesion: study of 73 epileptic patients with intracarotid Amytal test. *Neuropsychologia* 1988;26:167–72.
11. Zatorre RJ. Perceptual asymmetry on the dichotic fused words test and cerebral speech lateralization determined by the carotid sodium Amytal test. *Neuropsychologia* 1989;27:1207–19.
12. Loring DW, Meador KJ, Lee GP, et al. Cerebral language lateralization: evidence from intracarotid testing. *Neuropsychologia* 1990;28:831–38.
13. Snyder PJ, Novelly RA, Harris LJ. Mixed speech dominance in the intracarotid sodium Amytal procedure: validity and criteria issues. *J Clin Exp Neuropsychol* 1990;12:629–43.
14. Loring DW, Flanigin HF, Meador KJ, et al. Right hemisphere language representation determined by intracarotid sodium Amytal testing and functional cortical speech mapping. *Epilepsia* 1988;29:686 (abstract).
15. Loring DW, Meador KJ, Lee GP, et al. Crossed aphasia in a patient with complex partial seizures: evidence from intracarotid sodium Amytal testing, functional cortical mapping, and neuropsychological assessment. *J Clin Exp Neuropsychol* 1990;12:340–54.
16. Rosenbaum T, DeToledo J, Smith DB, et al. Preoperative assessment of language laterality is necessary in all epilepsy surgery candidates: a case report. *Epilepsia* 1989;30:712 (abstract).
17. Rausch R, Walsh G. Right-hemisphere language dominance in right-handed epileptic patients. *Arch Neurol* 1984;41:1077–80.
18. Jones-Gotman M. Commentary: psychological evaluation—testing hippocampal function. In: Engel J, ed. *Surgical treatment of the epilepsies.* New York: Raven Press, 1987:203–11.
19. Solomon PR, Solomon SD, Schaaf EV, et al. Altered activity in the hippocampus is more detrimental to classical conditioning than removing the structure. *Science* 1983;220:329–31.

20. Loring DW, Meador KJ, Lee GP, King DW. *Amobarbital effects and lateralized brain function.* New York: Springer-Verlag, 1992.

21. Penfield W, Mathieson G. Memory: autopsy findings and comments on the role of the hippocampus in experimental recall. *Arch Neurol* 1974;31:145–54.

22. Milner B, Branch C, Rasmussen T. Study of short-term memory after intracarotid injection of sodium Amytal. *Trans Am Neurol Assoc* 1962;87:224–6.

23. Kløve H, Grabow JD, Trites RL. Evaluation of memory functions with intracarotid sodium Amytal. *Trans Am Neurol Assoc* 1969;94:76–80.

24. Walker AE. Recent memory impairment in unilateral temporal lesions. *Arch Neurol Psychiatry* 1957;78:543–52.

25. Blume WT, Grabow JD, Darley FL, et al. Intracarotid amobarbital test of language and memory before temporal lobectomy for seizure control. *Neurology* 1973;23:812–19.

26. Rausch R. Psychological evaluation. In: Engel J, ed. *Surgical treatment of the epilepsies.* New York: Raven Press, 1987:181–95.

27. Snyder PJ, Novelly RA. An international survey of the administration and interpretation of the intracarotid sodium Amytal procedure (IAP). Paper presented at the annual meeting of the International Neuropsychological Society, Kissimmee, Florida, February 16, 1990.

28. Loring DW, Lee GP, Meador KJ, King DW. Does memory assessment during amobarbital testing predict postsurgical amnesia? *J Epilepsy* 1991;4:19–24.

29. Fedio P, Weinberg LK. Dysnomia and impairment of verbal memory following intracarotid injection of sodium Amytal. *Brain Res* 1971;31:159–68.

30. Rausch R, Fedio P, Ary CM, et al. Resumption of behavior following intracarotid sodium amobarbital injection. *Ann Neurol* 1984;15:31–5.

31. Milner B. Amnesia following operation on the temporal lobes. In: Whitty CWM, Zangwill OL, eds. *Amnesia.* London: Butterworths, 1966:109–33.

32. Milner B. Disorders of learning and memory after temporal lobe lesions in man. *Clin Neurosurg* 1972;19:241–46.

33. Milner B. Psychological aspects of focal epilepsy and its neurosurgical management. In: Purpura D, Penry J, Walter R, eds. *Neurosurgical management of the epilepsies.* New York: Raven Press, 1975:299–321. (Advances in neurology, vol. 8.)

34. Silfvenius H, Blom S. Results from intracarotid Amytal tests in epileptic patients. *Acta Neurol Scand* 1984;69(Suppl 99):77–8.

35. Silfvenius H, Blom S, Nilsson L, et al. Observations on verbal, pictorial and stereognostic memory in epileptic patients during intracarotid Amytal testing. *Acta Neurol Scand* 1984;69(Suppl 99):57–75.

36. Badour A, Kiss I, Dasheiff R, et al. Memory performance during Amytal testing: does it predict the side of temporal lobectomy? *Epilepsia* 1988;29:660 (abstract).

37. Walker JA, Laxer KD. Comparison of recall and recognition memory in the Wada test. *Epilepsia* 1989;30:712–13 (abstract).

38. Lesser RP, Dinner DS, Lüders H, et al. Memory for objects presented soon after intracarotid amobarbital sodium injections in patients with medically intractable complex partial seizures. *Neurology* 1986;36:895–9.

39. Loring DW, Lee GP, Meador KJ. The intracarotid amobarbital sodium procedure: false-positive errors during recognition memory assessment. *Arch Neurol* 1989;46:285–7.

40. Rausch R, Babb TL, Engel J, et al. Memory following intracarotid amobarbital injection contralateral to hippocampal damage. *Arch Neurol* 1989;46:783–8.

41. Loring DW, Lee GP, Meador KJ, et al. The intracarotid amobarbital procedure as a predictor of memory failure following unilateral temporal lobectomy. *Neurology* 1990;40:605–10.

42. Girvin JP, McGlone J, McLachlan RS, et al. Validity of the sodium amobarbital test for memory in selected patients. *Epilepsia* 1987;28:636 (abstract).

43. Jones-Gotman M. Reliability and validity of intracarotid sodium Amytal procedure for memory. *J Clin Exp Neuropsychol* 1992;14:71 (abstract)

44. Novelly RA, Williamson PD. Incidence of false-positive memory impairment in the intracarotid Amytal procedure. *Epilepsia* 1989;30:711 (abstract).

45. Lee GP, Loring DW, Meador KJ, et al. Severe behavioral complications following intracarotid sodium amobarbital injection: implications for hemispheric asymmetry of emotion. *Neurology* 1988;38:1233–6.

46. Lee GP, Loring DW, Meador KJ, et al. Hemispheric specialization for emotional expression. *Brain Cog* 1990;12:267–80.

47. Huh K, Meador KJ, Loring DW, et al. Attentional mechanisms during the intracarotid amobarbital test. *Neurology* 1989;39:1183–6.

48. McGlone J, MacDonald BH. Reliability of the sodium amobarbital test for memory. *J Epilepsy* 1989;2:31–9.

49. DeToledo J, Smith DB, Kramer RE. A proposed cause for the variability of memory lateralization in Amytal suppression (Wada) testing: role of the septal region. *Epilepsia* 1989;30:712 (abstract).

50. Rausch R. Survey on amobarbital testing procedures. Presented at the International Palm Desert Conference on the Surgical Treatment of the Epilepsies, 1992.

51. Loring DW, Meador KJ, Lee GP. Amobarbital dose effects on Wada memory testing. *J Epilepsy* 1992:5;171–4.

52. Jack CR Jr, Nichols DA, Sharbrough FW, Marsh WR, Petersen RC. Selective posterior cerebral artery Amytal test for evaluating memory function before surgery for temporal lobe seizure. *Radiology* 1988;168:787–93.

53. Engel J, Rausch R, Lieb JP, et al. Correlation of criteria used for localizing epileptic foci in patients considered for surgical therapy of epilepsy. *Ann Neurol* 1981;9:215–24.

54. Wyllie E, Naugle R, Chelune G, et al. Intracarotid amobarbital procedure: II. Lateralizing value in evaluation for temporal lobectomy. *Epilepsia* 1991; 32:865–9.

55. Dinner DS, Lüders H, Morris HH, et al. Validity of intracarotid sodium amobarbital (Wada test) for evaluation of memory function. *Neurology* 1987;37(Suppl 1):142 (abstract).

56. Teasdale G, Jennett B. Assessment of coma and impaired consciousness: a practical scale. *Lancet* 1974; 2:81–4.

57. Satz P, Fletcher JM. *Florida Kindergarten Screening Battery.* Odessa, FL: Psychological Assessment Resources, 1987.

Chapter 11

Neuroimaging in Evaluation of Patients for Surgery

WILLIAM H. THEODORE

There is a subtle but significant difference in the aim of neuroimaging in the evaluation of patients with partial as opposed to generalized seizures for possible surgery. In the former case, one assumes that a focus is likely to exist. The task is to identify it and, if possible, to eliminate the need for depth or subdural electrodes as part of the presurgical work-up. When patients have generalized seizures, on the other hand, imaging tests are performed as part of a fishing expedition to evaluate the possibility of surgery. This dichotomy should suggest that, when patients have partial seizures, study would be pursued more aggressively and the chance of gaining useful information from a procedure is high. But patients with seizure types not commonly thought of as being "localization-related" are increasingly subjected to complex procedures such as positron emission tomography (PET). Although perhaps paradoxical from an intellectual standpoint, this trend is not surprising, considering general tastes in American medicine. The risks involved are low enough that even if only a small amount of additional localizing information is obtained, and a few additional patients are thus afforded seizure relief through surgery, increased use of neuroimaging is certainly medically appropriate.

Earlier Imaging Techniques

The role of neuroimaging, which until recently had little application in epilepsy, in localizing epileptic foci has been enhanced dramatically by the availability of new techniques. Although pneumoencephalography (PEG) was used routinely in the evaluation of patients with seizures, results varied widely, and correlation between PEG and electroencephalographic (EEG) data was poor: ventricular dilatation was found contralateral to the EEG focus in up to 25% of patients [1].

Conventional radionuclide brain scans rarely detect epileptic foci unless a lesion such as a tumor or arteriovenous malformation (AVM) disrupts the blood-brain barrier. Computed tomography (CT) and magnetic resonance imaging (MRI) are abnormal in nearly all patients with seizures due to AVM; angiography is necessary only for performing Wada tests and planning invasive electrode implantation or the surgical approach itself [2–4]. Regions of focal hypoperfusion were reported on scans using ^{133}Xe and a variety of early detector systems, but poor resolution, the complexity of the equipment, and failure to obtain consistent results limited the clinical application of this technique.

Structural Imaging

MRI has proven to be a very valuable method for evaluation of patients for surgery. However, its yield is sensitive to details of technique. Proper choice of pulse sequences is essential. Neurologists should work closely with radiologists to review the protocols used for patient evaluation. T2-weighted sequences (e.g., TE 120, TR 3300, or TE 80, TR 2500) are most sensitive to the focal gliosis, low-grade tumors, and small hamartomas or AVMs seen in patients with seizures [5–7] (see Fig. 11-1). Abnormal regions of signal intensity appearing at TE 70 may not be detected at TE 35 [8]. Sections 5 to 7 mm rather than 10 mm thick also increase sensitivity [9]. Epileptogenic

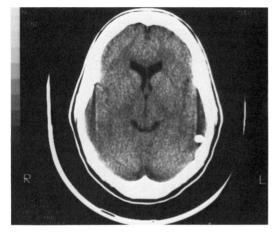

A

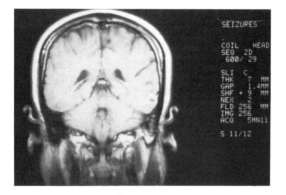

B

C

Figure 11-1. (A–C) Complex partial seizures: left temporal EEG focus. Technical factors make interpretation of location on CT (A) more difficult, but the pathologic nature of the lesion (a calcified "brain stone" without specific tissue identification) is more accurately reflected by CT (A) and T2-weighted MRI (C) than by T1-weighted MRI (B). The 1.5-Tesla MRI scan (C), although showing better anatomic detail, did not add information to the tissue diagnosis.

lesions may not be detected more readily at higher field strengths; T2-weighted studies performed at 1.5 Tesla (T) have not in general shown improved results [7,9–12]. Artifacts due to cerebrospinal fluid (CSF) flow become more prominent at high field strengths and in heavily T2-weighted images, and may cause confusion with regions of focal gliosis. However, the CSF artifacts share signal characteristics of ventricular CSF and overlap the temporal horns as shown on CT or T1-weighted sequences. Coronal images should provide more precise anatomic localization of regions of increased signal intensity and help exclude pulsation artifacts from flowing blood, since the blood vessel will be cut at 90 degrees to the transverse scan plane [5–9]. Cardiac gating can also be used to reduce such artifacts.

Enhancement with a paramagnetic contrast agent, Gd-DTPA, usually is performed on T1-weighted scans. Several studies have shown that Gd-DTPA does not aid in the detection of abnormalities when the unenhanced MRI scan is normal but may improve delineation of the structure and extent of mass lesions [13–14].

Attempts to perform quantitative imaging have been made in patients with complex partial seizures (CPS). Grant et al. found T1 13% and T2 14% higher in mesial temporal sclerosis and suggested that this technique might be more sensitive than conventional MRI [15]. In some patients the only abnormality is a small temporal lobe on the side of the lesion [7,12,16].

MRI temporal lobe volume measurements using thin sections and T1-weighted sequences, preferably at 1.5 T field strength, have proved to be a more sensitive and specific approach to quantitation in patients who are candidates for surgery [17,18]. Patients with reduced hippocampal volume ipsilateral to the resected temporal lobe were significantly more likely to have a good outcome [19]. This finding may be related to the hypometabolism and decreased perfusion seen on functional imaging tests (see below).

Both T2-weighted MRI for detection of increased signal and T1-weighted volumetry appear to be able to detect mesial temporal sclerosis and to be correlated with good outcome after temporal lobectomy

[19,20]. There is probably a close association between the two findings [20].

Not all lesions detected on MRI in patients with seizures may be of pathophysiologic significance. Regions of increased signal intensity on 5-mm T2-weighted scans have been reported in frontoparietal and periventricular white matter of patients with CPS [9,21]. Comparable CT findings are more common in patients with seizures beginning after the age of 50 years and have been interpreted as consistent with stroke [22]. However, similar abnormalities have been found in normal volunteers, especially in the elderly [23].

Although MRI has replaced CT as the primary neuroimaging test performed for initial evaluation of seizures, patients considered for surgery should have both tests performed. CT can offer valuable data in ascertaining the pathologic nature of epileptic lesions.

CT is helpful in evaluating the presence and degree of contrast enhancement in lesions that may be small tumors or AVMs or that contain calcium. The small additional risk of routine contrast administration is worth the information that can be obtained in most cases. Seizures, including status epilepticus, have been precipitated in patients with tumors given water-soluble contrast agents for CT [24]. The risk may be reduced by premedication with 5 mg of diazepam just before the procedure [25].

Quantitative CT approaches, combined with metrizamide infusion and thin (3-mm) sections, may help detect low-grade gliomas, temporal gliosis, and minimal degrees of uncal "herniation" [26–30]. These techniques have been largely superseded by MRI.

The relative yield of MRI and CT scanning depends on the patient population as well as on technical factors. From 20–70% of patients with normal CT scans have been reported to have focal regions of increased signal intensity on MRI scans, and a larger number have "atrophy" of one temporal lobe [5–11,31,32]. However, bilateral or multiple abnormalities may occur in some patients. Unless correlated with clinical and electrographic data, MRI findings by themselves do not identify seizure foci or account for the presence of epilepsy.

Patients with tumors, vascular malformations, or more intense gliosis are more likely to have abnormal CT or MRI [7,33] (see Fig. 11-2). Early reports suggested that MRI did not detect mesial temporal sclerosis, but more recent studies have shown increased signal intensity in about 30–50% of these patients [5,7,8,12]. Unfortunately, MRI findings may be nonspecific and may not distinguish between tumor and focal gliosis [7,33,34] (see Fig. 11-3). However, when both MRI and CT are normal, tumors may be less likely [5,7]. Patients with uncontrolled simple partial seizures (SPS) (more often extratemporal in origin than CPS) and with shorter seizure histories may be more likely to have tumors [35,36].

Even when a tumor or other space-occupying lesion is present, EEG findings may not always be localized to the region of the mass [4,31,35]. Sammaritano et al. reported that surface EEG recording falsely localized seizure onset to the hemisphere contralateral to a structural lesion in three patients, perhaps because epileptiform discharge amplitude on the side of the lesion itself was very low [37]. Depth electrode study was more reliable, all three patients showed seizure origin in the mesial temporal lobe ipsilateral to the radiographic findings, and the patients were seizure-free after surgery [37]. On the other hand, some investigators have suggested that

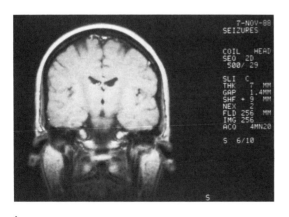

A

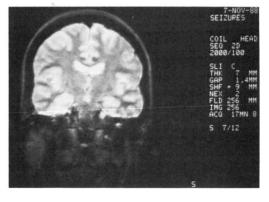

B

Figure 11-2. (*A* and *B*) Complex partial seizures: right temporal EEG focus. In the right mesial temporal region a small region of increased signal is seen on the T2-weighted scan, and decreased signal is seen on the T1-weighted scan. PET showed right temporal hypometabolism. A small ganglioglioma was present.

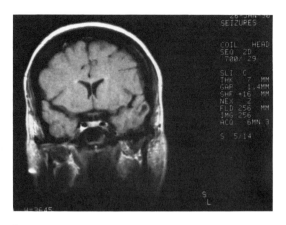
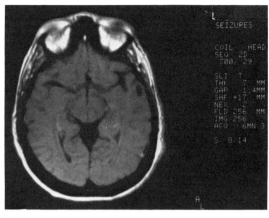

A

B

Figure 11-3. (*A* and *B*) Complex partial seizures: left temporal EEG focus. There is a region of decreased signal on the T1-weighted scan (also present on the T2-weighted scan [not shown]) that did not enhance with gadolinium and was consistent with prior history of trauma.

even when a mass is present, surgery should be based on EEG localization, and a nonprogressive lesion need not always be resected in patients operated on for uncontrolled seizures [38]. Fortunately, EEG and neuroimaging localization usually agree [5,7,33]. Nevertheless, it is clear that, even in patients with tumors, additional localizing data are needed for planning resections. It is important to perform surgery for seizure control as well as for tumor removal.

CT- and MRI-guided stereotaxic biopsies have been used to identify low-density lesions in patients presenting with seizures when tumors were suspected [39]. These data may help to plan a resection, especially when extratemporal surgery is being considered. MRI has been used as well for computer-assisted stereotaxic amygdalohippocampectomy for patients with posterior temporal EEG foci and seizures localized to mediobasolimbic structures [40]. Preliminary evidence suggests that the presence of increased magnetic resonance (MR) signal is not by itself correlated with good surgical results in patients with focal temporal gliosis [12].

Transient regional CT contrast enhancement or attenuation, as well as increased MR signal intensity, has been reported after seizure clusters or status epilepticus [41,42]. These tend to be larger than the foci of increased temporal signal on T2-weighted scans associated with focal gliosis or small tumors, but show no mass effect. They are more prominent in white than in gray matter and probably represent cerebral edema, but they may be mistaken for tumors, showing, on angiography, a capillary blush and early draining veins [41].

Cerebral Metabolism and Blood Flow in Partial Seizures

Positron Emission Tomography

Interictal studies

Positron emission tomography (PET) has become a routine part of preoperative evaluation at the centers where it is available. Using PET, interictal hypometabolism or reduced blood flow is found in 70–80% of patients with CPS [43–48] (see Fig. 11-4). Engel et al., in an early series, found 18 of 50 patients had unilateral temporal, six temporofrontal, three occipital, two frontal, two hemispheric, and four bilateral temporal hypometabolism [43]. Only eight of the patients had abnormal CT scans. Twenty-five patients had surgery; 19 of 22 with PET hypometabolism had a focal lesion [49]. The degree of PET hypometabolism was related to the severity of neuronal loss, but hypometabolic regions were larger than the area of pathologic abnormality. Three patients with normal scans had no pathologic findings [49]. Not all studies have suggested that hypometabolism is related to the degree of underlying gliosis [33,50]. Instead, PET hypometabolism could be due to reduced synaptic activity in projection areas of nonfunctioning inhibitory neurons [51]. Quantitative analysis of hippocampal cell loss, however, has shown that at least EEG seizure foci are associated with the region of maximal hippocampal sclerosis [52,53]. It is important to keep in mind the differences in resolution and technique between MRI and PET when attempting to interpret

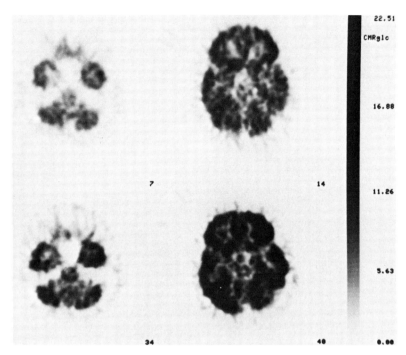

Figure 11-4. Interictal FDG-PET scan in a patient with complex partial seizures and left temporal EEG discharges. Left mesial temporal hypometabolism is present on the two lower cuts (7 and 34) but not on the higher slices (14 and 40).

the relation of the images. For example, the apparently wider extent of the hypometabolism seen on PET compared with the structural lesion seen on MRI may be due to the lower resolution of the functional imaging technique.

Interictal fluorodeoxyglucose PET appears to show abnormalities in more patients than either MRI or CT. Abou-Khalil et al. reported abnormal CT findings in only two, abnormal MRI findings in 10, and abnormal PET findings in 25 of 28 patients with CPS [48]. We saw abnormal PET findings in 21, abnormal MRI findings in eight, and abnormal CT findings in three of 26 patients [33]. Most reports agree that MRI is more sensitive for detection of lesions such as glioma and hamartoma, but PET is superior for

detecting focal gliosis [5,33,48,54]. Unfortunately, however, neither PET nor MRI can distinguish between low-grade tumors and focal gliosis (Tables 11-1 and 11-2).

Most studies have reported a good correlation between temporal lobe hypometabolism and EEG discharges [33,43–48]. Diffuse discharges are likely to be associated with nonfocal PET scans and focal EEG spikes with focal PET scans [48]. A significant proportion of patients with CPS, however, have frontal hypometabolism as well [48,55]. Moreover, well-localized hypometabolism may be frequent in patients with extratemporal EEG foci [55,56]. In a study of 22 patients with electroclinical features suggesting frontal lobe epilepsy, CT was abnormal in 32%, MRI

Table 11-1. Comparison of CT, PET, and MRI for Localization of Epileptic Foci

| | Studies with Pathologic Confirmation (% Abnormal) | | | | | |
| | CT | | MRI | | PET | |
Reference	Gliosis	Mass	Gliosis	Mass	Gliosis	Mass
Sperling et al. [5] (*n* = 21)	Excluded		0*	100	83	(0/1)
Ormson et al. [34] (*n* = 25)	0	60	0*	83		
Lesser et al. [11] (*n* = 11)	0	1/1	27	1/1		
Kuzniecky et al. [7] (*n* = 48)	0	66	80	100		
Theodore et al. [33] (*n* = 26)	5	66	22	100	83	66

*Related to techniques used.

Table 11-2. Comparison of CT, PET, and MRI for Localization of Epileptic Foci

| Reference | Studies without Pathologic Confirmation (% Abnormal) | | |
	CT	MRI	PET
McLachlon et al. [10] ($n = 16$)	44	75	
Latock et al.* [31] ($n = 50$)	26	46	
Abou-Khalil et al.* [48] ($n = 31$)	Excluded	36	81
Shorner et al. [8] ($n = 50$)	26	40	
Jabbari et al. [32] ($n = 30$)	33	43	
Swartz et al. [57] ($n = 22$; "frontal")	32	45	64

*These two studies included some of the same patients.

in 45%, and FDG PET in 64% [57]. The hypometabolic zones, although encompassing the region of probable seizure onset, tended to be regional or hemispheric. Engel et al. reported that when scalp-sphenoidal and PET localization agree, depth electrode studies did not provide additional information, and surgery could be performed on the basis of noninvasive data [58]. In a blinded prospective study, Theodore et al. found a significant association between PET hypometabolism and surgical outcome; all patients with an asymmetry of more than 25% were seizure-free after temporal lobectomy [59].

Several groups have detected thalamic and parietal hypometabolism in about 30% of patients ipsilateral to temporal EEG foci [60–62]. Patients with structural lesions in particular may have widespread associated metabolic deficits not necessarily predictable by their radiographic features [63]. Extension of hypometabolism to regions beyond the temporal lobe may depend on many factors, including the degree and extent of epileptiform discharges, underlying cerebral pathology, and the effect of antiepileptic drugs. Technical aspects of PET analysis such as employment of large regions of interest (ROIs), which increases the partial volume effect, and failure to exclude patients with tumors or abnormal CT may explain identification of extensive hypometabolic zones [46].

Interictal Cerebral Blood Flow and Oxygen Metabolism

Oxygen-15 (^{15}O) inhalation or ^{15}O-labeled water and PET have been used to study cerebral blood flow (CBF) and oxygen metabolism ($CMRO_2$) in patients with partial seizures. Several investigators found that CBF or $CMRO_2$ showed reductions comparable to FDG metabolism in epileptic foci [45,64,65]. Bernardi et al. reported more widespread reduction of $CMRO_2$ in 10 patients ipsilateral to temporal EEG foci, including temporal and frontal lobes, basal ganglia, and cerebellum, and reduced CBF in temporal lobes, basal ganglia, and cerebellum [66]. Contralateral temporal and cerebellar CBF and $CMRO_2$ were depressed as well. When CBF and FDG scans are compared in the same patient, generally similar patterns of abnormality are found. The zones of hypoperfusion are often less prominent and more diffuse than the hypometabolic regions, however, suggesting that interictal CBF measurements may be less valuable for surgical planning than FDG scans [45,65]. In patients who had both FDG and ^{15}O-labeled water PET studies before temporal lobectomy, focal hypometabolism but not reduced blood flow was correlated significantly with EEG lateralization and a good outcome [67].

No standardized methods of PET analysis exist. While some groups have taken a more or less purely "visual" approach, reading the PET pictures like x-ray films or nuclear brain scans, others have attempted to retrieve physiologic information in quantitative or quasiquantitative form. Widespread cerebral dysfunction may be a contraindication to surgery; with purely visual analysis, it may be more difficult to identify bilateral temporal or diffuse hypometabolism. However, qualitative PET analysis may be difficult to apply clinically. The normal variability in cerebral metabolic rate for glucose (CMRglc) and CBF is wide, and regions identified visually as hypometabolic often have absolute values within the normal range. "Asymmetry indices" (AI) can be used to compare side-to-side variation in patients and normal controls [40,48,63,68]. Using this approach, blood sampling is not needed. Although much information is lost, it may be appropriate for purely clinical PET applications, if any exist. Good agreement between quantitative and qualitative interpretation is usually found, but AIs may occasionally fail to show a significant difference from controls in qualitatively identified hypometabolic regions because of the normal range of side-to-side asymmetry [68]. The size and variability of the control population and the analytical method, such as the size and shape of the ROIs within which metabolic rates are measured, may affect the results.

Structural asymmetries in normal temporal lobes may be important for assessment of PET abnormalities. Several groups of investigators have attempted to map the anatomic information from MRI onto PET images in order to define the regions within which CMRglc or CBF will be measured. Two methods have the potential to include EEG data in the same reference system. One uses a common stereotaxic frame compatible with MRI, PET, and depth electrodes to obtain data [69]. The other performs a retrospective computer-based alignment of the data based on external head contour [70].

Ictal Studies

Ictal PET scans show increased metabolism and blood flow at foci of interictal hypometabolism [44,71–73]. Metabolic activation may spread beyond the region of the interictal abnormality, presumably depending on the extent and direction of seizure propagation. However, estimates of glucose metabolism, oxygen consumption, and blood flow are more difficult to make during seizures.

Clinical as well as theoretical issues affect accurate measurement of CMRglu during ictal PET scans. A seizure is usually a short event, compared to the 30- to 45-min FDG uptake period. "Ictal" scans include interictal, ictal, and postictal data, weighted in favor of events occurring soon after injection of the isotope. Combinations of hypo- and hypermetabolic regions, due to the influence of postictal depression and ictal activation, have been reported [44,71]. The lumped constant, which expresses the relation between deoxyglucose and glucose utilization, may change when the model assumption of steady-state glucose metabolism is violated.

$CMRO_2$ methods that require continuous or even bolus inhalation are obviously difficult to perform during seizures. Injection of ^{15}O-labeled water is a more practical approach, but even this technique underestimates flow at high values because of the progressive decrease in the fraction of water extracted from the blood by the brain [74]. Most ictal PET scans have been fortuitous, but attempts have been made to provoke seizures during CBF studies using pentylenetetrazole. Although the region of the EEG focus showed the greatest increase in blood flow, the method may not be specific enough to use for surgical localization [75].

Ictal metabolic alterations and increased CBF usually resolve within 30 min after a CPS [75] (Fig. 11-5). Elevated CBF and $CMRO_2$ have been reported to persist for up to a week after a seizure; the patients may have been having more frequent seizures than were detected clinically [73].

Single Photon Emission Computed Tomography

Single photon emission computed tomography (SPECT) is cheaper, easier to perform, and more widely available than PET. Stable, commercially available isotopes can be used, eliminating the need for an on-site or nearby cyclotron. Standard nuclear medicine cameras can produce the images, although higher resolution is obtained with specially designed SPECT equipment. SPECT has been treated as a routine nuclear medicine procedure, and the absence of the ritual surrounding PET has advantages and disadvantages. The main danger with SPECT is perhaps the tendency to take images at their face value. Moreover, the variety of imaging systems and tracers that have been used, including ^{123}I-MP, ^{123}I-HIPDM, ^{133}Xe, and ^{99m}Tc-HMPAO, makes the SPECT literature more difficult to evaluate [76–82].

SPECT detects interictal regions of hypoperfusion in about 50–60% of patients with CPS [76,77,81]. Increased interictal flow has been reported as well [83]. Quantitation is difficult to perform with current SPECT methods. The lower resolution, compared to PET, of most SPECT systems increases the partial volume effect and makes identification of focal defects in CBF more difficult. Within the past few years more centers have begun to perform SPECT than PET imaging, and data on its clinical utility should be obtained rapidly. "False localization" (the SPECT blood flow abnormality was not in the same region as the EEG focus) has been reported in 17–25% of patients [82,84].

Ictal SPECT scans can be performed much more readily than PET since longer-lived tracers are employed that may be held ready at a patient's bedside for immediate administration when a seizure occurs. Rowe et al. injected ^{99m}Tc-HMPAO an average of 6 min after CPS onset [81]. The combination of ictal and interictal data correctly identified epileptic foci, as judged by EEG, in 72% of patients. Lee, et al. and Shen, et al. reported that increased ictal flow agreed with EEG localization in 90% of their patients, using either HMPAO or ^{123}I-IMP [77,85].

Several studies have now compared SPECT and PET. Stefan et al. used FDG-PET and ^{99m}Tc-HMPAO SPECT in 10 patients with complex partial seizures who may have been selected for positive PET scans [78]. All had focal PET abnormalities, eight had abnormal MRI findings, five had abnormal SPECT findings, and three had abnormal CT lesions. One patient had decreased blood flow on SPECT in a region contralateral to abnormalities detected by CT, MRI, PET, and EEG.

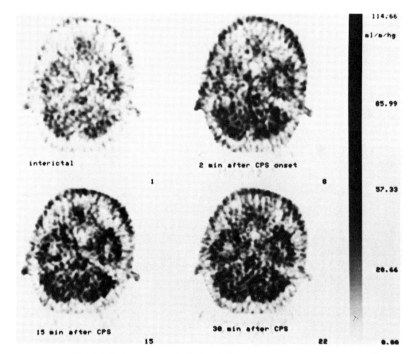

Figure 11-5. ^{15}O-labeled water cerebral blood flow scan in a patient with complex partial seizures and right temporal EEG focus. Interictal scan does not show obvious asymmetry. Injection 2 min after CPS onset shows increased right temporal flow, which becomes bilateral by 15 min and is persistent at 30 min. Note that cerebellar flow appears increased as well.

Data comparing ^{123}I-IMP SPECT and FDG were collected at the National Institutes of Health Clinical Center and Walter Reed Army Medical Center. Eight of 12 patients had a hypometabolic region on interictal PET, two showed hypoperfusion on interictal SPECT, and two additional patients had increased CBF during an ictal SPECT scan. MRI was abnormal in four patients. There was good localization agreement among EEG, MRI, SPECT, and PET; six patients had surgery (PET was abnormal in 5, SPECT and MRI were abnormal in 3), with good results (see Table 11-3). Ryvlin et al. found that PET was superior to SPECT in patients with normal MRI but not in those with abnormal MRI [86].

In all of these studies, the localization provided by PET was superior, even when blood flow abnormalities were detected. Newer imaging systems with higher resolution will increase the attractiveness of SPECT, which will inevitably be used more widely than PET, whatever the relative merits of the two technologies.

Xenon-Enhanced CT

Xenon-enhanced CT detected decreased blood flow in a region corresponding to the EEG focus in six of 12 patients with CPS [87]. Flow reduction was greater in lateral than in medial temporal regions, but distortion induced by movement artifact impaired resolution of mesial temporal structures. Regions of interest were defined on routine CT images. Four of five patients with CPS had a greater than 30% side-to-side asymmetry (lower on the side of the EEG

Table 11-3. Comparison of CT, MRI, PET, and SPECT for Localization of Epileptic Foci

Reference	CT	MRI	SPECT	PET
Stefan et al. ($n = 10$)	3	8	5(1 contralateral)	10
Theodore et al. ($n = 12$)	0	4	4(2 ictal)	8
Ryvlin et al.				
Normal MRI [10]			2	8
Abnormal MRI [10]			10	9

focus) in xenon-enhanced CT flow estimation, compared to a mean of 7.5% in normal volunteers [88].

Neuropsychological Activation

Hypometabolic regions on PET (or hypoperfused on SPECT) in patients with CPS may represent regions of nonepileptic cerebral dysfunction. There is a correlation between right and left metabolic rate asymmetry and performance on neuropsychological tasks [89]. Inferior left temporal hypometabolism was accentuated during a phoneme-monitoring task in patients with left temporal EEG foci [90]. PET performed during memory- and language-specific activation tasks might replace the Wada test for assessing hemispheric dominance [91].

Significant CMRglc increases have been reported only contralateral to the stimulated side in some studies but bilaterally in others [92,93]. Patterns of activation and involvement of extratemporal regions such as frontal and parietal cortex depend on the stimulus presentation paradigm and type of material used, such as understandable or incomprehensible (e.g., foreign language) speech. Spontaneous speech by the subject during PET has been reported to lead to widespread metabolic activation and, in epileptics, to increased definition of temporal lobe foci. The latter failed to show normal functional increases at the site of the "epileptic focus" and had greater relative hypometabolism than on the resting scan [94]. The demonstration of localized cerebral dysfunction in a patient with seizures, even if not in the same region as the EEG focus, may still be important for surgical planning.

Functional activation studies performed with ^{15}O-labeled water have a much shorter time resolution and the capacity to measure the effect of transient functional activation. These studies may be able to detect regions of relative dysfunction and to supplement, or eventually even to replace, procedures such as the Wada test and subdural electrode implantation for presurgical evaluation. MRI anatomic correlation is crucial for the proper use of these PET procedures [95].

"Nonfocal" Epilepsy

Although CT abnormalities, including agenesis of the corpus callosum, infarctions, and arachnoid and porencephalic cysts, have been reported in up to 80–90% of some series of patients with infantile spasms, diffuse atrophy and ventricular enlargement are the most common findings, and little evidence of

localized seizure onset is obtained (Fig. 11-6). Patients with a normal CT are more likely to have normal neurologic examinations and to be seizure-free at follow-up [96]. In a small group of patients with infantile spasms, however, whose MRI scans showed either diffuse atrophy or were normal, FDG-PET studies revealed focal hypometabolism [97]. Electrocorticography (ECoG) confirmed localization of the epileptic foci, and early results of resection are promising in three of the patients. SPECT using ^{133}Xe revealed focal hypoperfusion in 11 of 15 patients with infantile spasms and normal CT, which were felt to correlate with patterns of neuropsychological dysfunction, but none of the patients in this study has had surgery as yet [98]. These results suggest that there may be a subgroup of patients with infantile spasms due to focal cerebral dysfunction and who may be surgical candidates.

In patients with Rasmussen's encephalitis, CT or MRI studies are frequently abnormal. Regions of increased MR signal intensity may fluctuate with clinical evolution. SPECT showed hypoperfusion more extensive than structural lesions in five patients, which increased in size on repeat scans [99]. Extensive but unilateral hypometabolism has been found on FDG-PET scans in some patients with Rasmussen's encephalitis, providing physiologic support for hemispherectomy. Patients with refractory neonatal seizures and infantile hemiplegia, who had normal or nonfocal structural imaging studies, have been shown to have regions of focal dysfunction on PET; preliminary results of excision of these regions are promising [100].

Cerebral atrophy has been reported to occur in up to 70% of patients with Lennox-Gastaut Syndrome (LGS) but focal changes occur in only one third [101]. The variety of radiologic findings, including tuberous sclerosis, agenesis of the corpus callosum, infarctions, and arachnoid and porencephalic cysts, in patients with the stereotyped EEG and clinical features of LGS suggest that the lesions seen on CT may not be directly responsible for the clinical problems. The incidence of scans showing cerebral atrophy increases with age. Atrophy might be a consequence of the seizures, rather than being related to their cause [96].

Interictal FDG metabolic abnormalities reported in LGS include unilateral focal, bilateral multifocal, and diffuse hypometabolism [102,103]. The hypometabolic regions in some but not all of the patients were related to structural abnormalities. However, PET hypometabolism or SPECT hypoperfusion in patients with tuberous sclerosis or similar lesions is often more extensive than detected by CT or MRI [63,104]. Frontal and diffuse hypometabolism has

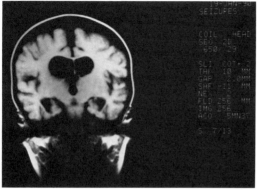

A

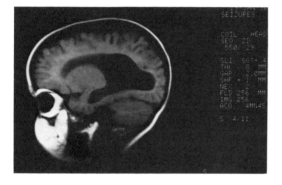

B

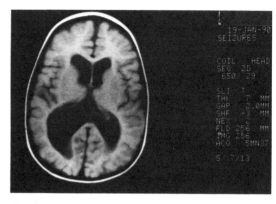

C

Figure 11-6. An 18-month-old child with atonic and myoclonic seizures with no obvious etiology. MRI shows diffuse ventricular enlargement.

been found in patients without abnormalities on CT [103].

Selected patients with LGS may benefit from section of the corpus callosum. Spencer et al. reported that focal, but not hemispheric, CT lesions were associated with a favorable outcome [105]. CPS increased postoperatively in some patients. In another small group of patients, the presence of a focal lesion on MRI predicted poor results [106]. Bladin et al. found 10 adults with LGS who had large, but nonprogressive, focal structural lesions [107]. Depth electrode studies suggested that seizure onset correlated with lesion location in four of these patients, but none improved after focal resection. Gur et al. [108] reported profound unilateral temporal hypometabolism in two patients with LGS. The hypometabolism resolved after clinically successful section of the corpus callosum (1 case), but persisted if the procedure was unsuccessful. The two patients in the study by Gur et al. had partial seizures, however, and the exact classification of their epilepsy was uncertain. The role of neuroimaging in selection of patients with LGS for surgery needs further study.

The Role of Neuroimaging in the Evaluation of Patients for Surgery

Although EEG, PET, SPECT, and MRI provide different information, some may be redundant, and it is unlikely that all these studies need to be performed to localize epileptic foci accurately. Detection of an interictal imaging abnormality is neither necessary nor sufficient for resection of an epileptic focus. Identification of ictal hyperperfusion or metabolism in the same region as interictal hypoperfusion or metabolism does strongly suggest the presence of an epileptic focus, however (Table 11-4).

Engel et al. [109] found that patients with and without focal hypometabolism were equally likely to improve after temporal lobectomy. All the patients had well-defined EEG localization. Detection of mesial temporal sclerosis or focal gliosis on routine pathologic examination of temporal lobe tissue specimens was not, in their study, associated with a favorable outcome. In contrast, Falconer et al. [110] reported that patients with these findings were more likely to be improved by surgery. Engel suggested that

Table 11-4. Comparison of MRI, PET, and SPECT in the Evaluation of Epileptic Foci

	MRI	PET	SPECT
Modality	Structure	Metabolism, flow	Flow
Resolution	2 mm	6 mm	10 mm
Complexity	Routine	High	Moderate
Ictal studies		Fortuitous	Reasonable
Quantitation	Experimental	Reasonable	Problematic
Risk	Gadolinium	Radiation	Radiation
		Arterial·line	
Sensitivity	30–50%	70–80%	50–70% (?)
Specificity	High	High	Unknown

degrees of cell loss too mild to be detected by routine pathologic or neuroimaging techniques could still be epileptogenic [109]. Other investigators have reported that the presence of focal PET hypometabolism was predictive of good surgical outcome [59,111]. In the study by Gur et al., patients with well-localized focal surface EEG spikes were more likely to have focal PET hypometabolism than those who needed subdural electrode placement.

Nevertheless, sufficient data exist to suggest that patients with uncontrolled seizures of presumed focal origin who are candidates for epilepsy surgery may benefit from interictal FDG-PET scans as well as from MRI. PET must be placed in the context of the range of tests used to evaluate patients for possible surgery, including neurologic examination; routine EEG, MRI, and CT; neuropsychological tests; intensive video/EEG monitoring; and invasive studies.

The detection of unilateral temporal hypometabolism ipsilateral to the EEG focus appears to be highly specific and is a valuable confirmatory procedure for the location of the seizure focus. A small region of increased MRI signal intensity ipsilateral to the EEG focus also appears to confirm its location; unfortunately, MRI does not reliably identify the underlying pathology. The yield of PET is higher than that of MRI. Interictal focal hypometabolism is present in a smaller proportion of patients with CPS of extratemporal origin, and its reliability in localizing seizure foci is less certain. In conjunction with neuropsychological tests, PET may help to assess possible adverse cognitive effects of surgery by revealing the presence of bilateral or multifocal hypometabolism. The presence of widespread PET hypometabolism in a patient with apparently well-localized EEG discharges suggests more diffuse cerebral dysfunction and may reduce the chance of surgical success. MRI may show severe structural abnormalities, which usually are associated with diffuse EEG discharges in patients without well-localized seizures. The correlation between CBF abnormalities, as measured by ^{15}O-PET, SPECT, or xenon-CT, and epileptic foci must still be regarded as under investigation.

Most patients who have had PET or SPECT scans have had uncontrolled seizures, and thus the influence of focal dysfunction on seizure prognosis is uncertain. Further studies will be needed to evaluate whether these tests can be used to select patients who are unlikely to respond to antiepileptic drugs and should be considered for surgery. Denays et al. reported that children with normal SPECT scans were more likely to have infrequent seizures and normal neuropsychological function than those who had hypoperfused regions [104].

Although it is not yet established that focal PET hypometabolism is a valid indication for surgery in a patient whose seizure origin is nonlocalized by surface EEG, the PET findings will help to plan invasive electrode evaluation. Preliminary studies indicate that a proportion of children with uncontrolled neonatal seizures and infantile spasms may have focal PET hypometabolism even when all other studies are nonlocalizing, thus allowing surgery to be performed in a group of patients for whom no other effective therapy exists.

Uncontrolled epilepsy is an important medical and social problem. PET contributes to its solution by increasing the number of patients who can be treated surgically, helping to plan the surgical approach in a safer and more cost-effective manner and, in some cases, suggesting that surgery might not be an appropriate therapy.

References

1. Theodore WH. Neuroimaging. In: Porter RJ, Theodore WH, eds. Epilepsy. *Neurol Clin* 1986;4:645–68.
2. Leblanc R, Feindel W, Ethier R. Epilepsy from cerebral arteriovenous malformations. *Can J Neurol Sci* 1983;10:91–5.

3. Gomori JM, Grossman RI, Goldberg HI, Hackney DB, Zimmerman RA, Bilaniuk LT. Occult cerebrovascular malformations: high field MR imaging. *Radiology* 1986;158:707–13.

4. Kucharczyk W, Lemme-Pleghos L, Uske A, Brant-Zawadzki M, Dooms G, Norman D. Intracranial vascular malformations: MR and CT imaging. *Radiology* 1985;156:383–9.

5. Sperling MR, Wilson G, Engel J Jr, Babb TW, Phelps M, Bradley W. Magnetic resonance imaging in intractable partial epilepsy: correlative studies. *Ann Neurol* 1986;20:57–62.

6. Theodore WH, Dorwart R, Holmes M, et al. Neuroimaging in refractory partial seizures: comparison of PET, CT, and MRI. *Neurology* 1986; 36:750–9.

7. Kuznicky R, de la Sayette V, Ethier R, Melanson D, Andermann F, Berkovic S, Robitaille Y, Olivier A, Peters T, Feindel W. Magnetic resonance imaging in temporal lobe epilepsy: pathological correlations. *Ann Neurol* 1987;22:341–7.

8. Schorner W, Meencke HJ, Felix R. Temporal lobe epilepsy: comparison of CT and MR imaging. *AJR* 1987;149:1231–9.

9. Triulzi F, Franceschi M, Fazio F, Del Maschio A. Nonrefractory temporal lobe epilepsy: 1.5T MR imaging. *Radiology* 1988;166:181–5.

10. McLachon RS, Nicholson RL, Black S, et al: Nuclear magnetic resonance, a new approach to the investigation of refractory temporal lobe epilepsy. *Epilepsia* 1985;26:555–62.

11. Lesser RP, Modic MT, Weinstein MW, Duchesneau PM, Lüders H, Dinner D, Morris HH III, Estes M, Chou S, Hahn J. Magnetic resonance imaging (1.5 Tesla) in patients with intractable focal seizures. *Arch Neurol* 1986;43:367–71.

12. Barbaro MM, Dillon WP, Dowd CF, Bluestone DL, Laxer KD. Magnetic resonance imaging evaluation of patients with pathologically proven mesial temporal sclerosis. *Epilepsia* 1989;30:711.

13. Cascino GD, Hirschorn KA, Jack CR, et al. Gadolinium-DTPA-enhanced magnetic resonance imaging in intractable partial epilepsy. *Neurology* 1989; 39:1115–8.

14. Wheless JW, Figueroa-Artiz RE, Binet EF, et al. Role of gadolinium-EDTA enhanced magnetic resonance imaging in presurgical evaluation for intractable partial epilepsy. *Epilepsia* 1989;30:675.

15. Grant R, Hadley DM, Condon E, Doyle D, Patterson J, Bone I, Galbraith SL, Teasdale GM. Magnetic resonance imaging in the management of resistant focal epilepsy: pathological case report and experience of 12 cases. *J Neurol Neurosurg Psychiatry* 1987; 50:1529–32.

16. Zimmerman RA, Sperling M, Bilaniuk LA, O'Connor M, Hackney DB, Grossman RI, Goldberg HI, Gonatas N. MR imaging findings in patients with mesial temporal sclerosis. *Radiology* 1987;165(Suppl):249.

17. Sharbrough FW, Jack CD, Cascino GR. Presurgical quantitative magnetic resonance based hippocampal volume measurements in patients undergoing tempo-

ral lobectomy for medically intractable seizures. *Epilepsia* 1989;30:675.

18. Jack CR, Gehring DG, Sharbrough FW, Felmlee JP, Forbes G, Hench VS, Zinsmeister AR. Temporal lobe volume measurement from MR images: accuracy and left-right asymmetry in normal persons. *J Comput Assist Tomogr* 1988;12:21–9.

19. Jack CR, Sharbrough FW, Cascino GD, Hirschorn KA, O'Brien PC, Marsh WR. Magnetic resonance image-based hippocampal volumetry: correlation with outcome after temporal lobectomy. *Ann Neurol* 1992; 31:138–46.

20. Berkovic SF, Andermann F, Olivier A, Ethier R, Melanson D, Robitaille Y, Kuzniecky R, Peters P, Feindel W. Hippocampal sclerosis in temporal lobe epilepsy demonstrated by magnetic resonance imaging. *Ann Neurol* 1991;29:175–82.

21. Mauguiere F, Ryvlin P, Froment JC, Revol M, Fischer C. Magnetic resonance imaging in patients with refractory partial seizures and normal computed tomography scan: a study of 100 cases. *Epilepsia* 1989; 30:674.

22. Shorvon SD, Gilliatt RW, Cox TC, et al. Evidence of vascular disease from CT scanning in late-onset epilepsy. *J Neurol Neurosurg Psychiatry* 1984;47:225–30.

23. Hunt AL, Orrison WW, Yeo RA, et al. Clinical significance of MRI white matter lesions in the elderly. *Neurology* 1989;39:1470–4.

24. Avrahami E, Weiss-Peretz J, Cohn DF. Focal epileptic activity following intravenous contrast material injection in patients with metastatic brain disease. *J Neurol Neurosurg Psychiatry* 1987;50:221–3.

25. Pagani JJ, Hayman LA, Bigelow RHJ, et al. Prophylactic diazepam in prevention of contrast media associated seizures in glioma patients undergoing cerebral computed tomography. *Cancer* 1984;54:2200–4.

26. Oakley J, Ojemann GA, Ojemann LM, et al. Identifying epileptic foci on contrast enhanced computerized tomographic scans. *Arch Neurol* 1979;36:669–71.

27. Hekster REM, Zapletal BJ, Marticali B. Comparison of CT and conventional neuroradiological procedures in lesions in the proximity of the tentorial hiatus. *Neuroradiology* 1978;6:510–11.

28. Turner DA, Wyler AR. Temporal lobectomy for epilepsy: mesial temporal herniation as an operative and prognostic finding. *Epilepsia* 1981;22:623–9.

29. Bolender NF, Wyler AR. CT measurements of mesial temporal herniation. *Epilepsia* 1982;23:409–16.

30. El Gammal T, Adams RJ, King DW, So E, Gallagher BB. Modified CT techniques in the evaluation of temporal lobe epilepsy prior to lobectomy. *AJNR* 1987;8:131–4.

31. Latock JT, Abou-Khalil BW, Siegal GJ, Sackellares JC, Gabrielson TO, Aisen AM. Patients with partial seizures: evaluation by MR, CT, and PET imaging. *Radiology* 159:159–63, 1986.

32. Jabbari B, Gundersen CH, Wippold F, Citrin C, Sherman JK, Bartoszek D, Daigh JD, Mitchell MH. Magnetic resonance imaging in partial complex epilepsy. *Arch Neurol* 1986;43:869–72.

33. Theodore WH, Katz D, Kufta C, Sato S, Patronas N, Smothers P, Bromfield E. Pathology of temporal lobe foci: correlation with CT, MRI, and PET. *Neurology* 1990;40:797–803.
34. Ormson MJ, Kispert DB, Sharbrough FW, Houser OW, Earnest F, Scheithauer BW, Laws ER. Cryptic structural lesions in refractory partial epilepsy: MR imaging and CT studies. *Radiology* 1986;160:215–9.
35. Spencer DD, Spencer SS, Mattson RH, et al. Intracerebral masses in patients with intractable partial epilepsy. *Neurology* 1984;34:432–6.
36. Angeleri F, Provinciali L, Salvolini U: Computerized tomography in partial epilepsy. In: Canger R, Angeleri F, Penry JK, eds. *Advances in Epileptology*. Eleventh Epilepsy International Symposium. New York: Raven Press, 1980:53–64.
37. Sammaritano M, de Lotbiniere A, Andermann F, Olivier A, Gloor P, Quesney LF. False lateralization by surface EEG of seizure onset in patients with temporal lobe epilepsy and gross focal cerebral lesions. *Ann Neurol* 1987;21:361–9.
38. Wyllie E, Luders H, Morris HH III, et al. Clinical outcome after complete or partial cortical resection for intractable epilepsy. *Neurology* 1987;37:1634–41.
39. Wilden JN, Kelly PJ. Computerized stereotactic biopsy for low density CT lesions presenting with epilepsy. *J Neurol Neurosurg Psychiatry* 50:1302–5.
40. Kelly PJ, Sharbrough FW, Kall BA, Goerss SJ. Magnetic resonance imaging-based computer-assisted stereotactic resection of the hippocampus and amygdala in patients with temporal lobe epilepsy. *Mayo Clin Proc* 1987;62:103–8.
41. Sammaritano M, Anderman FA, Melanson D, et al. Prolonged focal cerebral edema associated with partial status epilepticus. *Epilepsia* 1985;26:334–8.
42. Kramer RE, Luders H, Lesser RP, et al. Transient focal abnormalities of neuroimaging studies during focal status epilepticus. *Epilepsia* 1987;28:528–32.
43. Engel J Jr, Kuhl DE, Phelps ME, et al. Interictal cerebral glucose metabolism in partial epilepsy and its relation to EEG changes. *Ann Neurol* 1982;12:510–7.
44. Theodore WH, Newmark ME, Sato S, et al. 18-F Fluorodeoxyglucose positron emission tomography in refractory complex partial seizures. *Ann Neurol* 1983;14:429–37.
45. Ochs RF, Yamamoto Y, Gloor P, et al. Correlation between the positron emission tomography measurement of glucose metabolism and oxygen utilization with focal epilepsy. *Neurology* 1984;34(Suppl 1):125.
46. Sadzot B, Salmon E, Maquet P, et al. Assessment of the interest of PET and MRI in complex partial seizures. *J Cereb Blood Flow Metab* 1987;7(Suppl 1):432.
47. Franck G, Sadzot B, Salmon E, Depresseux JC, Grisar T, Peters JM, Guillaume M, Quaglia L, Delfiore G, Lamotte D. Regional cerebral blood flow and metabolic rates in human focal epilepsy and status epilepticus. In: Delgado-Escueta AV, Ward AA Jr, Woodbury DM, Porter RJ, eds. *Basic mechanisms of the epilepsies: molecular and cellular approaches*. New York: Raven Press, 1986:935–48.

48. Abou-Khalil BW, Siegel GJ, Sackellares JC, et al. Positron emission tomography studies of cerebral glucose metabolism in chronic partial epilepsy. *Ann Neurol* 1987;22:480–6.
49. Engel J Jr, Brown WJ, Kuhl DE, et al. Pathological findings underlying focal temporal lobe hypometabolism in partial epilepsy. *Ann Neurol* 1982;12:518–29.
50. Henry TR, Engel J Jr, Babbs TE, Phelps ME. Correlation of neuronal cell loss with degree of interictal focal temporal hypometabolism in complex partial epilepsy. *Neurology* 1988;38(Suppl 1):156.
51. Engel J Jr: Metabolic patterns of human epilepsy: clinical observations and possible animal correlates. In: Baldy-Moulinier M, Ingvar DH, Meldrum BS, eds. *Cerebral blood flow, metabolism and epilepsy*. London: John Libby, 1983:6–18.
52. Babb TL, Brown WJ. Pathological findings in epilepsy. In: Engel JP, ed. *Surgical treatment of the epilepsies*. New York: Raven Press, 1987:511–40.
53. Sagar HJ, Oxbury JM. Hippocampal neuron loss in temporal lobe epilepsy: correlation with early childhood convulsions. *Ann Neurol* 1987;22:334–40.
54. Henry TR, Engel J Jr, Sutherling WW, Risinger MR, Phelps ME. Correlation of structural and metabolic imaging with electrographic localization and histopathology in refractory complex partial epilepsy (abstract). *Epilepsia* 1987;28:601.
55. Holmes MD, Kelly K, Theodore WH. Complex partial seizures: correlation of clinical and metabolic features. *Arch Neurol* 1988;45:1191–3.
56. Radke KA, Coleman MW, Hanson TS, et al. Positron emission tomography in extratemporal epilepsy. *Neurology* 1989;39(Suppl 1):301.
57. Swartz BE, Halgren F, Delgado Escueta AV, et al. Neuroimaging in patients with seizures of probable frontal origin. *Epilepsia* 1989;30:547–58.
58. Engel J Jr, Henry TR, Risinger MW, Mazziotta JC, Sutherling WW, Levesque MF, Phelps ME. Presurgical evaluation for partial epilepsy: relative contributions of chronic depth-electrode recordings versus FDG-PET and scalp-sphenoidal ictal EEG. *Neurology* 1990; 40:1670–7.
59. Theodore WH, Sato S, Kufta C, Balish MB, Leiderman DB. Temporal lobectomy for uncontrolled seizures: the role of positron emission tomography. *Ann Neurol,* 1992;32:789–94.
60. Henry TR, Engel J, Phelps ME. Subcortical hypometabolism on interictal PET in complex partial seizures. *Neurology* 1989;39(Suppl 1):299.
61. Balish M, Leiderman DB, Bromfield E, Theodore WH. Subcortical metabolism in partial epilepsy patients as measured by fluorodeoxyglucose positron emission tomography. *Epilepsia* 1989;30:707.
62. Gur RC, Sussman NM, Gur RE, et al. Regional hypometabolism in focal epilepsy: a positron emission tomographic study. *Neurology* 1987;37(Suppl 1)327.
63. Theodore WH, Holmes MD, Dorwart RH, et al. Complex partial seizures: cerebral structure and cerebral function. *Epilepsia* 1986;27:576–82.

64. Franck G, Salmon E, Sadzot B, Maquet P. Epilepsy: the use of oxygen-15-labelled gases. *Semin Neurol* 1989; 9:307–16.

65. Leiderman D, Balish M, Bromfield EB, Sato S, Theodore WH. Comparison of interictal FDG and ^{15}O-H$_2$O PET scanning in patients with uncontrolled complex partial seizures. *Neurology* 1989;39(Suppl 1):301.

66. Bernardi S, Trimble MR, Frackowiak RSJ, et al. An interictal study of partial epilepsy using positron emission tomography and the oxygen-15 inhalation technique. *J Neurol Neurosurg Psychiatry* 1983;46:473–7.

67. Leiderman DB, Balish M, Sato S, Kufta C, Reeves P, Theodore WH. Comparison of PET measurements of cerebral blood flow and glucose metabolism for the localization of human epileptic foci. *Epilepsy Res*, 1992;13:153–8.

68. Theodore WH, Fishbein D, Dubinsky R. Patterns of cerebral glucose metabolism in patients with partial seizures. *Neurology* 1988;38:1201–6.

69. Henry TR, Engel J, Mazziotta JC. PET studies of functional cerebral anatomy in human epilepsy. In: Meldrum BS, Ferrendelli JA, Wieser HG, eds. *Anatomy of Epileptogenesis*. London: John Libby 1988: 155–78.

70. Levin DN, Pelizzari CA, Chen GTY, Chen C-T, Cooper MD. Retrospective geometric correlation of MR, CT, and PET images. *Radiology* 1988;169:817–23.

71. Engel J Jr, Kuhl DE, Phelps ME, et al. Patterns of human local cerebral glucose metabolism during epileptic seizures. *Science* 1982;218:64–6.

72. Engel J Jr, Kuhl DE, Phelps ME, et al. Local cerebral metabolism during partial seizures. *Neurology* 1983;33:404–13.

73. Depresseux JC, Frank G, Sadzot B. Regional cerebral blood flow and oxygen uptake in human focal epilepsy. In: Baldy-Moulinier M, Ingvar DG, Meldrum BS, eds. *Cerebral blood flow, metabolism and epilepsy*. London: John Libby, 1983;76–81.

74. Raichle ME, Martin WRW, Herscovitch P, Mintun MA, Markham J. Brain blood flow measured with intravenous H$_2$S$_O$15: II. Implementation and validation. *J Nucl Med* 1983;24:790–8.

75. Balish M, Leiderman D, Bromfield E, Sato S, Herscovitch P, Theodore WH. The effect of seizures on cerebral blood flow measured with ^{15}O-H$_2$O. *Neurology* 1989;39(Suppl 1):299.

76. Bonte FJ, Devous MD Sr, Stokely EM, et al: Single photon tomographic determination of regional cerebral blood flow in epilepsy. *AJNR* 1983;4:544–6.

77. Lee BI, Markand ON, Siddiqui AR, Park HM, Mock B, Wellman HH, Worth RM, Edwards MK. Single photon emission computed tomography (SPECT) brain imaging using N, N, N′-trimethyl-N′-(2 hydroxy-3-methyl-5-^{123}I-iodobenzyl)-1,3-propanediamine 2 HCl (HIPDM): intractable complex partial seizures. *Neurology* 1986;36:1471–7.

78. Stefan H, Pawlik G, Bocher-Schwarz HG, Biersack HJ, Burr W, Penin H, Heiss W-D. Functional and morphological abnormalities in temporal lobe epilepsy: a com-

79. Homan RW, Paulman RG, Devous MD, et al. Neuropsychological function and regional cerebral blood flow in epilepsy. In: Porter RJ, Mattson RJ, Ward AA, et al., eds. *Advances in Epileptology*. Fifteenth International Symposium. New York: Raven Press, 1984:115–20.

80. LaManna MM, Sussman NM, Harner RH, et al. Initial experience with SPECT imaging of the brain using I-123 p-iodoamphetamine in focal epilepsy. *Clin Nucl Med* 1989;14:428–30.

81. Rowe CC, Bewrkovic SF, Sia STB, et al. Localization of epileptic foci with postictal single photon emission computed tomography. *Ann Neurol* 1989;26:660–8.

82. Bluestone DL, Engelstad BL, Barbaro NM, Laxer KD. Tc-PAO SPECT imaging for intractable complex partial seizures of temporal lobe origin. *Epilepsia* 1989; 30:690.

83. Homan RW, Devous MD, LeRoy RF, Bonte FJ. Interictal blood flow elevations in partial seizures. *Neurology* 1989;39(Suppl 1):300.

84. Stefan H, Kuhnen C, Biersack HJ, Reichman K. Initial experience with 99m-Tc hexamethylpropylene amine oxime (HMPAO) single photon emission computed tomography (SPECT) in patients with focal epilepsy. *Epilepsy Res* 1987;1:134–8.

85. Shen W, Lee BI, Park HM, et al. HIPDM-SPECT brain imaging in evaluation of intractable epilepsy for temporal lobectomy. Neurology 1989;39(Suppl 1):132.

86. Ryvlin P, Philippon B, Cinotti L, Froment JC, Le Bars D, Mauguiere F. Functional neuroimaging strategy in temporal lobe epilepsy: a comparative study of ^{18}FDG-PET and ^{99m}Tc-HMPAO-SPECT. *Ann Neurol* 1992;31:650–6.

87. Fish DR, Lewis TT, Brooks DJ, Zilka E, Wise RJS, Kendall BE. Regional cerebral blood flow of patients with focal epilepsy studied using xenon-enhanced CT brain scanning. *J Neurol Neurosurg Psychiatry* 1987; 50:1584–8.

88. Scheurer M, Belo J, Nordli D, Pedley T. Xenon-enhanced CT in partial epilepsy. *Neurology* 1989; 39(Suppl 1):115.

89. Berent S, Sackellares JC, Abou-Khalil B, Gilman S, Siegal G, Hichwa R, Hutchins G. PET studies of cerebral glucose metabolic activity in temporal lobe epilepsy: the functional implications of lateralized hypometabolism. *Neurology* 1986;36(Suppl 1):337.

90. Bromfield EB, Ludlow CL, Bassich CJ, Theodore WH. Cerebral activation during speech perception in temporal lobe epilepsy. *Neurology* 1988;38(Suppl 1):278.

91. Fox PT, Peterson S, Psoner M, Raichle ME. PET assessment of hemispheric dominance for language. *Neurology* 1988;38(Suppl 1):365.

92. Mazziotta JC, Phelps ME, Carson RE, Kuhl DE. Tomographic mapping of human cerebral metabolism: auditory stimulation. *Neurology* 1981;31:503–16.

93. Kushner MJ, Schwartz R, Alavi A, Dann R, Rosen M, Silver F, Reivich M. Cerebral glucose consumption following verbal auditory stimulation. *Brain Res* 1987;409:79–87.

parison of interictal and ictal EEG, CT, MRI, SPECT, and PET. *J Neurol* 1987;234:377–84.

94. Heiss W-D, Pawlik G, Hebold I, Herholtz K, Wagner R, Wienhard K. Metabolic pattern of speech activation in healthy volunteers, aphasics, and focal epileptics. *J Cereb Blood Flow Metab* 1987;7(Suppl 1)299.

95. Levin DN, Pelizzari CA, Chen GTY, Chen C-T, Cooper MD. Retrospective geometric correlation of MR, CT, and PET images. *Radiology* 1988;169:817–23.

96. Curatolo P, Pelliccia A, Cotroneo E: Prognostic significance of CT finding in West syndrome. In: Akimoto H, Kazamatsuri H, Seino M, Ward AA Jr, eds. *Advances in Epileptology*. Thirteenth Epilepsy International Symposium. New York: Raven Press, 1982: 191–4.

97. Chugani HT, Shields WD, Shewmon DA, Olson DM, Phelps ME, Peacock WJ. Infantile spasms: I. PET identifies focal cortical dysgenesis in cryptogenic cases for surgical treatment. *Ann Neurol* 1990;27:406–13.

98. Chiron C, Dulac O, Raynaud C, Jambarquet I, Plouin P. [133]Xe brain SPECT imaging in cryptogenic West syndrome. *Epilepsia* 1989;30:654.

99. English R, Soper N, Shepstone BJ, Hockaday JM, Stores G. Five patients with Rasmussen's syndrome investigated by single photon emission computed tomography. *Nucl Med Commun* 1989;10:5–14.

100. Chugani HT, Shewmon DA, Peacock WJ, Shields WD, Mazziotta JC, Phelps ME. Surgical treatment of intractable neonatal-onset seizures: the role of positron emission tomography. *Neurology* 1988;38:1178–88.

101. Gastaut H, Pinsard N, Genton P: Electroclinical correlations of CT scans in secondary generalized epilepsies. In: Canger R, Angeleri F, Penry JK, eds. *Advances in epileptology*. Eleventh Epilepsy International Symposium. New York: Raven Press, 1980:45–52.

102. Chugani HT, Engel J Jr, Mazziotta JC, Phelps ME. The Lennox-Gastaut syndrome: metabolic subtypes determined by 2-deoxy-2-{18F}-fluoro-D-glucose positron emission tomography. *Ann Neurol* 1987;21:4–13.

103. Theodore WH, Rose D, Patronas N, et al. Cerebral glucose metabolism in the Lennox-Gastaut syndrome. *Ann Neurol* 1987;21:14–21.

104. Denays R, Rubenstein M, Ham H, Piepsz A, Noel P. Single photon emission computed tomography in seizure disorders. *Arch Dis Child* 1988;63:1184–8.

105. Spencer SS, Spencer DD, Williamson PD, Sass K, Novelly RA, Mattson RH. Corpus callosotomy for epilepsy. 1. Seizure effects. *Neurology* 1988;38:19–24.

106. DeToledo J, Smith DB, Kramer RE, et al. Anterior corpus callosotomy section results: factors associated with outcome. *Neurology* 1989;39(Suppl 1):150.

107. Bladin PF. Adult Lennox-Gastaut syndrome: patients with large focal structural lesions. *Clin Exp Neurol* 1985;21:105–14.

108. Gur RE, Sussman NM, Alavi A, et al. Positron emission tomography in two cases of childhood epileptic encephalopathy (Lennox-Gastaut syndrome). *Neurology* 1982;32:1191–4.

109. Engel J, Babb TL, Phelps ME. Contribution of positron emission tomography to understanding mechanisms of epilepsy. In: Engel JP, Ojemann GA, Luders HO, Williamson PD, eds. *Fundamental mechanisms of human brain function*. New York: Raven Press, 1987;209–18.

110. Falconer MA, Serefetinides EA, Corsellis JAN. Aetiology and pathogenesis of temporal lobe epilepsy. *Arch Neurol* 1964;19:23–40.

111. Theodore WH, Sato S, Kufta C, Bare M, Porter RJ, Ito B, Rose D, Devinsky O. Strategy for surgical selection of patients with partial seizures: the role of positron emission tomography. *Ann Neurol* 1987;22:133.

PART THREE
SURGICAL
PROCEDURES

Chapter 12
Focal Cortical Resections

ALLEN R. WYLER

General Considerations

The goal of this chapter is to summarize focal cortical resections in the treatment of partial seizure disorder. However, to do so would require a monograph rather than a chapter, because our understanding of the basic mechanisms of focal epilepsy is incomplete and therefore multiple approaches and techniques can be justifiably applied to its treatment. Because of this complexity, I will focus this discussion on just one type of focal resection, anterior temporal lobectomy (ATL), which is used as a prototype from which generalizations to other focal resections can be made. To be more specific, I will devote my discussion to focal epilepsy without obvious structural lesions, (space-occupying masses) because, more often than not, structural lesions and their immediate surroundings constitute the epileptogenic focus and are fairly straightforward in diagnosis and treatment. On the other hand, idiopathic partial epilepsy is much more difficult to understand and deal with surgically. The reason for focusing on ATL is that it is the most common focal resection that is done for epilepsy. In fact, Rasmussen [1] has reported that at the Montreal Neurological Institute two thirds of all cortical resections for focal epilepsy due to nontumoral epileptogenic lesions are within the temporal lobe. The surgical approach for ATL was pioneered by Penfield and Baldwin [2]. Follow-up of Penfield's patients from 1939 to 1949 demonstrated a success rate (defined as either seizure-free or significantly improved) of 53%. Long-term follow-up of the Montreal series after 1949 indicated a success rate of nearly 66% [1]. With the advent of newer brain-imaging techniques such as x-ray computed tomography (CT), magnetic resonance imaging (MRI), and positron emission tomography (PET), and long-term monitoring with and without intracranial recording techniques, the success rate from tempo-ral lobectomy has improved to approximately 70%. What is so surprising is the differing outcomes reported by various surgical centers. Some obvious reasons for these differences are: various selection criteria for surgical candidates, dissimilarity in surgical techniques and approaches, and extremes of opinion concerning which structures need to be removed from the temporal lobe to optimize a seizure-free outcome. Some of these issues will be discussed below.

The Pathologic Lesion

The fundamental concept underlying a focal cortical resection is that there exists a finite region of brain tissue, the focus, that contains the epileptogenicity capable of generating all of the patient's seizures. Hence, if this epileptogenic focus can be accurately identified and resected, the seizures will cease. The epileptogenicity is assumed to derive from neurons and their dendrites, but not axons, and thus is thought to be a problem of gray matter rather than of white matter. Numerous pathologic studies have been done of epileptogenic tissue removed from human brain. The most characteristic and ubiquitous changes are the presence of gliosis, loss of neurons, and dendritic abnormalities [3,4]. When dealing with typical idiopathic temporal lobe epilepsy, these changes can be quite characteristic in and around the hippocampus and can often be diagnosed as mesial temporal sclerosis. However, it is not at all clear whether mesial temporal sclerosis is the cause or the result of seizures. This confusion exists because similar gliotic changes can be found in the mesial temporal lobe of patients who have generalized (nonfocal) epilepsy and in patients who clearly have an epileptogenic focus outside the temporal lobe. What role, if any, the abnormal glia play in the generation of seizures also is not clear.

The electrophysiologic hallmark of epilepsy is the epileptiform spike. The spike is assumed to be an electrical potential that is generated from ensembles of neuronal soma and dendrites. However, the exact mechanisms that underlie the spike are not known with certainty. To make matters more confusing, whatever elements generate scalp-recorded spikes are not necessarily the same as those that generate cortically recorded spikes. For example, a subdural strip electrode will not record the same spikes as recorded from an electrode placed on the scalp directly overlying it. Furthermore, the relationships between epileptiform spikes and the epileptogenic focus are too often overstated or assumed to be highly correlative, which they are not. The correlative relationships between the two phenomena become less clear if one considers the following facts. First, spikes can be recorded from the scalp of a small percentage of nonepileptic subjects, and if one records from depth electrodes, spikes can be found in the region of the temporal lobe pole and orbital frontal cortex of almost all nonepileptic subjects [5]. Second, chronic recordings from depth or subdural strip electrodes implanted in the brains of epileptics have demonstrated that interictal spikes routinely occur at multiple sites distant as well as contralateral to the region of the focus [6,7]. In our own surgical experience we record either acutely or chronically from the surface of the brain, and we have found that epileptogenic spiking may often occur centimeters distant from the lesion and not from cortex directly involved with the lesion. Yet the seizures will stop when the lesion and not the spiking cortex is removed. Surgeons who routinely do acute electrocorticography (ECoG) at the time of surgery know that little correlation exists between the presence or absence of postresection spikes and clinical outcome. For example, we conducted a prospective study that measured the incidence of orbital frontal spiking at the time of ATL. We found that no correlation existed between the presence of preresection or postresection spiking and postoperative seizure outcome (Wyler, unpublished data). Thus, it is clear that although the epileptiform spike is often associated with the phenomenon of epilepsy, its existence within the brain does not provide a precise physiologic marker that can identify the location and limits of an epileptogenic focus.

The results of other diagnostic tests, such as a PET scan, will often correlate with the location of an epileptogenic focus [8]. Of interest is the finding that abnormalities on PET scans seem to be larger than the volume of cortex that needs to be removed for the patient to become seizure-free. The diagnostic test that seems to have the highest reliability for localizing an epileptogenic focus is chronic intracranial ictal EEG monitoring. However, none of our diagnostic tests is completely accurate in localizing or delimiting the epileptogenic focus 100% of the time, a fact that is probably responsible for several observations. First, most surgical epileptologists use a number of tests for localizing an epileptogenic focus and make prognostic decisions based on the degree of concordance among the tests. Second, even with the best presurgical evaluations, no surgical series of any magnitude has a postoperative seizure success rate of 100%. Third, the lack of knowledge concerning the basic mechanisms of focal epilepsy is why different surgeons may remove different structures during ATL, yet have similar results.

The ambiguity in knowing the location and limits of an epileptogenic focus in turn impacts on our efforts to illuminate the basic mechanisms of focal epilepsy. For example, we know that the hippocampus is the region from which 98% of seizures begin electroencephalographically in patients with idiopathic temporal lobe epilepsy. But for those patients is the hippocampus actually the epileptogenic focus? Several possibilities exist. First, because of its intrinsic neuronal circuitry [3,9] and the damage that can occur from seizures *per se* [4], the hippocampus may have a lower threshold for initiating seizures, which are actually being incited or driven from another region of the temporal lobe. Second, because the hippocampus and amygdala involve a great deal of circuitry for the temporal lobe, removing the hippocampus may profoundly affect the occurrence of clinically apparent seizures, yet not remove the focus (the pacemaker of the epileptogenic process). However, because the seizures may stop after a region of cortex has been removed, we often assume the focus has been removed. The second hypothesis could explain the clinical observation that there is a spectrum of responses to ATL even though the same operation is done for what is believed to be the same type of seizure disorder. Some patients are seizure-free from the day of surgery; other patients may have only occasional seizures under various conditions; and still other patients may have very little response to surgery. Because of our ambiguity and uncertainty in knowing exactly where an epileptogenic focus resides, it is not difficult to understand why so very little has been learned about the cellular mechanisms involved in focal epileptogenesis. If a surgeon supplies an investigator with human hippocampal samples, how is he to know if it really is the epileptogenic focus? And are any changes found in such tissue samples the cause or the effect of the epilepsy?

Preoperative Evaluation

No consensus has defined what constitutes an adequate presurgical evaluation before proceeding with a focal resection. That void was emphasized in the proceedings of the International Conference on the Surgical Treatment of Epilepsy [10]. Clinicians from 50 surgical centers worldwide were asked to submit their criteria for a surgical evaluation. No consensus existed on several crucial points. For example, some centers relied only on interictal EEG recordings, whereas other centers accepted only ictal recordings. Many centers never used intracranial monitoring, whereas others would not consider surgery without it. For those centers using intracranial monitoring, no opinion existed concerning the best type of monitoring, that is, with depth electrodes [11,12], subdural strip electrodes [13], or epidural grid electrodes [14]. Even with the same recording method, considerable disagreement may exist in interpretation of recordings. For example, Spencer et al. [15] had 144 scalp ictal EEGs from 54 patients analyzed by three independent electroencephalographers. The accuracy of these interpretations was correlated with subsequent depth EEG for localization of side and lobe of seizure onset. They found approximately 60% agreement among observers for lobe and 64–74% for side of onset when scalp EEGs were compared. They found 21–38% agreement for lobe and 46–49% agreement for side of seizure onset when observations with depth electrodes were compared. Their study points out the fact that interpretation of ictal onset from EEG or ECoG recordings can vary considerably. Such interobserver variability will influence crucial surgical decisions such as whether to remove a temporal or frontal lobe (two cortical regions that can generate complex partial seizures, yet have almost identical interictal and ictal recordings with scalp electrodes), which in turn can markedly influence surgical outcome.

Selection Criteria

Numerous factors have some prognostic value in identifying who will or will not do well following ATL: the presence of a correlative structural lesion, the patient's intelligence quotient (IQ), lateralized neuropsychological findings, long-term EEG monitoring, the presence of bilateral epileptiform discharges, the presence of generalized discharges, evidence of a single focus, and etiology and duration of seizures have all been reported as variables that can influence sur-

gical seizure outcome [16]. If a surgical center selects only patients with average intelligence, unilateral discharges, a work history, and a structural lesion in the mesial temporal lobe, the surgical results should be excellent. However, this combination is infrequent, and more commonly patients have idiopathic epilepsy with bilateral epileptiform discharges or otherwise complicated EEGs. Thus, one center may turn away patients who do not have clear unilateral interictal foci on scalp EEG but who, at other centers, would be invasively monitored and found to be excellent surgical candidates. Some surgeons may elect to operate on patients who demonstrate bitemporal foci, whereas other surgeons would never do so. These biases would obviously affect the outcome statistics of any surgical center.

Surgical Techniques

Several issues concerning surgical techniques may influence outcome but have never been evaluated critically. For example, some surgeons do ATL using the operating microscope because they feel it generates improved results since it provides improved visualization and hence allows a more complete resection of mesial temporal structures [17]. Other surgeons use no magnification for a similar operation. Another area of controversy is whether ATL should be done under local or general anesthesia [17]. Proponents of local anesthesia claim one can map temporal lobe cortex for active epileptiform spiking and function, thereby tailoring the resection to maximize removal of epileptogenic cortex while preserving eloquent cortex [18]. Other surgeons feel that for the routine temporal lobectomy only a minimal amount of lateral temporal cortex needs to be removed, which does not endanger speech cortex and yet allows the surgery to be done equally safely under general anesthesia.

There is no clear understanding as to what temporal lobe structures need to be removed for a successful ATL. For example, Wieser and Yasargil [19] reported a 93% success rate from selective amygdalohippocampectomy in which only medial temporal structures were resected. In direct contrast, Coughlan et al. [20] reported an excellent success rate from removing only lateral temporal cortex while leaving hippocampus intact. Spencer et al. [21] reported 20% of their patients showed epileptogenic foci caudal to the usual limits of temporal lobe resection and so propose treating patients with a modified temporal lobectomy wherein the hippocampus, parahippocampus, uncus, and fusiform gyri are resected. Spencer et al. leave the superior temporal gyrus and amygdala intact, whereas I always remove both these structures with similar surgical seizure results. In contrast to all of the above reports, Ojemann [18] stated that optimal ATL results were achieved by resecting no more than 4.5 cm of hippocampus and that further mesial resection added little to the seizure outcome of ATL. Many of the approaches to ATL have been reviewed in detail by Crandall [22].

Thus, for the most common focal resection performed worldwide (ATL) we do not know which structures should be removed for optimal seizure outcome. The reason we lack such knowledge is that we do not have a firm understanding of the basic mechanisms of focal epilepsy. The controversy surrounding ATL emphasizes only the same problems that surround focal resections of other lobes of the brain. In fact, our lack of understanding of frontal lobe epilepsy is mirrored by its poor surgical seizure outcome.

Preoperative Care

Once a patient has been identified as a surgical candidate and has elected to undergo surgery, we advise the patient of the potential need for blood transfusion during surgery. Because of concern for acquired immunodeficiency syndrome (AIDS) and other blood-borne infections, the patient is asked to consider banking 1–2 units of blood a month or more prior to surgery. The patient is then placed on a good multiple vitamin with iron supplement and allowed to rebuild his or her hematocrit. For pediatric patients we request directed blood donation from family members if possible.

The night before surgery the patient is asked to shampoo three times with povidone-iodine (Betadine) soap. If ECoG is to be used during surgery no benzodiazepine sleeping medication is prescribed that night. The morning of surgery an intravenous set-up of dextrose and lactated Ringer's solution is started and the patient is given a 10-mg dose (IV) of dexamethasone. Although the routine use of prophylactic antibiotics is debated, we have given 1 g of cefazolin sodium (Ancef) (IV) 1 hour before the patient is taken into the operating room. No further antibiotic medication is given.

Anticonvulsant Medication. At our center it is routine for patients who will undergo focal resection to be taking either phenytoin (Dilantin) or carbamazepine (Tegretol) as monotherapy or in combination with phenobarbital (as either phenobarbital or primidone). We feel there is no place for the treatment of partial seizures with any of the suxamide drugs or with valproic acid. Our bias against the preoperative use of valproic acid is twofold. First, we feel the drug is not particularly effective for focal seizures, although it is often excellent for treating primary generalized epilepsy. Second, valproic acid can provoke bleeding disorders. The patient's usual morning dose of drugs is given orally with a few sips of water on the day of surgery even though the patient has been allowed no intake by mouth (NPO) since midnight.

Steroids. These are begun the morning of surgery. For most adults a 10-mg dose of dexamethasone (Decadron) is given intravenously at 6 AM when the intravenous drip is initiated. Decadron is then continued every 6 h for the next 48 h. It is then replaced with ibuprofen (Motrin) 600 mg qid for the next 10 days as needed for pain control.

Choice of Anesthesia

A great deal of controversy remains as to whether patients should be operated on under local or general anesthesia for routine focal resections. The rationale for operating under local anesthesia was largely defined by Penfield and Jasper [23] and included the need to use electrical stimulation to delineate cortical function (such as language), to measure afterdischarge threshold, and to localize the epileptogenic focus by direct ECoG. Because general anesthesia will preclude direct cortical function mapping and different anesthetic agents will augment or suppress ECoG, it was believed that more precise data could be obtained with the patient awake. However, the need for much of the above-mentioned data has been nullified by present-day preoperative evaluations.

The Need for Acute Cortical Stimulation

The purpose of mapping cortex by electrical stimulation is to locate functional cortex with respect to the epileptogenic focus. Most commonly this is aimed at defining the cortex serving language function and the primary motor cortex or to determine afterdischarge thresholds.

Advocates of acute intraoperative mapping point out that, from person to person, speech function may reside a variable distance along the superior temporal gyrus. Therefore, speech cortex should be identified and spared to avoid postoperative speech damage. This argument makes two unsubstantiated assumptions. First, it assumes that most temporal lobe epileptogenic foci involve lateral temporal cortex, and second, a tailored resection of the lateral temporal epileptogenic focus is necessary for seizure control. Ictal monitoring data indicate that for nonlesional temporal lobe epilepsy, 98% of seizures begin from mesial temporal and not from lateral temporal cortex. For this reason, Wieser and Yasergil [19] and Spencer et al. [21] have pointed out the importance of removing mesial temporal structures for treatment of most temporal lobe epilepsy. The debate between a tailored or standard temporal lobe resection is more difficult to judge because there are no prospective studies that have compared outcome from each surgery. However, there are good data to evaluate language function outcome following a standard ATL. Hermann and Wyler [24] compared preoperative language function with 6-month postoperative language function in patients who underwent ATL of the dominant ($n = 15$) or nondominant ($n = 14$) hemisphere. Language dominance was confirmed by intracarotid sodium amobarbital test. Using a standardized language and aphasia battery, they found a significant trend of worse preoperative language function in patients with dominant hemisphere temporal lobe foci in comparison with patients with nondominant foci. Following ATL, neither group showed any significant losses in language function, whereas the dominant hemisphere temporal lobe group showed significant improvement in receptive language comprehension and associative verbal fluency. Thus, as a group, those patients who have dominant temporal lobe foci have poorer preoperative language function when compared with a comparable group of nondominant temporal lobe patients, and this factor should be considered when comparing outcomes from surgery. In another prospective study, Hermann and Wyler [25] asked whether surgery under local anesthesia with language mapping and ECoG mapping of the epileptogenic focus generated improved language outcome in comparison with patients operated on without language mapping and under general anesthesia. They studied 26 consecutive patients with dominant temporal lobe epileptogenic foci. All patients were evaluated by the same preoperative protocol and had, in addition to the usual neuropsychological tests, 16 tests of verbal abilities including formal evaluation of multiple aspects of language function. With the same surgeon and same surgical techniques, 13 patients underwent ATL with general anesthesia and 13 with local anesthesia. All surgeries were done within the same year. Patients were followed for at least 1 year (and have been followed continuously since then) and underwent neuropsychological reevaluation 6 months after surgery. Those patients operated on under general anesthesia had better seizure-free outcomes than those operated on under local anesthesia. The general anesthesia group showed more significant gains across a diversity of language skills but manifested a mild dysnomia. The generally superior neuropsychological outcome shown by the general anesthesia group was attributable to a higher probability of a totally seizure-free outcome, suggesting that more complete removal of the epileptogenic focus has beneficial effects on multiple aspects of cognitive functioning.

The seizure outcome of 50 patients who underwent ATL under local anesthesia was then compared with a demographically similar group of 50 patients who underwent ATL under general anesthesia [17]. The outcome for the two groups was statistically significant: the seizure outcome associated with surgery under general anesthesia was significantly better than for those patients operated on under local anesthesia. Hermann and Wyler ascribe the improved outcome to the fact that a surgeon can have a more controlled surgical field (less patient movement, better visualization of structures because of the operating microscope and its superior light source, more controlled retraction, and less morbidity) and obtain a more complete resection of hippocampus when operating under general anesthesia. Thus, for the routine case of idiopathic temporal lobe epilepsy, temporal lobectomy can be carried out successfully even within the dominant hemisphere under general anesthesia without any significant impairment to language function. In fact, our data suggest that surgery under general anesthesia with the operating microscope will provide improved seizure outcome than surgery under local anesthesia.

The Need for Identifying Central Sulcus

The central sulcus needs to be identified during some focal resections. This can be accomplished by electrically stimulating the cortical surface while observing for contralateral evoked muscle responses. Local anesthesia is preferred because general anesthesia will suppress evoked motor responses in a significant number of patients. However, an alternative to direct cortical stimulation is to record somatosensory evoked potentials (SSEP) directly from the cortical surface at the time of craniotomy [26]. The advantage of SSEP is that positive results can be obtained more reliably than cortically evoked motor responses, especially when using general anesthesia. The disadvantage of SSEP is that it requires bringing an evoked potential unit plus personnel into the operating room. For the routine ATL it is unnecessary to identify motor cortex.

The Need for Determining Afterdischarge Thresholds

Penfield and Jasper [23] felt that cortical stimulation is a helpful indicator of the epileptogenic focus when it elicits afterdischarge associated with the patient's habitual aura. In addition, they felt that measurement of afterdischarge threshold originally described by Walker [27], could help localize the epileptogenic focus. However, this tactic was created in the days before long-term ictal monitoring. Presently, if the seizure focus has been determined by long-term intracranial ictal monitoring, afterdischarge threshold measurements are not necessary. Moreover, the technique probably has little, if any, accuracy in localizing epileptogenic foci because of the fact that different cortical regions have different intrinsic afterdischarge thresholds, which have never been normalized. Also, the original concept that afterdischarge threshold is lower within the cortical region of the focus is not universally accepted. In fact, Engel [28] feels that afterdischarge thresholds of epileptogenic cortex are elevated (thus indicating hypoexcitability) rather than lowered.

Occasional situations do require mapping cortical function prior to resecting an epileptogenic focus. In my experience this most often involves removal of a lesion in or near the speech or motor cortex and seldom involves nonlesional epilepsy. The cortical mapping can be done acutely during surgery under local anesthesia or accomplished by using short-term grid electrode implantation [14]. Large-grid electrode arrays can provide the capability of mapping cortical function while monitoring the same region of cortex to determine site of ictal onset. Advantages of using grids over acute intraoperative mapping are as follows. Direct relationships can be formed between those cortical areas of ictal onset and cortical function, a point that cannot be made with acute interictal recordings. In most cases, the observations can be repeated to ensure validity over time. Finally, the testing is less stressful to the patient and not constrained to a small time period. Disadvantages are that it requires two surgeries, thereby increasing the risk of infection at the time of resection.

The Need for Acute Electrocorticography

There are perhaps two reasons for using acute ECoG during the course of surgery. The first is to locate the region of the epileptogenic focus, and the second is to determine the extent of focal resection once the location of the focus is determined.

In the early days of epilepsy surgery, seizure foci were localized by first looking for structural lesions rather than electrical abnormalities. The presurgical evaluation consisted of skull x-ray studies, a pneumoencephalogram, an arteriogram, a neuropsychological test battery, and a series of interictal scalp EEGs. The skull x-ray film and pneumoencephalogram were replaced by CT scans and, more recently, by MRI scans. There is no question that these newer imaging techniques provide much more data than did the standard skull x-ray film. More importantly, interictal scalp recordings have been replaced with long-term EEG/video ictal monitoring. Again, there is considerable evidence to indicate that ictal monitoring is superior to interictal monitoring for localizing epileptogenic foci. In addition, data from multiple centers show that intracranial monitoring (whether done with depth electrodes or strip electrodes) provides more accurate localization of the seizure focus than does scalp monitoring [12]. Intracranial monitoring decreases ambiguities in localization within one hemisphere. For example, frontal lobe foci may have a predominantly temporal EEG pattern, and *vice versa*. Or, occasionally, occipital foci may be mistaken for temporal lobe foci, or *vice versa*. To make matters worse, the discrimination between a frontal lobe focus and a temporal lobe focus cannot be made solely by observation of the clinical seizure phenomenology. Invasive monitoring gives additional essential information for selecting surgical candidates. For example, the time for interhemispheric spread of seizures is important in selecting candidates for ATL [29]. Therefore, it is no longer necessary to localize the epileptogenic focus by acute ECoG if the patient has already undergone such localization by intracranial long-term ictal monitoring.

The second reason some surgeons use acute ECoG is to define the extent or margins of a cortical resection, or, in other words, to help guide a tailored cortical resection. With that strategy the surgeon first maps out the extent of focal epileptiform abnormalities and then resects cortex. A post-resection ECoG recording is then made, and further resection is done if additional epileptogenic spiking is found. This tactic makes the following assumptions: first, that the epileptiform spike always correlates with epileptogenic brain; second, that the spike will always vanish immediately on removal of epileptogenic brain; and third, that the spike is indicative of continued epileptogenic potential. As noted in an earlier section of this chapter, none of these assumptions has been proven. In fact, there is no clear correlation between the presence or absence of spiking in the postresection ECoG and postoperative seizure outcome. In addition, there is no evidence that the seizure outcome from "tailored" resections (those done using acute ECoG to define the limits of resection) is any better than the seizure outcome of standardized focal resections. Thus, there is little support for the notion that acute ECoG is required or necessary in the course of routine focal resections.

From the above discussion, it seems that much of the rationale for doing focal resections, and especially temporal lobectomy, under local anesthesia is founded more in pioneering tradition than in scientific fact, and local anesthesia was thought to be helpful in the past when less information was available to the surgeon than is the case today. In reality, local anesthesia has very genuine limitations because it cannot be used for children, the mentally retarded, or people with significant psychiatric problems; local anesthesia is more stressful for the patient and the operating room personnel; and surgery under local anesthesia is performed more slowly in our experience and therefore results in higher operating room and anesthesia costs.

Operative Technique

General anesthesia is induced with intravenous thiopental (at a dosage of 1–3 mg/kg) and intravenous fentanyl (at a dosage of 50–150 μg) in an average adult. A nondepolarizing muscle relaxant, pancuronium bromide (Pavulon) (dose of 0.1–0.15 mg/kg), is given intravenously to facilitate endotracheal intubation. Anesthesia is maintained with nitrous oxide and oxygen supplemented with isoflurane (in low concentrations, 0.5–1.0% inspired). The proposed incision is infiltrated with a mixture of (equal volumes) 1% lidocaine with epinephrine 1:1000,000 and 0.5% bupivacaine (Marcaine). This mixture provides a rapid onset of local anesthesia that will last throughout the case if ECoG recordings are needed with relative light anesthesia or if the entire case is planned under local anesthesia. Arterial blood pressure and body temperature are maintained at normal levels; arterial pCO_2 is maintained near 40 mm Hg. Mannitol or other diuretics are not used. If ECoG is required, isoflurane is discontinued 10 minutes before beginning the recordings, and the patient is maintained on nitrous oxide and oxygen with supplemental fentanyl (50–150 μg) and Pavulon as necessary. If

electrical stimulation of the cortex is anticipated to identify motor cortex, Pavulon must not be given. Following cortical mapping, administration of isoflurane is resumed and continued as in any other surgical patient. Another combination that has also worked is 50% N_2O and O_2 and halothane up to 2%. If this is used, the concentration is reduced to 0.5% during cortical stimulation.

If surgery is to be done under local anesthesia, we inject a field block with the local anesthesia before beginning the skin prep. The areas injected include the supraorbital, preauricular, postauricular, and greater occipital nerves. The patient's head is then scrubbed and draped while this injection is becoming effective. The proposed incision is then injected with the remainder of the local anesthetic; the total volume is between 40–50 ml. After the cortical resection, supplemental narcotic anesthesia can be employed.

The positioning of the patient, type of incision, and exposure of the cortex all depend on the proposed resection, choice of anesthesia, and requirements for ECoG. However, there are a few general considerations that may be helpful.

1. An ultrasonic dissector is extremely useful for most focal resections, especially when dealing with a structural lesion or removing cortex along the sylvian fissure.
2. The operating microscope should be used for all but the largest resections (i.e., frontal lobe resections or hemispherectomies). This is most important when removing mesial temporal structures during routine anterior temporal lobectomy.
3. In nondominant frontal lobectomies, the posterior resection margin should be the gyrus in front of precentral sulcus. This must be modified when dealing with the dominant hemisphere to avoid the speech cortex.
4. Anterior temporal lobectomy for idiopathic epilepsy should include resection of hippocampus posterior to the cerebral peduncle.
5. For focal resections, all cortical margins should be produced using a subpial dissection technique. In addition, whenever possible, make the depth of the sulcus (rather than the middle of a gyrus) the margin of a resection.
6. Hemostasis should be controlled with the bipolar rather than with the unipolar cautery. Hemostatic agents such as Gelfoam with thrombin should not be used if possible.
7. In most cases, a structural lesion that involves the gray matter will be the epileptogenic lesion. This is usually the case even if the interictal scalp EEG or acute intraoperative ECoG localizes to adjacent cortex.

8. When removing structural lesions thought to be epileptogenic, one must also remove sufficient adjacent cortex. This usually requires resecting cortex to the nearest sulcus.

Postoperative Care

Routine postoperative neurosurgical care is given to the patient. Usually the patient is observed overnight in the neurosurgical intensive care unit. The Foley urinary catheter can be removed immediately on awakening, and the arterial catheter can be removed as soon as the blood pressure is stable. The patient should be out of bed the day of surgery for optimal pulmonary care. Dexamethasone (Decadron) is continued for 48 hours and then stopped without tapering. We routinely discharge the patient within 4 days of surgery and remove the staples on about the seventh postoperative day.

Complications

Hemiparesis. Hemiparesis following focal resections occurs most commonly following routine temporal lobectomy. The cause for this has been speculated to be the result of manipulation of the middle cerebral artery, and thus Penfield et al. [23] coined the term *manipulation* (or *traction*) *hemiplegia*. The mechanism for this complication has not been determined with assurance but may be due to inadvertent damage to the anterior choroidal artery during dissection of the mesial temporal structures or various vessels, including the middle cerebral artery. The complication is usually present within the first hour after the patient awakens from anesthesia, or it can occur acutely during the temporal lobectomy under local anesthesia. It is reversible in approximately 50% of cases, which could support the possibility that some cases represent vasospasm. The incidence of this complication is about 5% in the older literature (reviewed in Helgason et al. [30]), with little being written about this in more recent literature. Quite possibly the incidence could be declining as more surgeons rely on microsurgical techniques for removal of mesial temporal structures. The surgeon is urged to become familiar with the anatomy around the region of the tentorial notch, which has been extensively reviewed by Rhoton's group [31].

Visual Field Defects. It is common for temporal lobectomy patients to have a contralateral superior quadrantanopia because of damage to Meyer's loop. The incidence of this complication varies with amount and type of temporal resection. In addition, extensive homonomous hemianopia can occur from damage to the vessels feeding the geniculate body [32] following temporal lobectomy. Again, the incidence of this larger visual-field complication can be reduced if the surgeon uses the operating microscope during the mesial hippocampal resection.

Aseptic Meningitis. After most craniotomies, there is an elevation of temperature for the first few days. However, if fever continues longer than approximately 72 hours, aseptic (or chemical) hemogenic meningitis [33] should be suspected. In certain cases, there may be a smooth convalescence with a sudden attack of headache associated with a sharp rise in temperature, perhaps of a relapsing type. The diagnosis can be made by lumbar puncture, which will demonstrate a varying degree of xanthochromic spinal fluid under pressure. The CSF may have from several hundred to several thousand leukocytes per cubic millimeter. Although some authors believe that the relatively low pressure and leukocytosis can discriminate this condition from bacterial meningitis, the diagnosis can be made only with negative aerobic and anaerobic CSF cultures and thus is a diagnosis of exclusion.

Penfield [23] believed this syndrome was due to blood in the subarachnoid space. However, the complication occurs more often from operations that have opened the ventricular system, for example, temporal lobectomy. The offending agent has been ascribed to the presence of bilirubin in the CSF rather than to the intact red blood cells. In fact, the resolution of the clinical symptoms correlates directly with a decrease in CSF bilirubin.

The treatment is to minimize fever with an antipyretic and has, in the past, required keeping the patient on dexamethasone. I have not found the newer nonsteroidal anti-inflammatory drugs as effective as dexamethasone in minimizing symptoms. Some symptomatic relief can be obtained with twice-daily lumbar puncture in very symptomatic patients.

Aseptic meningitis can be prevented by making every attempt to keep the operative field as bloodless as possible, preventing blood from entering the ventricular system, and closing the dura as carefully and completely as possible so that there is no passage of subaponeurotic fluid into the resection site.

Significance of Postoperative Seizures

The significance of acute postoperative seizures (i.e., seizures within the first week of surgery) on long-term outcome is not entirely clear. In 1954 Penfield and

Jasper [23] wrote, "Convalescent seizures, which occur in the first days after operation, give a definitely gloomy prognosis of complete cessation of seizures later." Lüders et al. [34] have followed a group of 71 patients and found that those who had seizures during the first postoperative week had only a 33% chance of remaining seizure-free, whereas those without seizures during the first week had a 77% chance of a seizure-free outcome.

Summary

In this chapter I have used anterior temporal lobectomy as a prototype for a more general discussion of cortical resection as a treatment for partial epilepsy. The rationale for focal cortical resection is straightforward; if one can find the cortical region responsible for the seizures and then remove it, the patient will be free of seizures. As simple as this concept sounds, the fact of the matter is that results from such operations are not as good as they should be if our fundamental hypotheses are correct. The conclusion is that we know less about the basic mechanisms of focal epilepsy than we may think we do, and we should continue to challenge well-established ideas, such as the relevance of the interictal epileptiform spike, until our surgical results warrant complacency.

References

1. Rasmussen T. Surgical treatment of patients with complex partial seizures. In: Purpura DP, Penry JK, Walter RD, eds. *Neurosurgical management of the epilepsies.* New York: Raven Press, 1975:415–49. (Advances in neurology; vol 8.)
2. Penfield W, Baldwin M. Temporal lobe seizures and the technique of subtotal temporal lobectomy. *Ann Surg* 1952;136:625–34.
3. Schwartzkroin PA, Wyler AR. Mechanisms underlying epileptiform burst discharge. *Ann Neurol* 1980;7:95–107.
4. Auer RN, Siesjo BK. Biological differences between ischemia, hypoglycemia, and epilepsy. *Ann Neurol* 1988;24:699–707.
5. Kendrick JF, Gibbs FA. Interrelations of mesial temporal and orbital frontal areas of man revealed by strychnine spikes. *Arch Neurol Psychiatry* 1958;79:518–24.
6. Engel J Jr, Crandall PH. Intensive neurodiagnostic monitoring with intracranial electrodes. *Adv Neurol* 1987;46:85–106.
7. Lange HH, Lieb JP, Engel J Jr, Crandall PH. Temporospatial patterns of pre-ictal spike activity in human temporal lobe epilepsy. *Electroencephalogr Clin Neurophysiol* 1983;56:543–55.
8. Engel J Jr, Brown WJ, Kuhl DE, Phelps ME, Mazziotta JC, Crandall PH. Pathological findings underlying focal temporal lobe hypometabolism in partial epilepsy. *Ann Neurol* 1982;12:518–28.
9. Schwartzkroin PA, Turner DA, Knowles WD, Wyler AR. Studies of human and monkey "epileptic" neocortex in the in vitro slice preparation. *Ann Neurol* 1983; 13:249–57.
10. Engel J Jr. *Surgical treatment of the epilepsies.* New York: Raven Press, 1987.
11. Talairach J, Bancaud J. Stereotactic approach to epilepsy. *Prog Neurol Surg* 1973;5:297–354.
12. Spencer SS. Depth electroencephalography in selection of refractory epilepsy for surgery. *Ann Neurol* 1981; 9:207–14.
13. Wyler AR, Ojemann GA, Lettich E, Ward AA Jr. Subdural strip electrodes for localizing epileptogenic foci. *J Neurosurg* 1984;60:1195–200.
14. Goldring S, Gregorie EM. Surgical management of epilepsy using epidural electrodes to localize the seizure focus. Review of 100 cases. *J Neurosurg* 1984;60: 457–66.
15. Spencer SS, Williamson PD, Bridgers SL, Mattson RH, Cicchetti DV, Spencer DD. Reliability and accuracy of localization by scalp ictal EEG. *Neurology* 1985; 35:1567–75.
16. Dodrill CB, Wilkus RJ, Ojemann GA, et al. Multidisciplinary prediction of seizure relief from cortical resection surgery. *Ann Neurol* 1986;20:2–12.
17. Wyler AR, Hermann BP. Comparative results of temporal lobectomy under local or general anesthesia: seizure outcome. *J Epilepsy* 1988;1:121–5.
18. Ojemann GA. Surgical therapy for medically intractable epilepsy. *J Neurosurg* 1987;66:489–99.
19. Wieser HG, Yasargil G. Selective amygdalohippocampectomy as a surgical treatment of mediobasal limbic epilepsy. *Surg Neurol* 1984;17:445–57.
20. Coughlan A, Farrell M, Hardiman O, Moore BO, Staunton H. The results of removal of temporal lobe neocortex in the treatment of epilepsy in 40 patients (abstr). In: *Meeting abstracts.* Meeting of the Association of British Neurologists with the American Neurological Association, London, England, November 1-2, 1985.
21. Spencer DD, Spencer SS, Mattson RH, Novelly RA, Williamson PD. Access to the posterior temporal lobe structures in the surgical treatment of temporal lobe epilepsy. *Neurosurgery* 1984;15:667–71.
22. Crandall PH. Cortical resections. In: Engel J Jr, ed. *Surgical treatment of the epilepsies.* New York: Raven Press, 1987:377–404.
23. Penfield W, Jasper H. *Epilepsy and the functional anatomy of the human brain.* Boston: Little, Brown, 1954.
24. Hermann BP, Wyler AR. Effects of anterior temporal lobectomy on language function: a controlled study. *Ann Neurol* 1988;23:585–8.
25. Hermann BP, Wyler AR. Comparative results of dominant temporal lobectomy under general or local anesthesia: language outcome. *J Epilepsy* 1988;1:127–34.
26. Wood CC, Spencer DD, Allison T, McCarthy G, Williamson PD, Goff WR. Localization of human

sensorimotor cortex during surgery by cortical surface recording of somatosensory evoked potentials. *J Neurosurg* 1988;68:99–111.

27. Walker AE. Electrocorticography in epilepsy. *Electroencephalogr Clin Neurophysiol* 1949;2 (Suppl):30–7.

28. Engel J Jr, Rausch R, Lieb JP, Kunl DE, Crandall PH. Correlation or criteria used for locating epileptic foci in patients considered for surgical therapy or epilepsy. Ann Neurol 1981;9:215–224.

29. Lieb JP, Engel J Jr, Babb TL. Interhemispheric propagation time of human hippocampal seizures. I. Relationship to surgical outcome. *Epilepsia* 1986;27:286–93.

30. Helgason CM, Bergen D, Bleck TP, Morrell F, Whisler W. Infarction after surgery for focal epilepsy: manipulation hemiplegia revisited. *Epilepsia* 1987;28:340–5.

31. Ono M, Rhoton AL, Barry M. Microsurgical anatomy of the region of the tentorial incisura. *J Neurosurg* 1984;60:365–99.

32. Lende RA. Local spasm in cerebral arteries. *J Neurosurg* 1960;17:90–103.

33. Penfield W, Finlayson A. Acute postoperative aseptic leptomeningitis. *Arch Neurol Psychiatry* 1941;46:258–87.

34. Lüders H, Murphy D, Dinner D, Morris H, Wyllie E, Godoy J. Prognostic value of epileptic seizures occurring in the first week after surgery of epilepsy. *Epilepsia* 1988;29:679.

Chapter 13
Corpus Callosotomy

ALLEN R. WYLER

Background

Van Wagenen and Herren [1] were the first to describe the use of hemispheral commissurotomy for the treatment of uncontrolled seizures. In an article published in 1940, they reported 10 patients who were operated on in early 1939 and then followed for only a few months. Their data have been criticized because of the exceedingly short follow-up period. Their rationale for the surgery was based on personal clinical observations. They had noticed that early in the course of tumors that involved the corpus callosum, patients usually had generalized seizures. But, as the tumor grew the patient's convulsions became less frequent and were often unilateral and/or did not involve loss of consciousness. As destruction of the corpus callosum continued, the seizures diminished further. Thus, they reckoned that destruction of the corpus callosum and other commissures in epileptics should help in seizure control. The postoperative seizure control in their first group of patients was mixed but was encouraging enough to suggest they should continue with further evaluation of the surgery. Van Wagenen subsequently reported on an additional 14 operated patients. The surgical approach used by Van Wagenen and Herren was varied because, besides the corpus callosum, they occasionally included sectioning the anterior commissure and/or the fornical commissure in some patients.

Interest in callosotomy remained dormant until the 1960s when Bogen and colleagues [17] published a series of articles on the clinical and neuropsychological outcome from the surgery. Then in 1970 Luessenhop et al. [2] reported a group of patients with infantile hemiplegia on whom they had done corpus callosotomies as an alternative to hemispherectomy. In 1975 Wilson et al. [3,4] began a series of reports on the Dartmouth experience with callosotomies. Since then a renewed interest in epilepsy surgery in general has caused an increase in articles dealing with callosotomy for treatment of epilepsy [5–16].

Rationale

The aim of corpus callosotomy is to disrupt one or several of the major central nervous system (CNS) pathways that are suspected to contribute to generalization or spread of seizures. The rationale assumes that if these pathways are destroyed, seizures will not be allowed to spread between hemispheres to the point of producing either primary or secondary generalized seizures. Thus, the rationale is fairly nonspecific, and the operation has been applied to almost all types of seizures that have not responded to anticonvulsant control.

Indications

Unlike anterior temporal lobectomy for complex-partial seizures, there are no clear and consistent indications for corpus callosotomy other than medically refractory seizures (with either primary or secondary generalization). Although certain seizure types seem to respond more favorably than others, having a particular seizure type does not guarantee a good result. For example, those seizures that seem to be helped by callosotomy are classified as generalized (i.e., tonic, clonic, tonic-clonic, and atonic). Atonic seizures have been reported to be helped significantly by callosotomy, but having atonic seizures does not guarantee a successful outcome from surgery. Complex-partial seizures can be helped, but this result is more unreliable.

One of the reasons the indications for this operation are so poorly defined is that many of the earlier surgical series were done without benefit of the patients having long-term electroencephalography (EEG)/video monitoring. Thus, the surgery was done without clear knowledge of the patient's seizure type. Moreover, surgeons have done various degrees of midline sections that have included some or all of the corpus callosum and then some or all of the various other midline structures. Finally, until the recent introduction of magnetic resonance imaging (MRI), there has been no way of determining how much of the corpus callosum had been sectioned on any patient. Thus, when the literature is reviewed, it is often difficult to know what surgery was actually done, how much of the callosum was actually sectioned, and what type(s) of seizure the patients had. All of these factors make the literature somewhat problematic to interpret.

Some epileptologists feel that mentally retarded epileptics should not be considered for surgery, especially not for corpus callosotomy. One reason is that the callosotomy seldom renders patients seizure-free. In general, patients with mental retardation do not have as good postoperative seizure outcome from any type of epilepsy surgery as do mentally normal patients. Thus, why submit to the risk of surgery a patient who has little significant potential for vocational and social rehabilitation? However, mental retardation does not guarantee a poor surgical outcome, and in fact we have mentally retarded patients who have been seizure-free after callosotomy. Furthermore, callosotomy is often done not for social or vocational rehabilitation but rather to decrease the risk of seizure-related injury and morbidity.

Surgical Approaches

In spite of renewed interest in epilepsy surgery in general and corpus callosotomy in particular, there has been a great variation in reported outcome of corpus callosotomy from various centers. The variability is due to multiple factors, which were mentioned above and which have never been systematically accounted for even within individual series of patients. Some of those factors are the midline commissures sectioned and the selection criteria used at various centers.

In Van Wagenen and Herren's [1] first report, they approached the corpus callosum through a large right frontal parietal craniotomy. Exactly which structures they resected were variable among patients. Their surgeries included partial and complete corpus callosum sectioning with and without unilateral division of the fornix. Their complete callosal section was done through one craniotomy. On the other hand, Bogen [17] made two separate craniotomies for cutting the anterior or posterior portions of the callosum. They often sectioned the anterior commissure in addition to all or some of the corpus callosum. In a later series of patients Bogen included complete section of the corpus callosum and division of the anterior and hippocampal commissures and the massa intermedia when present. Since 1962 numerous other surgical series have been published that have included sectioning various combinations of corpus callosum, massa intermedia, anterior commissure, hippocampal commissure, and unilateral fornix. The wide variability in CNS structures sectioned by different surgeons and within individual surgical series makes interpretation of results problematic.

Complete corpus callosotomy was endorsed in many of the early reports. During the past decade interest has developed for more limited callosal sections. For example, Marino and Ragazzo [8] reported that by the use of intraoperative electrocorticography, selective sectioning of only portions of the corpus callosum could result in excellent seizure outcomes. However, the tactic of limited callosal resection has not been confirmed nor widely accepted by other surgeons. The strategy of using intraoperative EEG has been suggested by the Minnesota group [13]. They place a group of electrodes on the scalp before surgery for intraoperative EEG recordings. They look for disruption of bilateral synchrony to help guide the extent of callosal resection. They have not yet reported their results using this technique. Other epileptologists [6] have advocated selective anterior callosotomy for patients thought to have frontal lobe epilepsy but in whom the lateralization of the focus could not be determined, or in whom the spread of epileptiform activity between the two hemispheres was too rapid to predict a good result with focal frontal lobe resection. We have attempted this strategy in six patients with not very encouraging results [18].

Some surgeons advocate that complete callosal sectioning should be done in two stages for the following reasons. First, it is thought to decrease the severity of the postoperative disconnection syndrome (characterized by mutism, a left-sided apraxia resembling hemiparesis, and bilateral frontal lobe reflexes) that is more severe following a complete callosal sectioning. In my experience this syndrome is not only quite variable from patient to patient but is also somewhat dependent on how much callosum is sectioned and the degree of retraction on the frontal lobe during surgery. The second reason for staging complete section is that anterior callosal section may provide a satisfactory outcome in some patients. When the surgery is staged, the first stage includes sectioning of the anterior two thirds of the callosum or whatever is easily approached by the initial surgical exposure. The second stage is done several months later, after a reasonable period of time has passed and the outcome from the first surgery can be determined accurately. During the second stage, the remainder of the corpus callosum is resected.

Thus, a review of the literature will show that surgeons have reported a variety of procedures that include staging a complete section of the corpus callosum with or without including sectioning of the anterior commissure, the hippocampal commissures, the massa intermedia (when present), and one fornix. The more extensive surgeries have been termed commissurotomy rather than callosotomy, and any comparison between surgical series should make this distinction. In other words, if only the corpus callosum is sectioned, either partially or in its entirety, the surgery should be called *corpus callosotomy*. If the callosum and other midline structures are sectioned, the procedure should be termed *commissurotomy*.

Preoperative Evaluation

The preoperative evaluation is the same for any person considered for epilepsy surgery. It is assumed the patient is refractory to reasonable trials of conventional anticonvulsants. An MRI scan is done regardless of the patient's age and age of seizure onset. The MRI scan excludes a causal structural lesion. The scan also helps the surgeon visualize the corpus callosum and the cavum septum pellucidum preoperatively. (In fact, close examination of enlarged coronal images can often tell the surgeon if the pericallosal arteries are bilateral or singular. This point is worth knowing prior to the dissection to the callosum.) Next, long-term EEG/video monitoring (with scalp electrodes) determines the patient's seizure type (i.e., complex-partial, tonic, atonic, etc.). At our center, patients with complex-partial seizures are not considered for corpus callosotomy unless invasive monitoring is done to show that a focal resection is clearly not indicated. However, if the patient's seizures are obviously tonic, tonic-clonic, or atonic, and no structural lesion is present, corpus callosotomy is considered without invasive monitoring.

If possible, all patients are given a routine neuropsychological test battery that includes various tests of memory, speech, and motor function. Tests of behavioral function, such as the Minnesota Multiphasic Personality Inventory (MMPI) and the Washington Psychosocial Inventory (WPSI) are also administered.

Finally, an intracarotid amobarbital (Amytal) test determines language laterality and (if possible) memory integrity. Sass et al. [19] have reported that patients with mixed cerebral speech dominance (e.g., a right-handed person with also right cerebral speech dominance) are at risk for post-callosotomy language impairments. This complication appears to involve primarily verbal output (speech and writing) and to spare verbal comprehension. It seems to be more common following complete callosotomy rather than an anterior callosotomy.

Surgical Procedure

A major complication of the operation is air embolism, which is most likely due to a tear in the superior sagittal sinus during the initial part of the craniotomy. In addition, bleeding from the sagittal sinus can cause a significant blood loss within a short period of time. Thus, our policy is not to begin surgery without transfusable blood being available in the operating room. Because of the concern of transfusion reaction, hepatitis, and transmission of acquired immunodeficiency syndrome (AIDS), we request adult patients to bank 1–2 units of blood 1 month prior to surgery. Thus, autologous blood is available if needed. For pediatric patients we request that family members be cross-matched, and if a suitable donor is available, a directed donation is made immediately prior to surgery.

In our experience patients who have undergone callosotomy with narcotic anesthesia are often slow to arouse after surgery and consequently are difficult to evaluate neurologically. We have therefore abandoned narcotic anesthesia in favor of inhalation agents. We induce anesthesia with an appropriate amount of thiopental sodium (Sodium Pentothal) followed by an inhalation agent of choice, oxygen, and nitrous oxide. After general anesthesia is induced, a Foley catheter is inserted and a lumbar cerebrospinal fluid (CSF) drain is implanted. CSF is drained from the time the cannula is placed until the callosum is sectioned. Many surgeons position the patient supine, but this requires the frontal lobe to be retracted laterally. To decrease frontal lobe retraction, use the lateral decubitus position. The lateral decubitus position will allow gravity to pull the dependent hemisphere gently away from the falx, so that with CSF drainage and hyperventilation (and mannitol only if needed) brain retraction should not be necessary. After the lumbar CSF drain is implanted, the patient is moved to the lateral decubitus position and secured with the Mayfield head holder. The neck is placed in a neutral position. The operating table is tilted at an incline (head up) of approximately 15 degrees. Hyperventilation is maintained for a pCO_2 of 25 mm Hg.

A rectilinear vertex scalp incision is centered over the junction of the coronal and sagittal sutures. A four-hole bone flap is elevated. The remainder of the operation is done using an operating microscope. I prefer to operate in the sitting position using a sterile draped Mayo stand to support my elbows. A self-irrigating bipolar cautery is used throughout the dissection. The dura over the dependent hemisphere is opened to the edge of the sagittal sinus. The dural flap is pulled tight with retention sutures to provide maximum exposure of the interhemispheric fissure. The midline adhesions between arachnoid and dura are lysed using the bipolar cautery. All attempts are made to not sacrifice bridging veins, but one or two veins (anterior to the coronal suture) can be taken if necessary. Moist cottonoid strips are placed over the medial frontal cortex of the dependent frontal lobe, and any additional adhesions between cortex and falx are broken with the bipolar cautery. Dissection is carried to the corpus callosum, which is identified after exposing both pericallosal arteries. Without identifying these structures, the cingulate gyrus can sometimes be mistaken for the callosum. After separating the two arteries the corpus callosum is opened in the midline, entering into the cavum septum pellucidum. Rarely, one major pericallosal artery supplies both medial cerebral regions. This situation makes the surgery more difficult because the single vessel must be manipulated during the callosal dissection without destroying vessels branching to either hemisphere. Care is taken to avoid opening the ventricular ependyma. The entire genu is divided, and then dissection is carried posteriorly until the splenium is the only structure that remains undivided. The entire callosum can be sectioned if desired. It is difficult intraoperatively to know exactly how much of the callosum has actually been destroyed. Awad et al. [20] have reported a method for estimating the extent of callosotomy in the operating room with simple lateral skull films.

After the callosum has been divided, the lumbar CSF drain is removed, the pCO_2 allowed to rise to 40 mm Hg, and the wound generously irrigated to replace most of the drained spinal fluid. If nitrous oxide anesthesia is used, it is stopped at this time. If mannitol was used earlier, intravenous fluid can partially replace what was lost during the diuresis. The dura is approximated, dural tack-up sutures are secured, and the craniotomy is closed in layers. Blood loss should be no more than 150 ml.

Postoperative Care

The patient is observed in the intensive care unit for the first 24 hours. During this time, the patient's neurologic signs may fluctuate and be compromised by the disconnection syndrome. The patient may not verbalize readily nor move much to stimulation, and may even have unexplained pupillary inequality. Because of these findings we often obtain a computed tomography (CT) scan during the evening of surgery to assure ourselves that the patient is not developing a space-occupying lesion. By the second postoperative day the patient should be returning to baseline neurologic status.

At a later time, should one wish to evaluate the extent of callosal sectioning, an MRI scan in midsagittal plane can provide an excellent method for doing so.

Seizure Outcome

The patient is maintained on the same anticonvulsant regimen as before surgery. During the first postoperative week there may be an increase in seizures, but this should be only transient. The seizure outcome from callosotomy is quite variable. Our results seem to be typical of what has been reported.

Between December 1984 and September 1989, we have done a total of 77 operations on 66 patients; 11 patients had completion of an anterior corpus callosotomy. Seven (11%) have been completely seizure-free since surgery, and 12 patients have not been helped by surgery (i.e., had less than a 50% reduction in seizures). Forty-five patients have had between 50% and 95% reduction in seizures, with the majority of these patients showing about 65% reduction in seizures. Of the 11 patients who had a completion of their callosotomies, none were changed from improved to seizure-free. In other words, although completing the callosotomy improved seizure control somewhat, it was, in our experience, not worth the risk of the second surgery. It was also the case that the patients who underwent completion of the corpus sectioning had a higher rate of complications than did those who had only anterior callosotomy. Because of these results we advocate a 80–85% sectioning initially (leaving only part of the splenium) and no longer consider completing the section at a later time.

In my view, the major problem with this surgery is that it has resulted in incomplete seizure control in the majority of patients. Even with good preoperative instruction to the patient and family, if the patient remains with seizures after surgery the patient and family are likely to be disappointed with the results of surgery. However, for patients who suffer from frequent seizure-related injuries, the surgery may be of benefit by simply decreasing the number of injuries.

Neurologic Outcome

The neurologic sequelae are very few, providing there have been no intraoperative complications. Transient left hemiparesis has been reported, but we have found that the lateral decubitus position has eliminated this problem. Temporary bladder incontinence has been associated with damage to the cingulate gyrus.

Numerous psychological studies [21,22] have been done on patients who have undergone various degrees of midline commissurotomies. Most of them indicate that although tests can be given that demonstrate problems in interhemispheric information transfer, these changes do not seem to hinder the patients in their activities of daily living. Many of the earlier studies, however, have been with patients who underwent more extensive commissurotomies and not just partial or complete callosotomies. There have been reports of memory difficulties after complete callosotomy [23].

We have observed some behavioral changes following callosotomy. This has occurred most often in retarded children. It is characterized by a deterioration of impulse control and increase in aggressive outbursts. Similar findings have been observed by the Yale group (SS Spencer, personal communication). Although we have no formal measures of this behavior, it seems that after surgery many of these patients are more alert and more aware of their surroundings. They also become more aware of their limitations and are more easily frustrated.

The EEG effects of callosotomy are primarily to disrupt bilateral synchrony. Callosotomy does not seem to eliminate the presence of active epileptogenic discharges [7,24]. Because callosotomy disrupts bilateral synchrony, the Minnesota group [25] has advocated monitoring the interictal EEG during the surgery. The callosal split is carried posteriorly until a significant disruption of the bilateral synchrony is seen. They use intraoperative intravenous methohexital to augment interictal discharges.

Purves et al. [6] have suggested that some cases of frontal lobe epilepsy may have too short an interhemispheric conduction time to be localized by standard EEG methods. They also suggest that an anterior corpus callosotomy might therefore stop contralateral spread of discharges from one frontal lobe so that subsequent EEG recording would allow localization of the epileptogenic lobe. We attempted that approach with six patients [18], but the postoperative seizure results were not good enough to continue this strategy for the present time.

Complications

From earlier series, a 50% incidence of hydrocephalus and chemical or bacterial meningitis was reported. This was probably due, in part, to opening the ependyma and can be avoided by staying within the cavum septum pellucidum for the majority of the dissection.

There have been language impairments in patients with crossed cerebral dominance [19]. All of the patients in Sass's series had problems of verbal output (speech and writing), with spared verbal comprehension. Written language skills (reading and spelling), verbal memory, and verbal reasoning abilities were impaired to varying degrees. Three patients with severe speech difficulties after surgery were right hemisphere dominant for speech and were also right handed. One left-hemisphere speech-dominant, left-handed patient was agraphic after surgery, but spoke normally.

There is an elevation of temperature for the first few days after most craniotomies. However, if the temperature elevation continues longer than approximately 72 hours, aseptic (chemical, or hemogenic) meningitis should be considered. In certain cases, there may be a smooth convalescence with a sudden attack of headache associated with a sharp rise in temperature, perhaps of a relapsing type. The diagnosis is made by lumbar puncture, which will demonstrate a varying degree of xanthochromic CSF under pressure. The CSF may have from several hundred to several thousand leukocytes per cubic millimeter. Although some authors believe that the relatively low pressure and leukocytosis can differentiate this condition from bacterial meningitis, the diagnosis can be made only with negative aerobic and anaerobic CSF cultures, and thus is a diagnosis of exclusion.

The treatment is to minimize fever with an antipyretic and has required keeping the patient on dexamethasone. I have found that the newer nonsteroidal anti-inflammatory drugs are not as effective in preventing or minimizing symptoms when this complication occurs. Some symptomatic relief can be obtained with twice-daily lumbar puncture in very symptomatic patients.

Spencer et al. [5] have reported an increase in focal seizures following corpus callosotomy, especially in patients who have asymmetrical bilateral epileptogenic foci. We have seen this in one case in which the patient developed focal myoclonic jerks in the right arm following an anterior corpus callosotomy.

We have had two postoperative clots, both epidural hematomas, in patients who were taking Depakote at the time. Divalproex sodium (Depakote) has been known to alter bleeding times and so this side effect of the drug should be considered when planning surgery.

Increased intracranial swelling or venous infarction of the frontal lobe can occur with damage to the sagittal sinus or when too many bridging veins are sacrificed during the initial exposure.

Mortality from this surgery is considerably greater than for focal cortical resections. Many of the earlier series have reported death from hydrocephalus and meningitis. In our own series we have had two deaths, one of which resulted from an air embolism due to a tear in the sagittal sinus during a second operation to complete the callosal sectioning. The second death was associated with an acute postoperative seizure.

Summary

Corpus callosotomy is regaining popularity in the treatment of seizures. The past literature concerning this surgery is somewhat problematic to interpret for several reasons. First, the surgery has never been standardized, and various combinations of midline structures have been sectioned, including fornix, anterior commissure, massa intermedia, and hippocampal commissure. Second, reported series have included combinations of partial and complete corpus callosal sectioning. Third, most series have mixed various epileptic syndromes as well as seizure types with the surgical procedures just mentioned, thus confounding the results. Fourth, the guidelines for presurgical evaluation have never been standardized. Nonetheless, the operation seems to provide the majority of patients with 50–95% seizure reduction, with the majority of patients having about 65% reduction. Although it has been reported that some seizure types respond to this surgery better than do others, this remains conjectural. Furthermore, the presence of one particular seizure type does not guarantee a good outcome. My experience suggests that optimal outcome can be gained from an anterior 80–85% callosal sectioning (leaving the splenium) and that little is gained from completing the callosal sectioning at a later time. The problem with this surgery is that such a small percentage of patients seem to be made completely seizure-free. This shortcoming could be decreased with improved selection criteria.

References

1. Van Wagenen WP, Herren RY. Surgical division of commissural pathways in the corpus callosum: relation to spread of an epileptic attack. *Arch Neurol Psychiatry* 1940;44:740–59.
2. Luessenhop AJ, Dela Cruz TC, Fenichel GM. Surgical disconnection of the cerebral hemispheres for intractable seizures. Results in infancy and childhood. *JAMA* 1970;213:1630–6.
3. Wilson DH, Culver C, Waddington M, Gazzaniga M. Disconnection of the cerebral hemispheres. *Neurology* 1975;25:1149–53.
4. Wilson DH, Reeves A, Gazzaniga M. Division of the corpus callosum for uncontrollable epilepsy. *Neurology* 1978;28:649–53.
5. Spencer SS, Spencer DD, Williamson PD, Sass K, Novelly RA, Mattson RH. Corpus callosotomy for epilepsy. I. Seizure effects. *Neurology* 1988;38:19–24.
6. Purves SJ, Wada JA, Woodhurst WB, et al. Results of anterior corpus callosum section in 24 patients with medically intractable seizures. *Neurology* 1988;38:1194–201.
7. Gates JR, Leppik IE, Yap J, Gumnit RJ. Corpus callosotomy: clinical and electroencephalographic effects. *Epilepsia* 1984;25:308–16.
8. Marino R Jr, Ragazzo PC. Selective criteria and results of selective partial callosotomy. In: Reeves AG, ed. *Epilepsy and the corpus callosum.* New York: Plenum Press, 1985:281–302.
9. Spencer DD, Spencer SS. Corpus callosotomy in the treatment of medically intractable secondarily generalized seizures of children. *Cleve Clin J Med* 1989;56:S69–78.
10. Murro AM, Flanigin HF, Gallagher BB, King DW, Smith JR. Corpus callosotomy for the treatment of intractable epilepsy. *Epilepsy Res* 1988;2:44–50.
11. Rappaport ZH, Lerma P. Corpus callosotomy in the treatment of secondary generalizing intractable epilepsy. *Acta Neurochir* (Wien) 1988;94:10–4.
12. Rappaport ZH. Corpus callosum section in the treatment of intractable seizures in the Sturge-Weber syndrome. *Childs Nerv Syst* 1988;4:231–2.
13. Gates JR, Mireles R, Maxwell R, Sharbrough F, Forbes G. Magnetic resonance imaging, electroencephalogram, and selected neuropsychological testing in staged corpus callosotomy. *Arch Neurol* 1986;43:1188–91.
14. Geoffroy G, Lassonde M, Delisle F, Decarie M. Corpus callosotomy for control of intractable epilepsy in children. *Neurology* 1983;33:891–7.
15. Harbaugh RE, Wilson DH, Reeves AG, Gazzaniga MS. Forebrain commissurotomy for epilepsy. Review of 20 consecutive cases. *Acta Neurochir* (Wien) 1983;68:263–75.
16. Avila JO, Radvany J, Huck FR, et al. Anterior callosotomy as a substitute for hemispherectomy. *Acta Neurochir Suppl* (Wien) 1980;30:137–43.
17. Bogen JE, Vogel PJ. Treatment of generalized seizures by cerebral commissurotomy. *Surg Forum* 1963;14:431–3.

18. Wyler AR, Hermann BP, Richey ET. Results of reoperation for failed epilepsy surgery. *J Neurosurg* 1989; 71:815–9.

19. Sass KJ, Novelly RA, Spencer DD, Spencer SS. Postcallosotomy language impairments in patients with crossed cerebral dominance. *J Neurosurg* 1990;72: 85–90.

20. Awad IA, Wyllie E, Luders H, Ahl J. Intraoperative determination of the extent of corpus callosotomy for epilepsy: two simple techniques. *Neurosurgery* 1990; 26:102–6.

21. Sass KJ, Spencer DD, Spencer SS, Novelly RA, Williamson PD, Mattson RH. Corpus callosotomy for epilepsy. II. Neurologic and neuropsychological outcome. *Neurology* 1988;38:24–8.

22. Gazzaniga MS, Risse GL, Springer SP, Clark DE, Wilson DH. Psychologic and neurologic consequences of partial and complete cerebral commissurotomy. *Neurology* 1975;25:10–5.

23. Zaidel D, Sperry RW. Memory impairment after commissurotomy in man. *Brain* 1974;97:263–72.

24. Harbaugh RE, Wilson DH. Telencephalic theory of generalized epilepsy: observations in split-brain patients. *Neurosurgery* 1982;10:725–32.

25. Maxwell RE, Gates JR, Gumnit RJ. Corpus callosotomy at the University of Minnesota. In: Engel J Jr. ed. *Surgical treatment of the epilepsies*. New York: Raven Press, 1987:659–66.

Chapter 14
Hemispherectomy

EILEEN P.G. VINING
JOHN M. FREEMAN
BENJAMIN S. CARSON

Historical Perspective

The concept of removing massive amounts of brain or even an entire hemisphere is not new. Dandy [1] pioneered the technique of hemispherectomy in 1923 in an attempt to control the spread of cerebral glioblastomas. Even this radical approach, however, proved futile, and the technique was generally abandoned until 1950 when Krynauw [2] reported its successful use for infantile hemiplegic epilepsy. He performed a total hemispherectomy in 12 patients (ages 8 months to 21 years) who were hemiplegic and experiencing ongoing seizures and/or mental changes. The etiologies in his cases were varied, ranging from birth trauma to later events in infancy (trauma, infection, embolism). In 10 of the 12 cases in which seizures were present, all seizures stopped. Krynauw also noted marked improvement in behavior and mental function while remarking that motor function in many patients either remained unchanged or improved slightly and that, surprisingly, functions usually associated with parietal cortex were undisturbed (spatial orientation, body image). The single death reported occurred in the immediate postoperative period.

Other indications for the procedure were subsequently developed. In 1958, Rasmussen et al. [3] reported the use of hemispherectomy to treat "chronic progressive epilepsia partialis continua of childhood," which has come to be known as Rasmussen's syndrome. Again, removal of the hemisphere led to virtually complete seizure control and improved function. The revival of the procedure is reflected in the 1968 review of 420 cases by Ignelzi and Bucy [4].

Although all series reported some mortality and morbidity, these risks appeared acceptable until the report of Laine et al. [5] in 1964 of serious late complications—hemorrhage, hydrocephalus, and he-

mosiderosis. Concerns that such complications could arise even 20 years after the procedure led to abandonment of the procedure [6].

A renewal of interest occurred in the early 1980s. This stemmed from many factors, including frustration that even the newest anticonvulsant agents were ineffective against these intractable forms of epilepsy, whereas the efficacy of hemispherectomy was indisputable [7,8]. Some physicians advocated changing the procedure in the hope that the long-term risks would be diminished. This included the functional hemispherectomy advocated by Rasmussen and his Montreal colleagues [9] in which the temporal and parietal regions are removed and the frontal and occipital regions are deafferented. Adams [10] also offered an alternative that involved tacking the dura to the midline structures and that created a large extradural, rather than subdural, cavity. At Johns Hopkins we resumed doing the standard full hemispherectomy, believing that improved hemostasis techniques and improved ability to monitor patients with computed tomography (CT) and magnetic resonance imaging (MRI) would lead to either a lack of long-term complications or the ability to readily deal with them [11].

In the past 5 years, many centers have resumed doing hemispherectomies because they are convinced that the benefits clearly outweigh the risks [12]. It must be recognized, however, that the term *hemispherectomy* encompasses many procedures. The essence and fundamental principle of hemispherectomy is that the primary hemispheric functions are eliminated by tissue removal—motor, sensory, and, in the case of the left hemisphere, language function. Hemispherectomy may mean any of the following: (a) hemispherectomy with preservation of about half the hemisphere (hemihemispherectomy); (b) removal of the majority of the hemisphere with preservation of small remnants of frontal or occipital lobes; (c) large or anatomically complete hemispherectomy; (d) complete hemispherectomy with tacking of the dura to cover the midline structures; and (e) functional hemispherectomy in which the frontal and occipital portions of the hemisphere are preserved but disconnected. There are also variations on the themes even within these descriptions. Another term that is frequently used is *hemidecorticectomy*, implying that predominantly cortex, rather than underlying white matter, is removed. The neurologic deficits that each of these procedures produces are uniform. They lead to a permanent hemiplegia and hemisensory defect, as well as hemianopsia. However, whenever morbidity, mortality, or results are discussed, it is important to realize that procedures may actually differ.

Choosing Appropriate Candidates

Hemispherectomy should be *considered* whenever there is extensive *unilateral* epileptiform activity. This implies that the other hemisphere appears to be functioning normally. Much effort is directed at trying to be sure that the other hemisphere is "normal." However, this is often difficult to ascertain since it is under the influence of a hemisphere that is markedly dysfunctional. This interrelationship was well articulated by Krynauw [2]: "It would appear reasonable, therefore, to suppose that the dysrhythmia encountered in the remaining hemisphere was due, in the first instance, to an overflow from the grossly abnormal high amplitude components from the opposite and pathological hemisphere via the interhemisphere communicating pathways . . . . I feel that if any part of the hemisphere is retained, it will continue to inflict its unruly patterns on the opposite anatomically normal side, with consequent disruption of its natural physiological activities, particularly those more especially concerned with the highest intellectual integration." Recognition of this problem forces us to look not only at the electroencephalogram (EEG), but also at the seizure types, neurologic function of the child, cause of the seizures, and imaging of the "good hemisphere." Sometimes we cannot be completely certain that the "normal" hemisphere is completely normal, and this needs to be considered as we weigh the risks and benefits possible for the child.

There are two main groups of children in whom hemispherectomy is generally considered: those with unilateral developmental abnormalities of the brain and those with Rasmussen's syndrome. Many different entities are subsumed under the rubric of unilateral development abnormalities, among them abnor-

malities in cell migration, heterotopias, pachygyria, polymicrogyria, porencephaly, vascular events affecting a single hemisphere, and Sturge-Weber disease.

Candidacy for hemispherectomy has traditionally been deferred until a child has a total hemiplegia, on the assumption that society and parents will not tolerate a procedure that creates a deficit or that they will forget the reason for the procedure and blame the physician for the handicap. However, when a substantial hemiparesis is already present, when frequent seizures are interfering with daily function, or when electrical activity and/or medication is interfering with intellectual function of the normal hemisphere, it seems that the creation of such a deficit is a reasonable price to pay for seizure control, for decrease in anticonvulsant toxicity, and for stabilization. After the procedure, improvement in overall function is frequently seen.

This approach, which some might refer to as anticipatory, has already gained acceptance with respect to children with Sturge-Weber disease [13]. The literature of temporal lobectomy in children also suggests that earlier surgery, once the intractability of the seizures is clearly established, seems to be associated with better outcomes than when surgery was deferred [14].

Establishing Unilaterality

Many children are referred for surgical management of intractable seizures. Two elements are critical when considering hemispherectomy as opposed to limited focal excision or corpus callosotomy. First, the abnormality must involve the majority of the hemisphere so that piecemeal resections are not valid, and second, the epileptogenic tissue must be confined to a single hemisphere.

The focal, unilateral nature of the seizures in Rasmussen's syndrome is usually apparent. The diagnosis of Sturge-Weber disease is readily made, and it is the rare child with this condition who has bilateral abnormalities. The young child who has experienced a vascular or traumatic event that damages only one hemisphere, with changes readily visualized by neuroimaging techniques, presents little problem in deciding that a hemispherectomy is appropriate. However, the determination of unilaterality is critical and often difficult in the young child with unilateral dysmigration and developmental patterns whose seizures begin in the first few months of life. These children frequently experience seizures that are difficult to classify with respect to their partial onset, and in fact some of these children experience infantile spasms. EEGs, although quite abnormal, are often difficult to lateralize or localize. Many children have initial EEGs that suggest unilateral abnormalities that rapidly evolve into generalized patterns, even hypsarrhythmia [15,16]. Such "generalized" abnormalities are frequently sufficient justification for many physicians to deny surgery to these children on the basis that the condition is bilateral.

Two EEG techniques may be helpful in confirming unilaterality. Intravenous diazepam can sometimes suppress the secondary focus, making the unilaterality more apparent. In addition, continuous video/EEG monitoring allows the recording of ictal, rather than interictal, EEG and leads to the realization that the bilateral activity is simply reflective of extensive unilateral abnormality and that the seizure onset is actually unilateral.

Modern neuroimaging techniques may also be helpful. These include MRI with contrast agents and other techniques that are even more functionally oriented. Positron emission tomography (PET) scans have occasionally suggested unilateral pathology, even in children with hypsarrhythmia. Unilateral tissue removal has led to seizure control [17]. Other techniques such as single photon emission computed tomography (SPECT) scans may prove to be helpful in determining whether a single hemisphere is abnormal or the entire brain is dysfunctional. Development of such techniques appears to be important to further understanding these processes and in helping to decide if a process is truly unilateral. These newer diagnostic approaches have exploded the myth that bilateral EEG abnormalities *always* indicate bilateral brain disease.

The clinical outcome of patients who have undergone hemispherectomy, even in the presence of concerns about the "normalcy" of the remaining hemisphere, bears mention. The vast majority of the children have had no further seizures and have usually experienced a normalization of the EEG over the remaining hemisphere.

Decision Making

The decision-making process preceding hemispherectomy is often quite complex and difficult for the physician, the patient, and the patient's family. The process is also somewhat different for children with Rasmussen's syndrome and those with developmental abnormalities.

Rasmussen's Syndrome

When Rasmussen's syndrome is suspected, and we believe the diagnosis can be made on the basis of the clinical history, the family knows that the child was previously normal. The family remembers the normally developing child who suddenly became abnormal, deteriorating over various periods of time, sometimes seeming to stabilize and perhaps even seeming to gain ground slightly. It is difficult in the early stages for the family to grasp how inexorable the process really is; to realize that the child is going to get continually worse; to realize that the seizures will never be completely controlled and that there will be progressive deterioration in both motor and intellectual function. The family does not have a crystal ball or the prior experience to see the future. Only the experienced clinician, familiar with this process, can help them realize that the progressive course is inevitable. The family must be helped to understand that their child cannot return to his or her prior state; that their best hope is for eradication of seizures and elimination of medication side effects, and to allow the remaining hemisphere to function well. Physicians must also be able to recognize this inexorable process before they can be certain that they are dealing with Rasmussen's syndrome. Physicians cannot rush to these conclusions, but rather must base their recommendations on observations over a period of time. This time frame and the perspective it gives on the course of Rasmussen's syndrome may be variable but are vital to the diagnosis. A family (the parents and the child) should not be forced to see this reality, but must come to terms with it in their own time frame. Each person may come to this realization at different points, and it is not until the entire family can see the inevitability of the process that surgery should occur. However, this does not mean that the child must be totally hemiplegic before the surgery. One of our cases illustrates this point. It does not mean that piecemeal surgery in trying to eliminate only the most epileptogenic tissue to temporarily produce motor function is acceptable [18].

CASE #13

BU was entirely healthy until 5¼ years of age when she experienced her first seizure after a fall from a seesaw. It was a right focal motor seizure lasting 2 hours. A CT scan at the time showed cortical atrophy on the left side. In spite of various medications, the seizures continued and occasionally generalized. Serial CT examinations showed progression of the atrophy, and over the period of a year, BU developed a mild right hemiparesis. During seizures, her family noted that her speech sometimes slowed and occasionally she was actually mute. Teachers at her school noted that her language skills seemed to wax and wane. By 6½ years of age (1 year into the illness) psychometric testing documented a WPPSI FS intelligence quotient (IQ) of 95, verbal 102, and performance 88. These scores were lower than prior estimates of her potential. Her EEG showed abnormally slow background on the left and three spike foci—left occipital, left frontal, and left central. She also was reported to show relatively frequent and often independent sharp waves over the right frontal region that were presumed to be secondary. The question of Rasmussen's syndrome had been raised at this point, and she was seen in several epilepsy centers. Surgery was considered but deferred because the left hemisphere was involved and no one wanted to risk the loss of speech.

By 7 years of age (2 years into the illness), an MRI showed atrophic changes on the left and she had increasing motor dysfunction on the right. Her seizure frequency was variable, but about 20 partial seizures were noted per day, involving myoclonic jerks or posturing on her right side. She was seen at Johns Hopkins, and surgery was proposed, relying on previous experience with left hemispherectomy and knowledge that if language had not already transferred it could be expected to do so. The family was not ready to accept the risks of surgery and elected to continue to try to optimize medical therapy. The child was still active and enjoying school and retained a wonderful sense of humor and determination. The family was hopeful that the process would simply stop at that point and her condition would not deteriorate further. They could all live with the problems that they were currently facing.

Over the next 6 months, the family and the child were able to acknowledge her gradual decline. IQ testing showed a further decline, with a FS IQ of 82, verbal 84, and performance 84. Her academic and language abilities actually appeared to be below these levels. The family saw her motor abilities slowly deteriorating. When she had a seizure on stage, playing an angel in a Christmas play, they all knew the time had come for surgery. At the time of surgery, the entire family was prepared. They felt that the risks were far outweighed by the potential benefits. And in spite of a very difficult postoperative period that eventually led to an excellent recovery, the parents were able to withstand the tensions because they believed they had made the right decision for their child and because they had made it together.

Developmental Problems

It is often easier for families with children who have unilateral development problems of the brain to accept surgery, sometimes even in the face of uncertainty that the remaining hemisphere is completely normal. The majority of these families never had a normal child; they have known constant seizures since the early months of life and a child who frequently has made little developmental progress. They can only foresee a future that appears bleak, with little meaningful interaction. Even feeding is often a problem because the seizures and medications have had such devastating effects. These families are willing to take the risks and accept the consequences of surgery because they see the benefits are potentially so great and the potential losses so small. They are less concerned about a permanent hemiplegia because they have a child who can do little with either hand. When faced with these children, physicians frequently are reluctant to offer hemispherectomy because they cannot give a guarantee that the remaining hemisphere will be normal. This is particularly true when EEG abnormalities suggest bilateral involvement. It is also true when subtle changes on the MRI suggest that there may be problems with the contralateral hemisphere. However, both the family and the physician must realize an important concept. The best that can happen is that seizures will be eliminated and the remaining hemisphere will be allowed to develop unhindered by the influence of the epileptogenic tissue and medication. The worst that can happen is the death of the child. And when families have reached the desperate point of considering hemispherectomy, the possibility of the child's death has been faced any number of times during his or her seizures, with the risks of aspiration and pneumonia. It is terrible to consider, but death is an acceptable risk given the quality of life the child is currently enduring. The next-worse fate to be considered is that seizures will continue because the contralateral hemisphere is abnormal and that it will eventually serve as the source of ongoing seizures. However, this situation is really not worse than their current situation with ongoing seizures. Once these two concepts are embraced, a hemispherectomy can be considered. Some of these dilemmas are illustrated by the following case.

CASE #7

MG was a young girl with a normal gestational history who began to experience seizures immediately at birth. The seizures were generally described as flexor spasms, but other seizures involved her head and eyes turning to the side, more frequently to the left than to the right. Her original EEG showed left parieto-occipital spike activity. She continued to have almost constant seizures throughout the day. Her EEG evolved to show a grossly abnormal pattern with features of hypsarrhythmia, high-voltage bursts of spikes, and then suppression. The CT scan showed left cortical dysgenesis, which was confirmed on MRI. Multiple medications including adrenocorticotrophic hormone (ACTH) had been tried. At 3 months of age her development had never progressed, and she was about to be institutionalized because of the difficulties involved in her daily care. In spite of the focal neuroimaging studies and an early EEG that suggested focal abnormalities, the flexor spasms and evolution of the EEG pattern suggested a bilateral process and surgery was not recommended.

She was then seen at Johns Hopkins. Another EEG was performed using diazepam and showing suppression of the bilateral activity with persistence of spike activity over the left parieto-occipital region. We believed that there was sufficient evidence of a unilateral process (our EEG findings and unilateral changes on the neuroimaging studies) and proposed a left hemispherectomy. This family readily accepted the potential risks of surgery because they saw no acceptable future for their child. They were willing to take the risk that the other hemisphere might be abnormal and that there might be no improvement in seizure control or in developmental progression. They had never known any normalcy and could only hope for an improvement.

Techniques

As described above, many different techniques are subsumed under the rubric of hemispherectomy. The classical hemispherectomy described by Krynauw [2] involved dividing the hemisphere into four segments by a vertical and transverse incision of the superolateral surface *extending* into the ventricle. Each quadrant was dissected out, working from within the ventricle. The choroid plexus was carefully removed, and the middle cerebral artery was removed just lateral to the anterior perforated substance. The thalamus and the caudate nucleus and its tail were left intact.

Ignelzi and Bucy [4], in reviewing the 420 cases in the literature, also reported on their own technique of hemidecortication. It involved the following procedure: The Sylvian fissure was opened and the middle cerebral artery identified, clipped, and divided just lateral to the basal ganglia. They proceeded medially on the undersurface of the frontal lobe, exposing the anterior cerebral artery, which was occluded distal to the anterior communicating artery. The occipital lobe was then retracted and the posterior cerebral artery was identified and clipped just before it

entered the calcarine fissure. The entire cerebral cortex was then removed *en bloc,* leaving the basal ganglia and thalamus more or less intact. This extirpation was carried out above the fibers extending laterally from the corpus callosum, leaving them as a covering over the anterior horn and body of the lateral ventricle. The choroid plexus of the lateral ventricle was removed. An opening was also made in the septum pellucidum connecting the cavity on the operated side with the opposite lateral ventricle. The dura mater was then closed tightly and sutured to the defect in the skull and to the bone flap to prevent a dead space that might provide for the accumulation of blood extradurally.

When the concerns about the long-term morbidity and mortality were raised, alternative surgeries were proposed. These included a subtotal hemispherectomy frequently performed by the Montreal group [9], consisting of removal of two thirds to four fifths of the damaged hemisphere, leaving remnants of those regions believed to reflect less epileptogenic potential based on EEG findings. It was postulated that this tissue would serve as a buttress, splinting the remaining hemisphere and decreasing the likelihood that minor head trauma would lead to small bleeds and the development of hemosiderosis. In patients with Rasmussen's syndrome, complete hemispherectomy led to complete or nearly complete seizure control in 85% of patients, while the subtotal procedure led to similar results in only 68% of patients.

Adams [10] proposed an alternative approach to prevention of late mortality and morbidity—elimination of the subdural cavity and creation of an epidural cavity. He performs a standard hemispherectomy, but the dura on the operated side is freed and sutured to the falx, tentorium, and floor of the anterior and middle cerebral fossae. The residual subdural collection, although small, is further isolated from the ventricular system by obstructing the ipsilateral foramen of Monro by a plug of muscle. Follow-up has not been long enough to determine if this procedure has significant advantage.

The Montreal Group has developed still another procedure, described as a functional hemispherectomy [19]. It has been used since 1974 and consists of removing the central part of the hemisphere (motor and sensory regions) and the temporal lobe, leaving behind the anterior half of the frontal lobe and the posterior third of the hemisphere. Care is taken to preserve the vasculature of these areas. These areas are then disconnected from the remaining "normal" hemisphere and from the upper brain stem by sectioning the white matter in front of the rostrum of the corpus callosum down to the medial leptomeningeal membrane of the falx and by also sectioning the white matter behind the splenium of the corpus callosum down to the leptomeningeal membrane on the falx and tentorium. The group has reported on 21 patients who have undergone this procedure [20]. Seventeen of them have been followed from 2–11 years (median 5 years). Reduction in seizure frequency is almost identical to the complete hemispherectomy group they reported earlier. It is premature to determine if the long-term problems will be reduced by this procedure.

The UCLA group advocates still another variation. They perform the traditional complete hemispherectomy, providing acute drainage of the cavity, and then proceed to do a prophylactic shunt from the cavity created to the peritoneal space.

The Johns Hopkins surgical team advocates subdural drainage and repeated lumbar punctures in order to remove considerable amounts of high-protein, bloody CSF. This may decrease the amount of postoperative symptoms (headaches, fever, vomiting) from an apparent aseptic meningitis. Shunting the cavity is done only if symptoms of pressure occur.

None of these variations on the traditional procedure have been used long enough or with sufficient follow-up to determine if the long-term morbidity ascribed to "superficial cerebral hemosiderosis" will be decreased. The pathogenesis of that phenomenon [21] and the mechanisms by which it caused mortality and morbidity remain obscure. Some feel that the hydrocephalus causing acute decompensation many years after the original surgery can now be detected by modern radiologic techniques and treated by shunt procedures. Patients are now being followed more closely at each of these centers, and symptoms of increased pressure can be immediately evaluated with CT and MRI. Shunts can be placed if problems do develop. In addition, MRI presumably would be able to detect the deposition of hemosiderin-containing material so that children at risk of hemorrhage could be detected and treated appropriately.

Outcome

The startling success reported by Krynauw [2] included not only significant reduction in seizures but also improvement in cognitive and behavioral function. When Krynauw published his paper in 1950, six of the 10 patients had experienced complete seizure control. One patient, a child of 2½ years, died in the immediate postoperative period. Three other children who had seizures had not been followed long enough, but Krynauw notes that their seizures were completely controlled. At least seven of the twelve children had experienced significant intellectual improvement from the point of view of performance in school and daily living, and seven had clear improvement in behavior. Two of the children also seemed to show evidence of improved motor function.

Ignelzi and Bucy [4], in their review of the literature on hemispherectomy in 1968, also included four of their own cases in which hemidecortication had been done. They reported complete seizure control and improved motor function in all four patients. Their review of the literature indicated that although 420 cases had been reported, only 240 had sufficient detail for any analysis, and even then follow-up was limited. Follow-up was reported in less than half the cases in the literature, and this ranged from 3 days to 10 years, with an average of 1.5 years. In the 198 cases in which motor function was well documented, 57.9% showed improved motor function, and one third had significant improvement. Seizures were abolished in 76% of the 171 cases reported, decreased in 18%, and worsened in only 2%. Personality improved in 95% of the 141 cases in which such changes could be determined. In the 131 cases in which intellectual function was documented, IQ improved in 82% and decreased in only 5%.

In the preliminary Johns Hopkins experience [11], 26 hemispherectomies have been followed 1.5–21.58 years (average 4.59 years). Overall, 68% (17 children) are seizure-free. This ranges from 75% for those with Rasmussen's syndrome to 61% for those with developmental abnormalities. The three patients with Rasmussen's syndrome who continue to have seizures include the one patient who had a hemidecorticectomy 23 years ago, leaving cortical tissue behind and connected in the hemisphere, and a second patient who had experienced exceptionally severe episodes of status and who was actually operated on after having been flown to us intubated, with status being controlled by barbiturate coma and paraldehyde. We believe she experienced damage to the previously normal opposite hemisphere prior to surgery. The third person was the oldest individual operated on who experienced a brief recurrence when her last antiepileptic drug was tapered. The children with developmental abnormalities who continue to have seizures include one youngster in whom we suspected bilateral problems prior to surgery, one who had a very long-standing seizure disorder before she was operated on, and the young woman who had experienced a vascular event in infancy and underwent only a subtotal hemispherectomy.

Psychological Testing and Function

The function of children preoperatively and postoperatively is shown in Table 14-1. Frequently, due to the severe debilitation and/or young age of the child, only an estimate of IQ or developmental quotient can be made.

Parents, with the exception of the family of the one child with bilateral developmental abnormalities who continues to experience seizures and the parents of one child with Sturge-Weber disease who had a stormy postoperative course and who continues to have significant neurologic handicap, uniformly have

Table 14-1. Functional Assessment of Hemispherectomy Patients

Patient	Etiology	Age at Operation	Preoperative Function	Age at Follow-Up	Postoperative Function
1	R	4.50	Bedridden IQ <50	25.25	Community residence IQ 60–70
2	R	16.25	Bedridden	29.83	Part-time work IQ 51
3	R	14.33	IQ 59	24.08	High school graduate Clerical work IQ 67
4	D	18.25	IQ 67	24.17	IQ 80 Married Licensed day-care worker Delayed
5	D	0.75	Delayed DQ 30	6.08	DQ 30
6	R	4.25	Nonambulatory DQ 50	8.08	IQ 77 Dances
7	D	0.25	Pre-institution Functions as newborn	3.92	Normal school IQ 80s Ambulatory IQ 60s
8	D	1.08	Tube fed DQ 25	4.58	IQ 82
9	R	3.83	IQ 81	7.25	IQ 52 In school
10	R	5.25	Bedridden Barely verbal	8.42	IQ 44 Ambulates
11	R	12.92	ICU-status Not testable	15.83	Regular school IQ 77
12	R	5.75	Nonambulatory DQ 50	8.75	IQ 98
13	R	7.67	IQ 82	10.00	Stable Junior college graduate
14	R	20.58	IQ 76	22.58	Deceased
15	D	0.83	DQ 30		Improved DQ 25
16	D	2.17	DQ 25	3.58	DQ 25
17	D	6.58	DQ 25	7.92	
18	D	0.58	DQ 20	1.67	DQ 10
19	R	6.92	IQ 70	8.00	IQ 65
20	D	1.58	DQ 30	2.58	No change
21	R	14.33	IQ 92	15.33	IQ 92
22	D	4.08	DQ 20	5.00	DQ 25
23	D	2.50	DQ 40	3.42	IQ 84
24	D	1.83	DQ 60	2.50	DQ 60
25	D	2.17	DQ 60	2.83	DQ 65
26	D	1.67	DQ 30	2.33	DQ 20

Key: R = Rasmussen's syndrome; D = development abnormalities; DQ = estimated development quotient; postoperative function measured June 1989.

informed us of the improved function and better quality of life seen in their children.

The Risks

With a surgical procedure of this magnitude, there is the obvious risk of mortality. A 6.6% postoperative mortality rate was found in the 269 cases reviewed by White in 1961 [22]. These patients had been followed a mean of 16 months. After Laine's 1964 report of long-term morbidity [5], several series documented the significant morbidity and mortality. Wilson's 1970 paper reported that 12% died of early complications and 20% died of late complications [23]. In the Montreal series of 29 patients who underwent anatomically complete hemispherectomy between 1952 and 1968, two (7%) died within the first postoperative year. Eleven of the surviving 27 patients (41%) developed superficial cerebral hemosiderosis 5–24 years after surgery. Five died, three made partial recoveries, and three who were diagnosed and treated early have restabilized and returned to their precomplication neurologic status. The total mortality rate in this population was therefore 24% [20].

In the Johns Hopkins series of 26 patients, many children have experienced perioperative and postoperative problems, the majority of which resolved or could be successfully treated. Thirty-five percent experienced significant aseptic meningitis, which we believe is related to the chemical/immunologic inflammation associated with resorption of blood and other byproducts of surgery. This problem may have decreased with the surgical intent of not entering the ventricular space and with aggressive lumbar puncture in the immediate postoperative period. Aseptic meningitis occurred in 56% of children operated on between 1980 and 1986 and in only 21% operated on in the past two years. Proven bacterial meningitis that responded well to antibiotics has occurred in 29% of the recent cases. Difficult-to-manage metabolic derangement problems in the immediate postoperative period occurred in some of our youngest children. Significant bleeding occurred in four children, and at times this is believed to have caused damage to the "good hemisphere." Death occurred in one child under 1 year of age who was operated on for the second time to complete the hemispherectomy because seizures had not been stopped by a previous, more conservative corticectomy.

Summary

Hemispherectomy can be a lifesaving procedure. In cases of Rasmussen's syndrome, when done early,

prior to "complete hemiplegia," it may result in children of normal intelligence, who are seizure-free and on no medication, who run and play, but whose paretic hand is only a helper hand. This motoric outcome is similar to that reported from Montreal and Toronto, but the intellectual outcome seems even better.

In children with unilateral developmental problems, the procedure has allowed for more normal intellectual outcomes, often approaching the mildly retarded range and continuing to improve years after surgery. The hemiparesis has not been the limiting function in any of the children.

The only major discrepancies among the centers performing this procedure is the technique by which it is done (a distinction without a proven difference) and the timing of the procedure. At Johns Hopkins we believe that earlier surgery decreases intercurrent morbidity and seems to produce better long-term outcomes.

References

1. Dandy W. Removal of right cerebral hemisphere for certain tumors with hemiplegia: preliminary report. *JAMA* 1928;90:823–5.
2. Krynauw RA. Infantile hemiplegia treated by removing one cerebral hemisphere. *J Neurol Neurosurg Psychiatry* 1950;13:243–67.
3. Rasmussen T, Olszewski J, Lloyd-Smith D. Focal seizures due to chronic localized encephalitis. *Neurology* 1958;8:435–45.
4. Ignelzi RJ, Bucy PC. Cerebral hemidecortication in the treatment of infantile cerebral hemiatrophy. *J Nerv Mental Dis* 1968;147:14–30.
5. Laine E, Pruvet P, Osson D. Resultats eloignes de l'hemispherectomie dans les cas d'hemiatrophie cerebrale infantile generatrice d'epilepsie. *Neuro-Chirug* 1964;10:507–22.
6. Wilson PJ. Cerebral hemispherectomy for infantile hemiplegia: a report of 50 cases. *Brain* 1970;93:147–80.
7. Goodman R. Hemispherectomy and its alternatives in the treatment of intractable epilepsy in patients with infantile hemiplegia. *Dev Med Child Neurol* 1986;28:251–8.
8. Lindsay J, Ounsted C, Richards P. Hemispherectomy for childhood epilepsy: a 36-year study. *Dev Med Child Neurol* 1987;29:592–600.
9. Rasmussen T. Hemispherectomy for seizures revisited. *Can J Neurol Sci* 1983;10:71–8.
10. Adams CBT. Hemispherectomy—a modification. *J Neurol Neurosurg Psychiatry* 1983;46:617–9.
11. Vining EPG, Freeman JM, Carson BS, Brandt J. Hemispherectomy in children, the Hopkins experience: 1968–1988. A preliminary report. *J Epilepsy*, 1990.

12. Duchowny MS. Surgery for intractable epilepsy: issues and outcome. *Pediatrics* 1989;84:886–94.

13. Hoffman HJ, Hendrick EB, Dennis M, Armstrong D. Hemispherectomy for Sturge-Weber syndrome. *Childs Brain* 1979;5:233–48.

14. Lindsay J, Ounsted C, Richards P, Ounsted C. Developmental aspects of focal epilepsies of childhood treated by neurosurgery. *Dev Med Child Neurol* 1984;26:574–87.

15. Vining EPG, Carson B, Freeman JM, et al. "Bilateral" epileptic abnormalities: a unilateral cure. *Epilepsia* 1987;28:591.

16. Vigevano F, Bertini E, Boldrini, et al. Hemimegalencephaly and intractable epilepsy: benefits of hemispherectomy. *Epilepsia* 1989;30:833–43.

17. Chugani HT, Shewmon DA, Peacock WJ, Shields WD, Mazziotta JC, Phelps ME. Surgical treatment of intractable neonatal-onset seizures: the role of positron emission tomography. *Neurology* 1988:38:1178–88.

18. Piatt JH, Hwang PA, Armstrong DC, Becker LE, Hoffman HJ. Chronic focal encephalitis (Rasmussen's syndrome): six cases. *Epilepsia* 1988;29:268–79.

19. Tinuper P, Anderman F, Villemure JG. Functional hemispherectomy for treatment of epilepsy associated with hemiplegia. *Ann Neurol* 1988;24:27–34.

20. Rasmussen T, Villemure JG. Cerebral hemispherectomy for seizures with hemiplegia. *Cleve Clin J Med* 1989;56(Suppl):S62–8.

21. Oppenheimer DR, Griffith HB. Persistent intracranial bleeding as a complication of hemispherectomy. *J Neurol Neurosurg Psychiatry* 1966;29:229–40.

22. White HH. Cerebral hemispherectomy in the treatment of infantile hemiplegia: review of the literature and report of 2 cases. *Confinia Neurol* 1961;21:1–50.

23. Wilson PJE. More second thoughts on hemispherectomy in infantile hemiplegia. *Dev Med Child Neurol* 1970;12:799–800.

Chapter 15

Selective Amygdalohippocampectomy

HEINZ GREGOR WIESER

Better knowledge of the electroclinical semiology of seizures, and in particular of the site of seizure initiation and spread, was gained from direct intracerebral depth recordings during presurgical evaluation of candidates for epilepsy surgery. These findings led us to classify complex-partial seizures (CPS) into five subtypes: (a) mesiobasal limbic, (b) temporal polaramygdalar, (c) temporal lateral (neocortical-posterior), (d) opercular-insular, and (e) frontobasal-cingulate [1]. By far the most frequent and therefore the most important subtype of CPS is the mesiobasal limbic one. In our series, 65% of seizures classified as mesiobasal limbic originated simultaneously in the hippocampus and amygdala (Fig. 15-1), 25% in the hippocampus only (Fig. 15-2), and about 10% in the amygdala. Of those with amygdalar origin approximately two thirds invade the hippocampus within 3 to 5 s [2].

Based on these findings, we have argued that in patients with seizures of mesiobasal limbic origin, the "classical" anterior temporal lobe (TL) resection is too crude a surgical operation. The need for a more selective resection of the mesiobasal limbic structure [3] was satisfied by G. Yasargil and resulted in the selective amygdalohippocampectomy (AHE), performed in our hospital since 1975. At the end of June 1992, a total of 293 patients had undergone this operation in Zürich. At the second Palm Desert Conference on the Surgical Treatment of the Epilepsies [4] it was reported that worldwide a total of 548 AHEs were performed during the period 1986–1990.

During the first years, the indication in Zürich for AHE was strictly confined to patients with focal seizure onset within the amygdala and hippocampal formation ("causal AHE"). Satisfying early results [5] led us then to offer this type of operation also to certain patients with a seizure origin in the lateral temporal cortex, in particular when located in the dominant hemisphere encroaching on indispensable language areas, but only if a secondary pacemaker role of the ipsilateral hippocampal formation could be proven ("palliative AHE"). Although the results of the palliative AHE were clearly less favorable compared with those obtained with a "causal indication" (Table 15-1), in general they were good enough to justify this approach. In turn, the sometimes unexpectedly good postoperative seizure control following palliative AHE led us to conceptualize the so-called amplifier role of the hippocampal formation, and in particular of the parahippocampal gyrus [1,6].

Although AHE is done today with a less restrictive indication than during the first decade of its use, it should be emphasized that in essence it remains a surgical treatment for drug-resistant temporal lobe epilepsy with a well-defined, unilateral mesiobasal limbic seizure onset *only* [2].

The principal objective of this chapter is to review the results obtained with this operation. A few remarks on the operative anatomy and surgical technique seem necessary, however. A more detailed description of the main surgical steps of this operation has been published elsewhere [7–9].

Principles of the Operative Technique

Parenthetically it should be noted that the term *selective amygdalohippocampectomy* is not entirely correct, since it does not denote the removal of the parahippocampal gyrus, which is partly resected also. During 1975–1980, the operative technique was slightly modified several times. Since then, however,

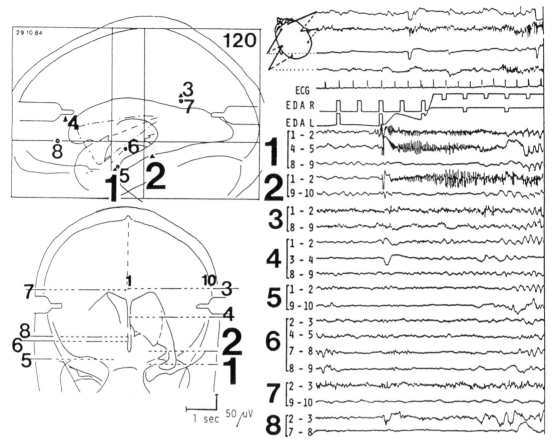

Figure 15-1. Combined scalp and stereotaxic depth (SEEG) recording at the beginning of a typical complex-partial seizure, showing the simultaneous seizure onset in the left amygdala (1/1–2 and 1/4–5) and hippocampus (2/1–2). There is a change in the electrodermal activity (EDA) measured at the right (*R*) and left (*L*) hands. (ECG, electrocardiogram). The localization of the depth electrodes (*large bold numbers*) is indicated in the stereotaxic reference scheme. Each hollow-core electrode has 10 contacts (*small numbers*), with contact 1 located at the tip of the electrode.

the AHE has become a fairly standardized operation, as described by Yasargil et al. [7,10]. Following a modified interfascial pterional craniotomy [11], the trans-sylvian route—with a cortical incision of 1–2 cm lateral to the M-1 segment and anteromedial to the M-2 segment into the superior temporal gyrus—has been adapted to gain access to the tip of the temporal horn and to the amygdala. The amygdala is removed piecemeal both by rongeur (to provide histologic specimens) and by gentle suction. By use of the

Table 15-1. AHE Series: Comparison of Results of "Causal" Versus "Palliative" Operations.*

| | | Seizure Outcome Categories | | | | | Follow-Up |
	n	I	II	III	IV	n.cl.	Mean ± SD† (Months)
Causal AHE	37	22 (73%)	6 (20%)	— (0%)	2 (7%)	7	50.4 ± 35.3
Palliative AHE	28	3 (12%)	— (0%)	8 (31%)	15 (58%)	2	55.7 ± 31.0

*Last available seizure outcome of "non-lesional" patients with either normal histologic findings (*n* = 34) or gliosis only (*n* = 37). For outcome classification, see Table 15-5.
†SD = standard deviation.

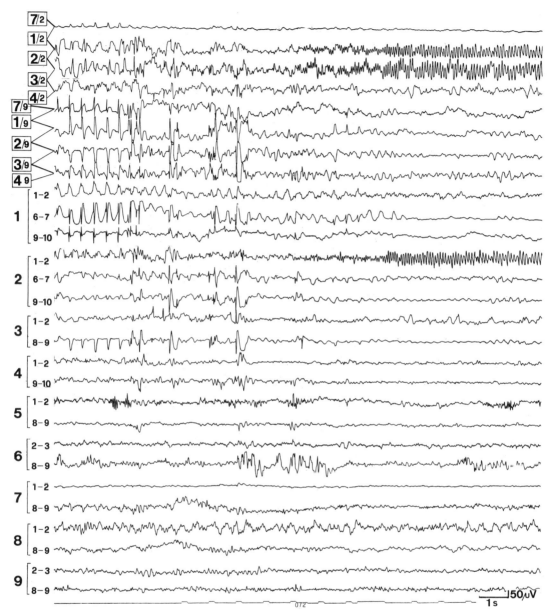

Figure 15-2. (*A*) Stereotaxic depth recording showing the transition from the preictal state (*left half*), with regional interictal epileptogenicity more pronounced in the lateral cortex, to a strictly localized seizure onset in the left hippocampus (2/1–2). Note that in addition to the orthogonal short-distance bipolar derivations (channels 9–28) two chains of bipolar long-distance derivations (channels 1–8) are used, which connect, in the parasagittal plane, either the contacts 2 or the contacts 9 of the electrodes 7-1-2-3-4. In the longer parasagittal chain the phase reversal of the ictal discharge is clearly at 2/2.

so-called keyhole technique, the hippocampus and the more anterior parts of the parahippocampal gyrus are then resected *en bloc*. The resected specimen measures approximately 3.5–4 cm in length, 1.5 cm in width, and 2 cm in depth. In the anteroposterior plane the posterior transection of the parahippocam-

pal gyrus is at the level of the bifurcation of the P-2 segment to form the P-3 segments. This is at the level of the lateral geniculate body, where the fimbria ascends to the splenium to form the crus of the fornix.

Figure 15-3 shows the extent of the resection in serial magnetic resonance imaging (MRI) scans and

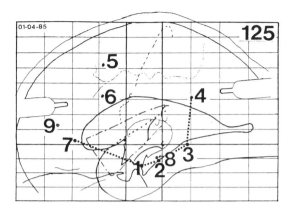

Figure 15-2. (*B*) This figure illustrates the importance of defining the primary epileptogenic zone by means of the ictal information, since this patient is seizure-free following a left AHE. Would one have relied on the interictal information, a more extensive temporal lobectomy with removal of the lateral cortex would have been suggested by the interictal EEG information.

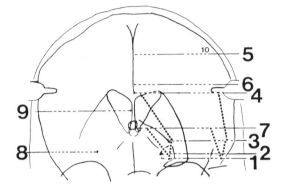

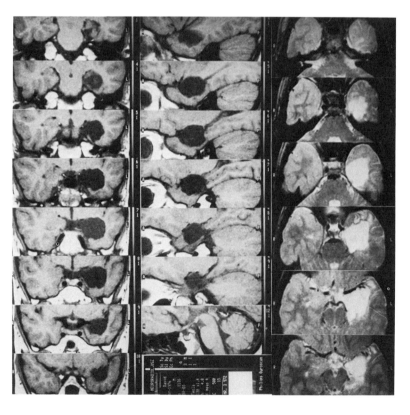

Figure 15-3. Composition of serial MRI scans in all three planes showing the resection following a left selective AHE in a patient evaluated with the multipolar foramen ovale electrode recording technique [32]. Coronal and sagittal images are T1-weighted, whereas the transverse images are T2-weighted (in order to improve visualization of suspected gliosis adjacent to the borders of the resection). The patient was operated on at age 11 years and remains seizure-free since the operation; postoperative follow-up was 4 years, and the patient has been off drugs since the end of the first postoperative year.

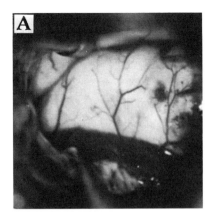

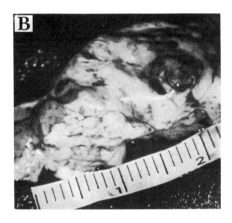

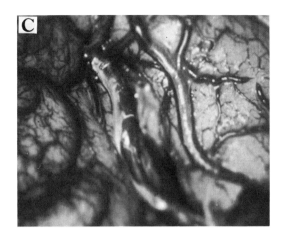

Figure 15-4. (*A*) Visualization of the pes hippocampi *in situ* through the microscope. (*B*) Removed hippocampus. (*C*) Situation after completion of a left selective AHE. From Yasargil MG, Wieser HG. Selective amygdalohippocampectomy at the University Hospital, Zürich. In: Engel J Jr. ed. *Surgical treatment of the epilepsies.* New York: Raven Press, 1987: 653–8. With permission.

The situation following the completed operation is shown in Figure 15-4.

Relationships between MR-Imaged Total Amount of Tissue Removed, Resection Scores of Specific Mesiobasal Limbic Subcompartments, and Clinical Outcome Following Selective Amygdalohippocampectomy

In a recently published study [12] my colleagues and I examined 30 patients in whom special preoperative and postoperative MRI was carried out and who had a follow-up of at least 1 year postoperatively. The mean total size of the resection was 7.2 cm^3 (range 2.1–17.7 cm^3). The extent of the removal with respect to anatomically defined specific limbic subcompartments [13] was rated by an estimation procedure involving three persons. The mean resection scores (in percentages) of the limbic subcompartments obtained from this study are amygdala 92%, pes hippocampi 92%, uncus 92%, hippocampus 46%, dentate gyrus 45%, parahippocampal gyrus 32%, and subiculum 40% (Fig. 15-5).

The main correlations with respect to the outcome are as follows: The seizure outcome tended to be the better the larger the resected volume. Since the resection scores of amygdala, pes hippocampi, and uncus are more or less the same in all outcome categories (I–IV; see Fig. 15-5), the seizure outcome correlated most distinctly with the extent of the resection of the parahippocampal gyrus and in particular with that of its subicular part.

Neuropathologic Findings

Table 15-2 shows the neuropathologic findings of the Zürich AHE series based on 215 patients. Tumors were classified according to the recommendations of the World Health Organization (WHO). In order to simplify further analyses, we grouped them into benign, semibenign, and malignant tumors. Arteriovenous malformations (AVM), cavernous angiomas, hamartomas and epidermoid cysts were classified together as dysontogenetic lesions (in all of these an abnormal ontogenesis is assumed). Hippocampal gliosis was differentiated into slight, moderate, and severe.

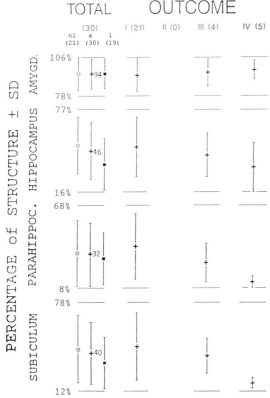

Figure 15-5. Percentage of removal per indicated limbic subcompartment for a total of 30 examined patients (*TOTAL*) and the split-up according to seizure outcome categories I–IV. The rubric TOTAL is further divided into nonlesional (*nl*) and lesional (*l*) cases. Note that the seizure outcome is better the more radical the removal of the parahippocampal gyrus, and in particular the subicular part. The numerical values of removal of the respective structures in percent of the anatomically [11] defined structure, are given with the figure as means for the respective group. Vertical bars represent ± standard deviation (SD). For definition of the outcome categories, see Table 15-6. Numbers in parentheses refer to the number of patients.

This grouping therefore resulted in nine histologic classes: benign ($n = 26$), semibenign ($n = 47$), and malignant ($n = 37$) tumors; dysontogenetic lesions ($n = 32$); sequelae of encephalitis ($n = 2$); slight ($n = 22$), moderate ($n = 9$), and severe ($n = 6$) gliosis; and no microscopic pathology ($n = 34$). This grouping was used for further analyses (Table 15-2).

Twenty-two patients underwent reoperations because of recurrence of tumor: 20 patients had one, one patient had two, and one patient had three reoperations. Thirty-nine patients have died: 37 patients had recurrence of tumors, and two patients died as a

consequence of having been inoculated with Creutzfeldt-Jakob disease. The circumstances of the latter extraordinary complication have been reported elsewhere [14]. The mean postoperative survival time of the 39 patients was 20.9 months.

Clinical Characteristics

In Zürich AHE series, more males ($n = 120$; 56%) than females ($n = 95$; 44%) were operated on. The AHE was on the right in 114 patients (53%) and on the left in 101 patients (47%).

The mean age at onset of epilepsy was 18.8 years. As might be expected, age at onset was the lowest in patients without a lesion or with gliosis compared with those with tumors. It is lower in patients with

Table 15-2. AHE Series: Neuropathologic Findings

Benign Tumors	**26**
Pilocytic astrocytoma, WHO I	11
Subependymal giant cell astrocytoma, WHO I, with tuberous sclerosis	4
Ganglioglioma, WHO I	9
Fibroblastic meningioma, WHO I	1
Meningotheliomatous meningioma, WHO I	1
Semibenign Tumors	**47**
Fibrillary astrocytoma, WHO II	23
Gemistocytic astrocytoma, WHO II	1
Oligodendroglioma, WHO II	16
Mixed oligo-astrocytoma, WHO II	6
Ganglioglioma, WHO II	1
Malignant Tumors	**37**
Anaplastic astrocytoma, WHO III	20
Anaplastic mixed oligo-astrocytoma, WHO III	1
Glioblastoma multiforme, WHO IV	12
Anaplastic ganglioglioma, WHO III	1
Anaplastic meningioma, WHO III	2
Primitive neuroectodermal tumor	1
Dysontogenetic Lesions	**32**
AVM	21
Cavernous angioma	4
Hamartoma	6
Epidermoid cyst	1
Sequelae of Encephalitis	**2**
Gliosis	
Slight	22
Moderate	9
Severe	6
No Microscopic Pathology	**34**
TOTAL	**215**

Table 15-3. AHE Series: Age at First Seizure (Years)

	n	Mean	SD*	Minimum	Maximum
Benign tumors	26	11.1	11.4	0.6	47.0
Semibenign tumors	47	23.6	15.3	0.3	57.8
Malignant tumors	37	33.6	17.5	4.0	73.9
Dysontogenetic lesions	32	22.0	12.0	0.2	47.0
Sequelae of encephalitis	2	12.3	11.8	4.0	20.7
Gliosis					
Slight	22	11.7	8.6	0.5	31.0
Moderate	9	10.4	5.5	1.0	19.0
Severe	6	5.3	4.3	1.0	12.0
No microscopic pathology	34	8.5	6.1	0.5	25.0
TOTAL	215	18.8	15.3	0.2	73.9

*SD = standard deviation.

benign than in those with malignant tumors. Furthermore, there was a good correlation between age at first seizure and severity of gliosis: patients with severe gliosis had their first seizure earlier in life than those with slight gliosis (Table 15-3).

The mean preoperative duration of seizure illness was 11.0 years. It was shorter in patients with malignant tumors than in patients with benign tumors; the more severe the gliosis, the longer the duration, and it was longer in patients without pathologic histologic findings compared with patients with tumors (Table 15-4).

The mean age at operation was 29.7 years. As can be seen from Table 15-5, patients with malignant tumors were older at operation than patients with benign tumors, and patients with slight gliosis were operated on at a younger age than patients with severe gliosis.

Postoperative Seizure Outcome

The epileptologic outcome was classified into four categories according to the recommendations of the International League Against Epilepsy Commission on Surgery for Epilepsy: I = seizure-free; II = rare seizures (not more than two per year); III = worthwhile improvement ($\geq 90\%$ seizure reduction and significant improvement in quality of life); and IV = no worthwhile improvement. A follow-up of at least 1 year was required. With this requirement, outcome classification was possible in 177 patients at the end of 1988.

The last available seizure outcome for the Zürich AHE series together with the follow-up period is given in Table 15-6 for each histology group. Of the 177 classified patients 105 (59%) are seizure-free; 7% have rare seizures; 11% have a worthwhile improvement; and 22% have no worthwhile improvement. The mean follow-up of these 177 patients was 47.0 months (range: 13 to 162 months).

At the second Palm Desert Conference [4] outcome data were available for 413 patients worldwide who had AHE within the period 1986–1990. The following numbers were reported: seizure-free, 68.8%; "improved," 22.3%; and "not improved," 9.0%.

Comparing the neuropathologic groups, three findings emerge: (a) in the tumoral groups (benign, semibenign, and malignant) the distribution within

Table 15-4. AHE Series: Preoperative Duration of Illness (Years)

	n	Mean	SD*	Minimum	Maximum
Benign tumors	26	9.0	7.1	0.1	28.0
Semibenign tumors	47	6.0	7.2	0.1	27.6
Malignant tumors	37	3.7	5.8	0.1	31.3
Dysontogenetic lesions	32	7.5	8.3	0.1	30.5
Sequelae of encephalitis	2	9.9	11.3	1.9	17.8
Gliosis					
Slight	22	18.5	8.1	6.1	41.1
Moderate	9	21.9	9.1	9.9	32.8
Severe	6	28.8	4.5	27.2	35.4
No microscopic pathology	34	19.5	9.1	1.8	36.7
TOTAL	215	11.0	10.2	0.1	41.1

*SD = standard deviation.

Table 15-5. AHE Series: Age at Operation (Years)

	n	Mean	SD*	Minimum	Maximum
Benign tumors	26	20.2	14.8	3.0	67.1
Semibenign tumors	47	29.6	13.8	0.8	62.8
Malignant tumors	37	37.3	16.7	7.5	74.0
Dysontogenetic lesions	32	29.5	12.6	0.3	53.9
Sequelae of encephalitis	2	22.2	0.5	21.8	22.7
Gliosis					
Slight	22	30.1	10.6	8.8	47.7
Moderate	9	32.2	9.6	19.9	42.2
Severe	6	34.1	7.3	28.3	43.4
No microscopic pathology	34	28.0	8.8	9.8	48.8
TOTAL	**215**	**29.7**	**13.7**	**0.3**	**74.0**

*SD = standard deviation.

the seizure-outcome categories is similar; (b) in patients with gliosis the operation was the more successful the more severe the gliosis; and (c) patients with a normal histology have a less favorable postsurgical seizure outcome than patients with tumors or dysontogenetic lesions.

The fluctuation of the epileptologic outcome rate was studied, classifying each patient at the end of each postoperative year. This year-by-year classification allowed determination of both the individual (Fig. 15-6) *and* population outcome status changes (Figs. 15-7 and 15-8).

In the 177 patients in the Zürich AHE series the seizure outcome was classified 1 year after the operation. With increasing postoperative follow-up period the number of patients naturally decreases, but 73 patients have a follow-up of at least 5 years and 10 patients were followed for 9–13 years.

Figure 15-6 depicts the year-by-year outcome classification for the individual patients together with the transition probabilities to move to another or to remain in the same outcome category. As can be seen, the probability of a patient staying within the same outcome category as that in which he or she was at the end of the third postoperative year is very high, that is, the likelihood of a substantial improvement in particular becomes very small. Within the first three postoperative years, there are, however, patients who show substantial improvement (e.g., from category III to category I) and *vice versa*, substantial worsening. The probability to change the outcome category is greatest for patients with rare seizures (category II).

Figure 15-7 shows the percentage of the AHE population in each of the four outcome categories on a year-by-year basis and compares these data with the figure given by Engel [15], who analyzed the UCLA

Table 15-6. AHE Series: Last Available Seizure Outcome and Follow-Up (Months)*

	n	Seizure Outcome Categories					Follow-Up Mean ± SD (Months)
		I	II	III	IV	n.cl.	
Benign tumors	26	13 (68%)	1 (5%)	1 (5%)	4 (21%)	7	66.7 ± 31.4
Semibenign tumors	47	28 (67%)	2 (5%)	5 (12%)	7 (17%)	5	46.1 ± 28.3
Malignant tumors	37	19 (63%)	2 (7%)	3 (10%)	6 (19%)	7	19.8 ± 16.2
Dysontogenetic lesions	32	20 (71%)	2 (7%)	2 (7%)	4 (14%)	4	51.4 ± 24.7
Sequelae of encephalitis	2	0 (0%)	0 (0%)	1 (50%)	1 (50%)	0	44.0 ± 11.3
Gliosis							
Slight	22	5 (31%)	2 (13%)	3 (19%)	6 (38%)	6	48.4 ± 31.4
Moderate	9	2 (40%)	1 (20%)	1 (20%)	1 (20%)	4	75.6 ± 54.1
Severe	6	4 (100%)	0 (0%)	0 (0%)	0 (0%)	2	45.5 ± 11.0
No microscopic pathology	34	14 (45%)	3 (10%)	4 (13%)	10 (32%)	3	52.4 ± 31.9
TOTAL	**215**	**105 (59%)**	**13 (7%)**	**20 (11%)**	**39 (22%)**	**38**	**47.0 ± 30.8**

*Seizure outcome is classified into categories I–IV: I, seizure-free; II, rare seizures (not more than 2 per year); III, worthwhile improvement (≥90% seizure reduction and marked improvement of quality of life); IV, no worthwhile improvement; n.cl., not classified; SD, standard deviation.

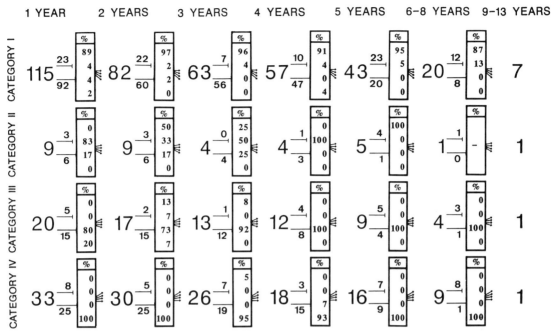

Figure 15-6. Year-by-year seizure outcome classification into categories I–IV of the Zürich AHE patients. This figure takes into account the length of follow-up and contains information on possible transition of each individual to other categories. The large numbers represent the patients falling into a given outcome category. The upper small number represents the number of patients not entering the next-year classification because of the conclusion of their follow-up. The lower small number (with termination into the boxes) represents those patients who are classified the next year. The numbers within the box indicate the new outcome distribution of those patients coming from one outcome category. This distribution is given in percentages within outcome categories I–IV (top to bottom). For example, this admittedly complex graph reads as follows: At the first postoperative year nine of the 177 patients are classified as having rare seizures (category II). Six of these nine patients can be evaluated at the end of the second postoperative year. Five of these six patients (83%) are still in the same category at the end of the second postoperative year; one patient (17%) worsened and is now classified as falling into category III. In addition, three patients (i.e., 4% from 92) arrive from category I, that is, they are classified as being outcome category II at the end of the second year. Therefore, outcome category II comprises a total of nine patients at the end of the second year. From these nine patients six can be classified at the end of the third postoperative year. Three patients became seizure-free (50%, category I), two remain in category II (33%, category II), and one patient is classified as being outcome category III (17%, category III). Newcomers to outcome category II within the third postoperative year are one patient from category I (2% of 60 patients) and one patient from category III (7% of 15 patients), and so on.

data on a year-by-year basis for the first 10 years following *anterior temporal lobectomy*. The seizure outcome classification of the AHE series remains fairly stable. In comparison with the UCLA series, the Zürich AHE series shows a slightly higher course of the curve depicting the seizure-free patients (category I). On the other hand, in the Zürich AHE series the curve of the patients without worthwhile improvement (category IV) is running slightly higher than the respective curve of the UCLA series.

The percentage of patients who were seizure-free during the first postoperative year and remained seizure-free for 5 postoperative years is the same in both series, that is, 78% (Fig. 15-8). From those patients

who had been seizure-free for 2 years, 81% in the UCLA series and 84% in the Zürich AHE series remained seizure-free for 5 postoperative years (Fig. 15-8).

Figure 15-9 shows a comparison between the two series (UCLA and Zürich AHE series) of the outcome classification on a year-by-year basis for patients who were classified as having rare seizures (category II; Fig. 15-9, left) and many seizures (categories III and IV, here lumped together; Fig. 15-9, right) during the first postoperative year. For patients in the Zürich AHE series, the "running-down phenomenon" [16] occurs later than in the UCLA series. This is true for both categories (category II, rare seizures, and categories III and IV, many seizures).

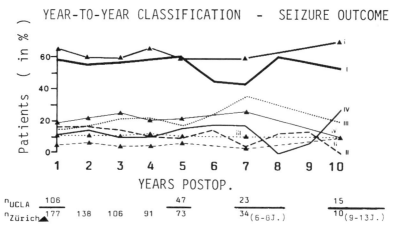

Figure 15-7. Percentage of a population of patients in each of the four outcome categories on a year-by-year basis. Comparison of the UCLA series (anterior temporal lobectomy), as published by Engel [15], with the Zürich AHE series. Patients of the AHE series with a postoperative follow-up of more than 5 years have been summed up into 6- to 8-year and 9- to 13-year follow-up groups.

Outcome with Respect to "Causal" Versus "Palliative" Amygdalohippocampectomies ("Nonlesional" Cases)

Seventy-one patients in the Zürich AHE series, who had either no histologic abnormality ($n = 34$) or only a gliosis ($n = 37$), were separately analyzed with respect to their preoperative classification into "causal" ($n = 40$) versus "palliative" ($n = 31$) operations. As can be seen from Table 15-6, patients in whom the AHE was performed with a "causal" indication (i.e., who had seizure onset within the resected

structures) did much better (73% seizure-free) than those in whom the operation was performed with a "palliative" indication (12% seizure-free).

Postoperative Antiepileptic Drug Treatment in the Zürich AHE Series

In order to rate the success or failure of the operation it is necessary to consider the changes in antiepileptic drug (AED) treatment. Whereas preoperatively all patients were drug-resistant and were taking, as a

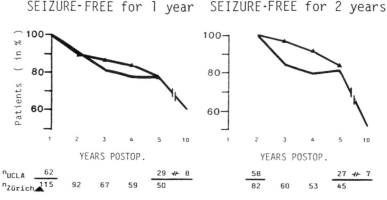

Figure 15-8. Comparison of the UCLA series (anterior temporal lobectomy), as published by Engel [15], with the Zürich AHE series. Year-by-year outcome classifications for patients who were classified as seizure-free for 1 year (*left*) and 2 years (*right*) after surgery.

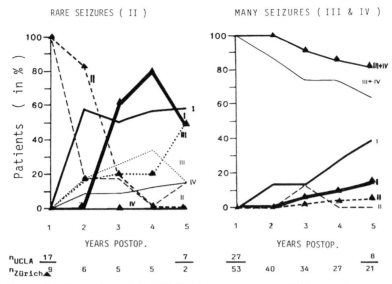

Figure 15-9. Comparison of the UCLA series (anterior temporal lobectomy), as published by Engel [15], with the Zürich AHE series. Year-by-year outcome classifications for patients who were classified as having rare seizures (category II; *left*) and "many" seizures (categories III and IV combined; *right*).

rule, high doses of AEDs in various combinations, postoperatively in many patients the AEDs could be withdrawn or dosages reduced. The AED regimen at 1 year after operation and the corresponding seizure outcome are given in Table 15-7. The generic names of the AEDs taken 1 year after operation are given in Table 15-8 for patients with monotherapy and for patients with a combination of two AEDs. The three most frequent combinations were phenytoin plus phenobarbital (23%); phenytoin plus carbamazepine (19%); and phenytoin plus valproate (19%).

Of the 177 patients, the AEDs could be withdrawn postoperatively in 49 patients (28%). The AEDs could be withdrawn in 42% of patients with a follow-up of at least 5 years ($n = 73$); in 43% of the patients with a follow-up of at least 6–8 years (n 34); and in 70% of patients with a follow-up between 9 and 13 years ($n = 10$). The mean postoperative

period before withdrawal was 20.0 months (range: 1–78). The further mean follow-up period without AEDs was 38.8 months (range: 6–60). Forty-six patients (94%) remained seizure-free following drug withdrawal (AED withdrawal 20.1 months postoperatively; follow-up without AEDs 40.2 months; means). Two patients (4%) experienced a recurrence of seizures after withdrawal: in one patient seizures persisted despite immediate *de novo* antiepileptic treatment (AED withdrawal after 6 months; follow-up with *de novo* treatment 6 months); the other patient once again became seizure-free following *de novo* AED treatment (AED withdrawal 6 months postoperatively; follow-up with *de novo* AED treatment 60 months). After the withdrawal of AED, one patient (2%), experienced rare auras with a frequency of 1–2/year. This patient preferred to remain without AED (AED withdrawal 42 months postoperatively; follow-up without AED 24 months) [17].

Table 15-7. AHE Series: Antiepileptic Drugs Taken 1 Year After Operation

		Seizure Outcome Categories			
Antiepileptic Drug Therapy	Number of Patients (%)	I	II	III	IV
No drug	28 (16%)	28	0	0	0
1 AED	82 (46%)	57	6	8	11
2 AEDs	43 (24%)	22	2	7	12
3 or more AEDs	24 (14%)	8	1	5	10
TOTAL	177 (100%)	115	9	20	33

Table 15-8. AHE Series: Type of Antiepileptic Drugs Taken in Monotherapy and Two-Drug Combinations 1 Year After Operation

	Monotherapy n (%)	Two-AED Combination n (%)
Type of Drug		
Phenytoin	46 (56%)	34 (79%)
Carbamazepine	17 (21%)	16 (37%)
Phenobarbital	15 (18%)	15 (35%)
Primidone	3 (4%)	4 (9%)
Valproate	—	11 (26%)
Diazepam and others	1 (1%)	6 (14%)
TOTAL	82 (100%)	43 (100%)

Neuropsychological Data

Several groups have reported on the detrimental effects of lesions in hippocampus and amygdala on learning and memory performance. Experiments in monkeys have shown that the hippocampus and amygdala are of great importance in learning and memory [18,19]. Horel [20,21] has reevaluated the role of the hippocampus for memory and has argued that the temporal stem is the decisive "structure" in learning and memory procedure. Therefore, it was of considerable interest whether and to what extent the unilateral, selective AHE influences postoperative neuropsychological performance. Earlier studies comparing the preoperative and postoperative neuropsychological performance showed that the neu-

ropsychological postoperative results were better in AHE patients than in patients who underwent an anterior temporal lobectomy. In AHE patients the greater the improvements in postoperative learning and memory performance, the better was the postoperative seizure outcome. Furthermore, it was found that the postoperative improvement was mainly due to the improvement of the nonoperated contralateral hemisphere, whereas the performance of the operated hemisphere remained more or less unchanged compared to the preoperative test performance [22–24]. In no case did we observe a severe memory deficit or an amnestic syndrome following AHE. Patients judged to be at risk for a worsening of their memory, however, are routinely submitted to a so-called selective temporal lobe amobarbital test [25–27].

Noninvasively, learning and memory were tested with three series of 15 items, each drawn or written in black ink on white cards (size, 15 × 10 cm). The items of the first series were nonsense designs (in the following called "designs"). Drawings of common objects (called "drawings") were used in the second series. The third series consisted of concrete nouns (called "nouns"). The items were presented until the subjects were able to reproduce at least 12 items, but for a maximum of five trials. The reproduction of as many items as possible of each series (designs, drawings, nouns) after a distraction interval of 30 min made up the memory performance. In order to avoid memory savings from preoperative to postoperative testing, parallel versions (A + B) of these tests were used. Half of the subjects were tested preoperatively

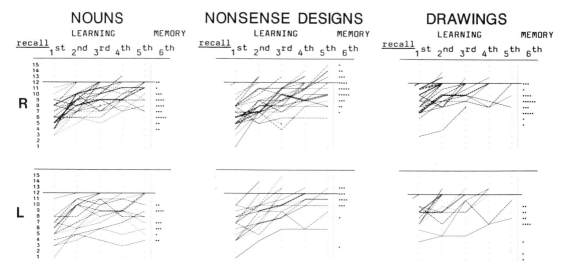

Figure 15-10. Preoperative learning curves and memory assessment using the Nadig test (see text and Table 15-9) in 43 candidates for AHE (27 with right, *R,* and 16 with left, *L*) mesiobasal temporal seizure onset.

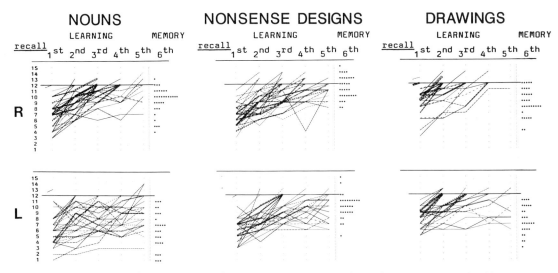

Figure 15-11. Postoperative learning curves and memory assessment using the Nadig test (see text and Table 15-9) in 67 patients operated by selective amygdalohippocampectomy (35 right, *R*, and 32 left, *L*).

with version A and postoperatively with version B, and *vice versa*.

This neuropsychological test [28] was performed in 43 patients (27 right-sided and 16 left-sided AHEs) before and in 67 patients (35 right-sided and 32 left-sided AHEs) after the operation. The results are displayed in Figures 15-10 and 15-11 and Table 15-9. Of the 27 patients with a seizure focus that was *right* mesiobasal temporal, preoperatively the learning criterion was reached with the verbal material by 14 (52%), with the figural material by 16 (59%), and with the pictorial material by 22 (81%) patients.

Of the 16 patients with a seizure focus that was *left* mesiobasal temporal, preoperatively the learning criterion was reached with the verbal material by eight (50%),with the figural material by 11 (69%), and with the pictorial material by 12 (75%) patients.

Postoperatively, of the 35 patients with a *right* AHE the learning criterion was reached with the verbal material by 30 (86%), with the figural material by 25 (70%), and with the pictorial by 34 (97%) patients.

Postoperatively, of the 32 patients with a *left* AHE the learning criterion was reached with the verbal material by 15 (47%), with the figural material by 18 (56%), and with the pictorial by 26 (81%) patients.

The means of the memory performance for the four groups (preoperative and postoperative, right and left) are given in Table 15-9. These values suggest that the verbal memory improves slightly after a right-sided AHE, whereas it worsens slightly after a left-sided AHE. There is no significant change in the figural memory following a right or left AHE, but the pictorial memory seems slightly improved following a left AHE.

Psychosocial Outcome

Together with Nadja Khan we have examined the psychosocial outcome of our AHE patients [29]. They were assessed for (a) psychosocial variables: emotional adjustment and coping abilities (depression, tension, fear, shame, disgust, guilt), interpersonal

Table 15-9. AHE Series: Material Specific Preoperative and Postoperative Memory Performance as Measured by the Nadig Test

Time of Testing	Side of Operations	Number of Patients	Memory Performance ($x \pm SD$) (Scores in Nadig Test)		
			Verbal	Figural	Pictorial
Preoperative	Right	27	7.8 ± 2.3	11.0 ± 2.0	8.8 ± 1.9
Postoperative	Right	35	9.3 ± 2.2	11.4 ± 1.9	8.8 ± 2.3
Preoperative	Left	16	7.2 ± 2.0	10.7 ± 2.5	6.9 ± 2.9
Postoperative	Left	32	6.0 ± 3.1	10.0 ± 2.0	7.7 ± 2.3

adjustment (social comfort, number of contacts and relationships), adjustment to seizures, and behavioral disturbances (along with the Bear-Fedio Personality Inventory; see reference 24); (b) vocational and employment career; and (c) "family support."

The following results emerged: *Postoperatively*, psychosocial functioning improved in 72% of AHE patients, remained unchanged in 15%, and deteriorated in 13%. All patients with a postoperative deterioration had persisting seizures, being classified in outcome categories III and IV. Probably even more important is the fact that all of them had preoperatively marked personality and behavioral changes in line with the original description of Waxman and Geschwind [30].

With reference to the vocational and employment career, the preoperative-to-postoperative comparison revealed the following: *preoperatively* 61% were employed and 39% unemployed (included in the unemployed group are children, housewives, and students). *Postoperatively,* with a mean follow-up of 3.4 (standard deviation 2.6) years, 59% were employed. One patient has lost his job because of the reappearance of a paranoid psychosis, and one claimed to have lost his job because of permanent headache associated with insomnia.

The employment status *postoperatively* was much better in 24%, better in 45%, unchanged in 23%, slightly worse in 5%, and markedly worse in 3% of patients, compared to the preoperative state.

There is a strong relationship between the scores of the "psychosocial variables," "employment status," "family support," and "seizure outcome." Patients with a good seizure outcome (categories I and II) improved postoperatively in all measured psychosocial variables and had significantly better family support. An improvement in the employment status, however, was observed nearly exclusively in only those patients who were completely seizure-free.

Concluding Remarks

The selective AHE is a technically difficult but appealing operation for carefully selected patients. This means for the "causal" indication: patients with medically refractory seizures with proven unilateral focal (i.e., well-localized) mesiobasal TL seizure onset. As a "palliative" operation, AHE can be offered in patients with a more widespread regional seizure onset with limbic predominance or, in certain cases, with a lateral temporal primary epileptogenic focus encroaching into indispensable language areas, but *only* if a "secondary pacemaker

role" of the ipsilateral mesiobasal TL structures has been ascertained.

In the hands of our neurosurgeon M. Gazi Yasargie, the complication rate in terms of lasting morbidity of this operation is 0.4%, that is, in only one patient an intraoperative spasm of the anterior choroidal artery resulted in a permanent slight hemiparesis. No visual field deficit was induced. There was no mortality related to AHE. No unexpected severe memory impairment and, in particular, no postoperative amnesia have been observed in our Zürich AHE series. It should, however, be emphasized that all candidates for AHE undergo exhaustive noninvasive neuropsychological examination and, if the patient is at risk, also invasive amobarbital (Amytal) testing. In order to better assess the possible risks in this regard, we have developed and use so-called selective TL amobarbital tests [25–27]. We have returned to and currently prefer the so-called balloon technique with a short-lasting balloon occlusion distal to the anterior choroidal artery and anterior circulation injection (into the anterior choroidal artery and posterior communicating artery).

With the help of modern neurophysiology, including radiotelemetric long-term seizure monitoring from many intracranial electrodes (stereotactic depth, foramen ovale electrode EEG) [32] and modern structural (MRI) and functional (single photon emission computed tomography, positron emission tomography) imaging methods, the seizure-generating structures can be precisely defined, at least as far as the mesiobasal TL seizure type is concerned.

The operative technique in AHE should be such that it prevents any harm to the normal brain tissue during operation, in particular with respect to its vascular supply. Concerning the question as to the exact borders of the resection of potentially epileptogenic tissue, our results suggest that a certain critical mass of epileptic pacemaker neurons [31] has to be resected in order to achieve good postoperative seizure control and that removal of the anterior parts of the parahippocampal gyrus, and particularly its subicular part, improves the results.

If careful presurgical evaluation and case selection are combined with an immaculate operative technique of a neurosurgeon thoroughly familiar with the operative anatomy of this region, the results of this selective operation are very rewarding. Performed with a "causal" indication, complete or almost complete seizure control (outcome categories I and II) can be expected postoperatively in 93% of patients according to our series. Associated with or as a consequence of postoperative seizure control, good to excellent neuropsychological and psychosocial outcome can be expected also. This, in turn, is linked with the early termination of, or at least considerable reduction in, antiepileptic drug treatment and the associated relief of the often severe side effects of high-dose AED treatment influencing neuropsychological and higher intellectual and emotional functions.

Since the mesiobasal limbic subtype of TL epilepsy often is resistant to AED treatment but responds well to adequate surgical treatment, an indicated selective AHE should not be unnecessarily delayed. There is now ample evidence that at least this type of epilepsy should be viewed as a potentially ongoing process rather than a stable condition, and that the operative results are better with earlier seizure control.

Acknowledgment

Professor M. Gazi Yasargil performed all selective amygdalohippocampectomies in this series. Mrs. C. Schmidt and Sepp Müller helped with artwork. Dr. Normann Cook improved the English.

I want to thank all my colleagues from the clinical, theoretical, and experimental side and the technicians and nursing personnel for their past and ongoing support of the Zürich Epilepsy Surgery Program.

References

 1. Wieser HG. *Electroclinical features of the psychomotor seizure.* London: Gustav Fischer-Butterworths, 1983: 1–242.
 2. Wieser HG. Selective amygdalo-hippocampectomy for temporal lobe epilepsy. *Epilepsia* 1988;29(Suppl 2): 110–3.
 3. Niemeyer P. The transventricular amygdalohippocampectomy in temporal lobe epilepsy. In: Baldwin M, Bailey P, eds. *Temporal lobe epilepsy.* Springfield, IL: Charles C. Thomas, 1958:461–82.
 4. Engel J Jr, ed. *Surgical treatment of the epilepsies.* (2nd ed.) New York: Raven Press, 1993.
 5. Wieser HG, Yasargil MG. Selective amygdalohippocampectomy as a surgical treatment of mesiobasal limbic epilepsy. *Surg Neurol* 1982;17:445–57.
 6. Wieser HG. Data analysis. In: Engel J Jr, ed. *Surgical treatment of the epilepsies.* New York: Raven Press, 1987:335–60.
 7. Yasargil MG, Teddy PJ, Roth P. Selective amygdalohippocampectomy: operative anatomy and surgical technique. In: Simon L, Brihaye J, Guidetti B, et al, eds. *Advances and technical standards in neurosurgery,* vol 12. Vienna: Springer, 1985:92–123.
 8. Yasargil MG, Wieser HG. Selective microsurgical resections. In: Wieser HG, Elger CE, eds. *Presurgical evaluation of epileptics.* Heidelberg: Springer, 1987:352–60.
 9. Yasargil MG, Wieser HG. Selective amygdalohippocampectomy at the University Hospital, Zürich. In:

Engel J Jr, ed. *Surgical treatment of the epilepsies.* New York: Raven Press, 1987:653–8.
10. Yasargil MG, Wieser HG, Valavanis A, et al. Surgery and results of selective amygdala-hippocampectomy in one hundred patients with nonlesional limbic epilepsy. *Neurosurg Clin North Am,* 4(2) April 1993 (pp 1–19).
11. Yasargil MG. *Microneurosurgery,* vol I. Stuttgart: Thieme, 1984.
12. Siegel AM, Wieser HG, Wichmann W, et al. Relationship between MR-imaged total amount of tissue removed, resection scores of specific mediobasal limbic subcompartments and clinical outcome following selective amygdalohippocampectomy. *Epilepsy Res* 1990; 6:56–65.
13. Duvernoy HM. *The human hippocampus: an atlas of applied anatomy.* Munich: JF Bergmann Verlag, 1988: 1–166.
14. Bernoulli C, Siegfried J, Baumgartner G, et al. Danger of accidental person-to-person transmission of Creutzfeldt-Jakob disease by surgery. *Lancet* 1977; 1:478–9, 569.
15. Engel J Jr. Outcome with respect to epileptic seizures. In: Engel J Jr, ed. *Surgical treatment of the epilepsies.* New York: Raven Press, 1987:553–71.
16. Rasmussen T. Cortical resection for medically refractory focal epilepsy: results, lessons and questions. In: Rasmussen T, Marino R, eds. *Functional neurosurgery.* New York: Raven Press, 1979:253–69.
17. Siegel AM. Nachuntersuchungen bei Patienten mit selektiver Amygdala-Hippokampektomie (thesis). Zürich: University of Zürich, 1990.
18. Mishkin M. Memory in monkeys severely impaired by combined but not separate removal of amygdala and hippocampus. *Nature* 1978;273:297–8.
19. Zola-Morgan S, Squire LR, Mishkin M. The neuroanatomy of amnesia: amygdala-hippocampus versus temporal stem. *Science* 1982;218:1337–9.
20. Horel JA. The neuroanatomy of amnesia. A critique of the hippocampal memory hypothesis. *Brain* 1978; 101:403–45.
21. Horel JA, Pytho DE. Behavioral effect of local cooling in temporal lobe of monkeys. *J Neurophysiol* 1982;47:11–22.
22. Birri R, Perret E, Wieser HG. Der Einfluss verschiedener Temporallappenoperationen auf das Gedächtnis bei Epileptikern. *Nervenarzt* 1982;53:144–9.
23. Gonser A, Perret E, Wieser HG. Ist der Hippokampus für Lern und Gedächtnisprozesse notwendig? *Nervenarzt* 1986;57:269–75.
24. Wieser HG. Selective amygdalohippocampectomy: indications, investigative technique and results. In: Symon L, Brihaye J, Guidetti B, et al, eds. *Advances and technical standards in neurosurgery,* vol 13. Vienna: Springer, 1986:39–133.
25. Wieser HG, Valavanis A, Roos A, et al. "Selective" and "superselective" temporal lobe Amytal tests I: neuroradiological, neuroanatomical, and electrical data. In: Manelis J, Bental E, Loeber J, et al., eds. *Advances in epileptology,* vol 17. New York: Raven Press, 1989;20–7.

26. Wieser HG, Landis T, Regard M, et al. "Selective" and "superselective" temporal lobe Amytal tests II: neuropsychological test procedure and results. In: Manelis J, Bental E, Loeber J, et al., eds. *Advances in epileptology*, vol 17. New York: Raven Press, 1989:28–33.
27. Wieser HG. Anterior cerebral artery Amobarbital test. In: Lüders H, eds. *Epilepsy surgery*. New York: Raven Press, 1990:515–23.
28. Nadig T, Wieser HG, Perret E. Learning and memory performance before and after unilateral selective amygdalohippocampectomy. In: Will BE, Schmitt P, Dalrymple-Alford JC, eds. *Brain plasticity, learning, and memory*. New York: Plenum Press, 1985:397–403.
29. Khan N, Wieser HG. Psychosocial outcome of patients with amygdalohippocampectomy. *J Epilepsy* 1992; 5:128–34.
30. Waxman SG, Geschwind N. The interictal behavioural syndrome of temporal lobe epilepsy. *Ann Gen Psychiatry* 1975;32:1580–6.
31. Wyler AR, Ward AA. Epileptic neurons. In: Lockard JS, Ward AA, eds. *Epilepsy: a window to brain mechanisms*. New York: Raven Press, 1980:51–68.
32. Wieser HG, Moser S. Improved multipolar foramen ovale electrode monitoring. *J Epilepsy* 1988;1:13–22.

Chapter 16
Pediatric Epilepsy Surgery: Special Considerations

MICHAEL S. DUCHOWNY

Medically resistant seizures that begin early in life are often associated with serious later handicap [1]. At least one third of children with chronic epilepsy suffer from a psychiatric disability, a rate that is increased fivefold over the general population and threefold over non-neurologically disabled children [2]. Even more disturbing is that almost 60% of children who have both chronic epilepsy and a neurologic handicap develop educational or psychiatric dysfunction [2]. The growing awareness of these and other disabilities and the benefits of early surgical intervention have spurred an increase in young patients being referred to centers for epilepsy surgery.

More refined concepts of early childhood seizure patterns and epilepsy syndromes also help facilitate early case selection. Many syndromes have a defined prognosis [3–5], allowing children with seizures that are unlikely to remit to be identified early. Variability in childhood electroencephalographic (EEG) patterns and the tendency for pediatric seizures to be age-dependent [6,7] do not limit case selection, and the majority of children will benefit from early surgical intervention [8–11].

Justifying Early Surgical Intervention

Functional Plasticity of the Immature Brain

The ability of the immature brain to recover more fully from injury is an important rationale for performing surgery at a young age. This special property has been recognized for many years and was quanti-

fied in a series of experiments comparing the consequences of ablating motor cortex in infant and adult monkeys [12]. Unilateral motor and premotor cortical excisions in infant monkeys were shown to induce relatively little functional impairment, whereas adult monkeys undergoing identical operations became permanently hemiplegic [12]. Contralateral ablation of previously lesioned young animals produced bilateral motor deficits, which indicated that restoration of function resided in the contralateral hemisphere. These observations showed convincingly that young animals are remarkably able to recover from early acquired lesions.

Repeated clinical observations confirm the existence of similar phenomena in humans. Except for complex language and motor function, many of the deficits from early acquired unilateral hemispheric damage are largely reversible. Hemispheric ablation is better tolerated in younger patients but in later life can still be associated with superior recovery if the pathologic substrate is acquired early. Thus, in the formative stages of postnatal human development, the cerebral hemispheres are able to compensate for the loss of specialized skills. With maturation, this capacity disappears as regions of specialized function become permanently established.

It is doubtful, however, that restoration of function is ever fully complete, even for lesions acquired in very immature brain. Anatomic asymmetries of the speech area are already present *in utero* [13,14], and language impairment is more typical of early dominant hemisphere disturbances [15], whereas early nondominant hemisphere lesions preferentially affect visuospatial performance [16]. Recovery from unilateral lesions may result in less severe but more widespread cognitive disturbances.

Long-Term Consequences of Medically Uncontrolled Childhood Epilepsy

Neuronal Development

Seizures in early life are deleterious to the developing nervous system. Mass stimulation of rat pups at 30-min intervals reduces brain protein and myelin and dissociates ribosomes [18–20]. Early status epilepticus [21] can delay neural maturation, and kindled rat pups have an increased susceptibility to seizures as adults [22,23].

Frequent seizures also produce cytotoxic damage. N-methyl-D-aspartate (NMDA) and glutamate are released by seizure-induced hypoxia and mediate a variety of cytopathic changes that ultimately culminate in cell death [24]. Experimental glutamate and NMDA administration also induces seizures, whereas valproic acid, a glutamate antagonist, decreases NMDA concentration [25].

Neuropsychiatric Morbidity

Neuropsychiatric disturbances in children with chronic epilepsy limit psychosocial adaptation and functional independence [26–28] and are often more debilitating than the actual seizures. Neuropsychiatric dysfunction is especially severe if seizures begin early, making normal neuropsychiatric status an important rationale for preadolescent surgery.

There is no single theory that satisfactorily explains neurobehavioral deterioration in children with longstanding epilepsy [29,30]. Since children with recurrent seizures are often brain damaged, it is difficult to prove that their seizures are responsible for the psychiatric deterioration. Drug toxicity also plays a role, although this too may be difficult to document. Taylor [31] has further hypothesized that seizure-induced limbic disturbances impair the child's ability to attach social or emotional significance to routine events, thereby distorting experience despite the appearance of normal behavioral function.

Behavior. Irritability, aggressiveness, hyperactivity, impulsiveness, attentional impairment, and temper tantrums are common in children with chronic epilepsy [32–34]. Behavioral abnormalities are more prevalent in brain-damaged children with early seizure onset, but similar disturbances are also found in nonepileptic brain-damaged children. Children with temporal lobe tumors show a particularly high incidence of behavioral pathology [35], suggesting that focal temporal dysfunction, rather than seizures, is responsible for behavioral deterioration. By contrast, healthy children with epileptiform EEGs [36] and normal children who later become epileptic [37] also manifest high rates of behavioral disturbance. Thus, any simple assignment of risk can be misleading, and prophylactic administration of antiepileptic drugs (AEDs) to at-risk children does not prevent later behavior problems [36].

Emotional Disorder. Over one third of young adults with temporal lobe seizures have psychological complications, and 11% experience overt psychotic disorders [38]. Emotional problems usually appear by adolescence, especially when seizures begin in the first decade.

The occurrence of psychotic thinking in children with temporal lobe seizures has been confirmed repeatedly [39–41], with only one study not reporting its occurrence [42]. Children with left-sided seizure foci display reflective personality styles and are at greatest risk for psychosis, whereas children with right temporal foci tend to be more impulsive, as has been reported in adults [43,44].

Cognition. Over 10% of children with seizures show a permanent decrease of 10 or more intelligence quotient (IQ) points. They often present with higher IQ scores and earlier seizure onset and exhibit poorer seizure control. Drug toxicity is believed to be an important contributor.

Early seizure onset and frequent seizures are independent risk factors for later cognitive impairment. Farwell et al. [28] found an inverse correlation between seizure duration and control and performance on the WISC-R and Halstead-Reitan batteries. This effect was even more severe for seizures that began before the age of 5 years [45]. Early seizure onset is also linked to lower intelligence in adulthood compared to late-onset seizures matched for duration and frequency [46,47].

It is not universally accepted that children with chronic epilepsy are more vulnerable to intellectual decline. Although their intelligence as a group is lower than that of the general population, the number of nonfebrile seizures does not explain the diminished IQ scores of these children [48]. Studies of cognition have also failed to differentiate children with acute from those with chronic seizure presentations.

There are also relatively few studies comparing the effects of AEDs and seizures on intelligence. AEDs impair cognitive function selectively [49], and global intellectual impairment is seen only in cases of extreme toxicity. As suggested by Loiseau et al. [50], the reasons for poor intellectual performance in children with epilepsy are complex, and parameters such as the type and frequency of seizures, duration of disease, and medication effects probably all contribute to the observed deficits.

Functional Outcome

The long-term consequences of childhood epilepsy were first reported by Ounsted et al. at the Park Hospital for Children, Oxford, England. In a prospective study begun in 1948, 100 children with clinical and electrographic evidence of temporal lobe epilepsy were investigated and followed into adulthood [51,52]. Eighty-six percent experienced seizure onset before the age of 11 years. Hyperactivity and aggressive behaviors ("catastrophic rage") were extremely frequent and caused many children to be excluded from normal schools and denied access to standard pathways of learning and socialization. By adulthood, fewer than half had remitted and one third were physically dependent with major handicaps [53]. There were nine deaths, all in the handicapped group, three of which were epilepsy-related [40]. Almost all medically resistant patients also manifested disturbances of behavior and cognition; early seizure onset was highly correlated with exclusion from normal schools.

One of the more disturbing findings of this study was that 30% of children with persistent seizures developed a major psychiatric disability [53]. Antisocial conduct disorders were particularly prevalent, and males with left temporal foci were especially vulnerable to psychotic thought disturbances and much less likely to marry [54]. Males also showed a higher incidence of sexual apathy [54]. These findings showed that chronic childhood epilepsy predisposes to profound disturbances in later life. Psychopathology is usually far advanced by adolescence and therefore must be alleviated early [55].

Psychological dysfunction in children with uncontrolled seizures may unwittingly be compounded by caretakers who have unrealistic fears or who place inappropriate sanctions. It is not unusual for adults to ascribe behavioral changes to the seizures or brain damage [56,59]. Behavioral deterioration and social dependency of children with chronic epilepsy thus often exceed those of children with chronic, nonepileptic illnesses [57,58].

Acute Consequences of Uncontrolled Seizures

Children with status epilepticus have high rates of subsequent neurologic impairment [60], but an episode of status should not be used to rationalize surgery, since children with chronic epilepsy are no more prone to recurrent status epilepticus than are medically controlled patients. Less than one fourth of infants and children who present in status epilepticus have even had a previous seizure [61], and fewer still have had more than one or two seizure episodes. However, the complications of status epilepticus remain highest in brain-damaged children, a group also at high risk for chronic epilepsy. Sudden unexpected death in epilepsy is an extremely rare event [62–64], and fear of this complication is better dealt with in counseling.

Compassionate Care

Approximately half of all adult surgery candidates experience seizure onset before the end of the first decade of life and one fourth present by age 5 years [65]. Since neurobehavioral deterioration typically begins by adolescence, surgery should be considered before puberty. Intolerance of neurobehavioral deterioration is being expressed more frequently by families, and pediatric epileptologists need to be sensitive to family concerns.

Timing of Surgery

The generally accepted rule that surgery should not be performed unless medically resistant seizures have been experienced for 2 years needs to be reinterpreted for younger patients. In the childhood epilepsies, timing of surgery should be considered in terms of long-term prognosis and potential for deterioration [40,53,54]. Eight risk factors—IQ below 90, early onset of seizures, five or more grand mal attacks, daily seizures, left hemisphere EEG focus, hyperactivity, behavioral disorder, and need for specialized schooling—predict poor outcome. The last factor is particularly significant since virtually all children who outgrow their seizures attend regular schools. An abnormal neurologic examination and the presence of structural brain damage are also prognostically unfavorable. Thus, any child who has uncontrolled seizures should be referred for surgery if these factors are present, and a final decision should be reached before adolescence.

Despite the clinical impression that surgery is more beneficial if performed in childhood, the superiority of early surgical intervention is difficult to prove. Temporal lobectomy is more successful if the preoperative seizure duration is 4 years or less [65–67], whereas seizure durations of 10 years or more are associated with poor psychosocial outcome. More than 60% of patients undergoing temporal lobectomy before age 17 years are gainfully employed at follow-up, compared with 30% of older patients [65].

Syndromes of Intractable Partial Childhood Epilepsy

Partial seizures in children are often caused by prenatally acquired lesions related to the abnormal growth or migration of neurons, glia, and supporting structural elements. These disorders are of considerable importance since many are associated with chronic epilepsy. Several of the more widely encountered syndromes are discussed below.

Neurocutaneous Disorders

Sturge-Weber Syndrome

The Sturge-Weber syndrome is characterized by venous angiomas of the leptomeninges and ipsilateral facial angiomatosis (port wine stain, nevus flammeus) in the ophthalmic division of the trigeminal nerve. Associated clinical features include glaucoma, mental retardation, and epilepsy. Cerebral hemiatrophy may be progressive, and both cerebral hemispheres are affected in approximately 15% of cases [68]. Intracranial manifestations can present without the facial abnormalities [69,70]. Intracranial calcifications usually appear in infancy (Fig. 16-1).

Patients with the Sturge-Weber syndrome are prone to partial seizures [68,71,72]. If controlled by medication, the prognosis for their intellectual function is generally favorable [68], but increasingly intense partial motor attacks are often associated with severe postictal hemiparesis and deteriorating psychosocial status.

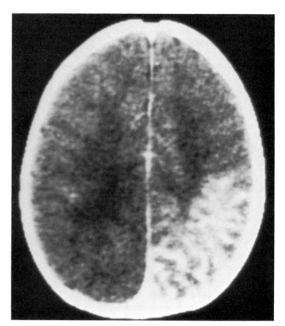

Figure 16-1. Contrast-enhanced CT scan in a child with the Sturge-Weber syndrome and chronic partial seizures. Note calcified gyral markings in the parieto-occipital cortex of the left hemisphere. This patient had a right hemisyndrome and obtained complete seizure freedom after functional hemispherectomy.

Hemispherectomy in the treatment of chronic epilepsy in young Sturge-Weber patients was first suggested by Polani [73]. Falconer and Rushworth [74] subsequently confirmed the effectiveness of this approach in five patients whose seizures began in the first year of life. All became seizure-free and achieved significant behavioral improvement. Before age 2 years, hemispherectomy results in comparably less motor and cognitive impairment and reverses the intellectual decline [75,76].

The timing of hemispherectomy in Sturge-Weber patients must be individualized [77]. The EEG is not prognostically useful although attenuated background is predictive of progressive calcification [78]. Positron emission tomography (PET) studies have been used to identify children who might benefit from earlier intervention [79].

Large excisions are not always required for seizure control. Rosen et al. [80] obtained permanent seizure remission after right occipital lobectomy in an infant experiencing multiple daily seizures, and favorable outcomes following excisions have been reported by others [81]. Excisional surgery is therefore indicated in less involved patients with circumscribed seizure foci, with hemispherectomy reserved for cases of more widespread involvement.

Tuberous Sclerosis

Patients with tuberous sclerosis (TS) manifest psychomotor delay, adenoma sebaceum, and seizures in conjunction with hypopigmented skin lesions and shagreen patches. Multiple organ systems may undergo neoplastic changes, whereas "formes frustes" of the disorder present with a single clinical feature [82]. Forme fruste patients are occasionally discovered by histologic analysis of tissue removed at epilepsy surgery [83].

Seizures occur in up to 80% of children with TS. They typically begin early, rarely remit, and may intensify in later childhood. Infantile spasms occur in one third to one half of TS patients [84], and partial seizures are also common. The EEG yields little definitive information; imaging studies reveal single or multiple calcified cortical tubers.

Excisional surgery has improved the status of many TS patients with focal epilepsy and is typically performed in early life [85,86]. Multiple cortical tubers are not a surgical contraindication when a single lesion is epileptogenic.

Dysplasias

Neuronal migration disorders are typified by irregular and often bizarre-appearing cellular elements. In the lissencephaly-agyria syndrome, the entire cortical mantle is dysplastic and lacks secondary and tertiary sulci. The Miller-Dieker syndrome consists of lissencephaly in association with a characteristic facies and may be produced by deletion of the distal short arm of chromosome 17 [87] or may be sporadically acquired. Virtually all patients with lissencephaly have chronic epilepsy [88].

Pachygyria (Macrogyria)

Focal pachygyria consists of grossly thickened gyri that are separated by shallow sulci and reduced white matter [89]. Similar abnormalities have been described in hemimegalencephaly and the hamartomatous lesions of TS [90].

Pachygyria often produces focal seizures of early onset. Children with bilateral central (rolandic) pachygyria present with atonic or mixed seizures, psychomotor delay, dysarthria, pseudobulbar palsy, and long tract signs [91] and resemble adults with acquired bilateral opercular infarction (Foix-Chavany-Marie syndrome) [92]. Medically resistant seizures begin early in children with bilateral perisylvian polymicrogyria [93], and there is one report of

improvement in the drop attacks and behavioral status of children with bilateral pachygyria after corpus callosotomy [91].

Focal Cortical Dysplasia

Although the earliest reports of focal cortical dysplasia in chronic epilepsy did not emphasize its onset in childhood [94], this presentation is now well established [95,96]. Cortical dysplasias show a predilection for rolandic cortex, in which they produce simple partial attacks with secondary generalization [90]. A generalized form of dysplasia has been reported in two unrelated retarded girls [97], both of whom experienced seizure onset and mental deterioration before age 4 years. Patients with the syndrome of rolandic dysplasia, early-onset focal myoclonus, and progressive hemiparesis have benefited from corticectomy [96].

Heterotopias and Microdysgenesis

Nodular and laminar heterotopias are frequent pathologic findings in chronic childhood epilepsy [98,99]. Microdysgenetic abnormalities are usually widespread and result from abnormal neuronal migration in the later part of gestation [100]. Microdysgenesis is especially common in temporal neocortex [101] but occurs at multiple brain regions in patients with primary generalized epilepsy [102]. Seizures due to microdysgenesis usually begin in the first or early second decade of life [101]. The pathologic significance of microdysgenesis has recently been questioned since similar cytoarchitectonic abnormalities exist in patients with nonepileptic disorders [103,104].

Hemimegalencephaly

Hemimegalencephaly is a rare congenital malformation consisting of unilateral enlargement of one cerebral hemisphere. Gyri are thickened and show bizarre giant neurons and heterotopias similar to the findings in TS and cortical dysplasia [105]. Hemispheric asymmetry is usually present at birth and progresses postnatally (Fig. 16-2). Mental deterioration, contralateral hemiconvulsions, and early death in status epilepticus are a virtual certainty in many affected children. The EEG reveals widespread disorganization and multifocal discharges; hemihypsarrhythmic patterns have also been reported [106].

The invariably fatal outcome of many patients has prompted aggressive surgical intervention [107].

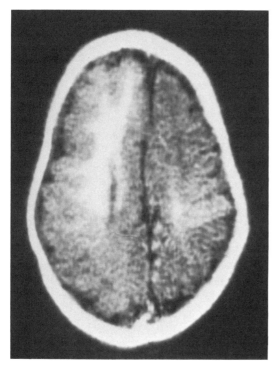

Figure 16-2. Axial magnetic resonance imaging (MRI) study in a child with hemimegalencephaly. Besides the hemisphere volume asymmetry, there is abnormal myelin production in both cerebral hemispheres.

Hemispherectomy significantly reduced seizure frequency in one infant who ultimately died 5 years later, but more favorable long-term outcomes have recently been achieved [107–109]. In a series of six children, two became seizure-free, two experienced infrequent attacks, and two obtained modest benefit, whereas only two of five medically treated patients were controlled and one infant died in cardiac failure [110]. Two additional infants showed striking improvement in psychomotor performance coincident to postoperative cessation of seizures and reduction of anticonvulsant therapy [111].

Dysplastic Gangliocytoma

Dysplastic gangliocytomas of the cerebral hemispheres are a rare but surgically treatable cause of early-onset seizures [112]. Believed to represent granule cells that undergo arrested migration, gangliocytomas are hamartomatous but can enlarge in later life [113–115].

Gangliocytomas of the cerebral hemispheres can produce partial seizures of unusual severity and very early onset [116,117]. Magnetic resonance imaging

reveals mixed signal-intensity abnormalities on T1-weighted images and proton-density images and decreased signal intensity on T2-weighted images (Fig. 16-3) [118].

Chronic Focal Encephalitis (Rasmussen's Syndrome)

In 1958, Rasmussen et al. described three children with chronic partial seizures and focal inflammatory changes of brain tissue [119]. Although relatively uncommon, this disorder has now been reported at multiple centers and typically has its onset in childhood [120–124].

Patients with chronic focal encephalitis (CFE) have focal or lateralized seizure patterns that may progress to epilepsia partialis continua. Contralateral hemiparesis and dementia ensue, and serial neuroimaging studies reveal hemispheric atrophy. The EEG demonstrates polymorphic slowing and spike discharges. A viral etiology has been proposed [125] but has not been confirmed. Most excisional procedures, including hemispherectomy, are of equivocal benefit [121–124,126], and CFE typically follows a biphasic course characterized by early deterioration and a plateau phase [125].

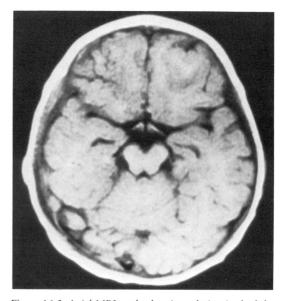

Figure 16-3. Axial MRI study showing a lesion in the left frontal pole without mass effect in an infant with medically resistant partial seizures. The pathologic diagnosis was dysplastic gangliocytoma.

Catastrophic Seizures in Infancy

Partial seizures may occur multiple times per day in some infants and be resistant to all medical therapy. The cumulative burden of the seizures and pharmacotoxicity raises significant concerns about long-term neurologic status. Interventional surgery is therefore an attractive option in the context of rapid deterioration. Hemispherectomy is advocated for infants with lateralized seizure patterns, hemiplegia, and hemianopia [126], but the optimal management of infants who are neither hemiplegic nor hemianopic is less well established. Many have extratemporal seizures and nonconvergent EEG and imaging findings [127]. In a single report of excisional surgery in five infants with very frequent partial seizures and deteriorating status [128], three became seizure-free and two improved significantly. Surgery did not impair neurologic or developmental status.

Contraindications to Early Surgery

Benign Focal Childhood Epilepsies

Several types of benign focal epilepsy are uniquely age-dependent and must be distinguished from more serious forms of partial seizures.

Benign Rolandic Epilepsy. This presents at the end of the first decade and accounts for as many as 23% of seizure disorders in school-age children [129]. Seizures typically consist of nocturnal simple partial motor or sensory events involving facial or oropharyngeal structures [130]. Secondary generalization is unusual, and permanent remission is the rule by age 15 years [131]. The disorder is familial, and the EEG reveals a characteristic centrotemporal spike field in drowsiness.

Benign Focal Epilepsy of Childhood with Occipital Spikes. This accounts for 4.3% of childhood seizures and has a uniformly favorable prognosis [132]. Elementary or complex visual hallucinations and migraine-like symptoms are typical, whereas other symptoms are rare [133]. The EEG demonstrates high-amplitude posterior-quadrant spike-and-wave discharges that attenuate with visual fixation. Imaging studies are unremarkable, and the EEG normalizes by adolescence. Seizures respond to most medications [134].

Landau-Kleffner Syndrome. This syndrome consists of acquired aphasia, seizures, and focal EEG abnormalities [135]. Markedly impaired receptive language abilities and verbal auditory agnosia characterize the majority of cases. Hyperactivity and personality disorders are also common, but there are few localizing signs other than the aphasia. Imaging studies are also unrevealing, and a smoldering encephalitis has been proposed as the underlying etiology [136]. Prognosis is variable, but older patients often recover more completely [137].

Seizures consist of simple partial, myoclonic, or generalized tonic-clonic attacks [138]. Complex partial seizures are distinctly unusual. Repetitive spikes and spike-waves occur in the posterior temporal and parietal regions [139], and occasional patients demonstrate multifocal EEG discharges.

AEDs will prevent seizures, and the disorder remits by late adolescence [139]. Therapy must therefore not be overly aggressive. Seizures and EEG disturbances are usually self-limited, whereas language deficits are often permanent, making the disorder "benign" only in terms of the epilepsy.

Benign Psychomotor Epilepsy. Dalla et al. [140] described an unusual benign form of childhood partial seizures consisting of attacks of fear or terror. Seizures usually last less than 2 minutes and motor manifestations are rare. The EEG reveals bilateral slow spike-and-wave discharges. Although seizures may be quite frequent early on, this disorder responds to AEDs and disappears by adolescence.

Neurodegenerative and Metabolic Disorders

Children with degenerative and metabolic conditions often have medically resistant epileptic seizures. A neurodegenerative etiology should therefore be suspected in any child with refractory seizures. Careful history and neurologic examination usually serve to identify most children, but progressive deficits become apparent within 1–2 years.

Degenerative and metabolic conditions in which seizures are either prominent or the first presenting signs are presented in Table 16-1.

Presurgical Evaluation

Noninvasive Monitoring

Most commercially available video/EEG systems can be used to monitor children [141–143]. Video/EEG monitoring is the cornerstone of the pediatric workup, and children adapt surprisingly well to the restrictive nature of the monitoring environment [8]. Prolonged recording is not a problem, but children

Table 16-1. Metabolic and Neurodegenerative Causes of Early Onset Intractable Epilepsy

Infancy
Adrenoleukodystrophy
Alper's disease
Amino acid disorders
- Argininosuccinic aciduria
- Homocystinuria
- Hyperprolinemia
- Phenylketonuria
Ceroid lipofuscinosis
Hereditary fructose intolerance
Kinky hair (Menkes') disease
Leucine sensitivity
Leukodystrophies
- Alexander's disease
- Canavan's disease
- Krabbe's disease
- Metachromatic leukodystrophy
Neurolipidoses
- GM_1 gangliosidosis
- GM_2 gangliosidosis
- Gaucher's disease
- Niemann-Pick disease
Subacute necrotizing encephalopathy

Childhood
Acute intermittent porphyria
Ceroid lipofuscinosis
Huntington's disease
Hypocalcemia
Metachromatic leukodystrophy
Mitochondrial encephalomyopathy
Progressive familial myoclonic epilepsy

should be allowed to visit a playroom or communal area at reasonably frequent intervals during the testing. Monitoring the hospital playroom will increase ictal capture rate.

Video/EEG recording of infants, toddlers, and brain-damaged children may present special difficulties. Very prolonged electrode placement is rarely tolerated, and EEG leads must be secured by occlusive dressings to prevent their removal or damage. A "rapid-release" EEG cable helps prevent dislodgement of the electrodes and ensures that data are not lost. Once these modifications are made, manual restraint is rarely necessary.

Crib siderails are a visual barrier to monitoring. Video cameras in pediatric units should therefore be mounted high enough to avoid such obstruction. Customized crib siderails of clear Persplex (Fig. 16-4) are a means of obtaining unobstructed viewing.

Teaching parents about video/EEG recording can yield important dividends. A satellite monitor at the bedside alerts parents to their child's being off camera. The video camera can be repositioned by the parents or they may seek assistance from the EEG technologist.

Special recording electrodes, including supraorbital, nasopharyngeal, and sphenoidal placements, and closely spaced electrode arrays are well tolerated by children and often yield valuable localization information [144]. Computerized EEG topographic mapping studies of the childhood epilepsies [145] reveal increased faster frequencies in the region of the epileptic focus [146].

PET studies of infants with nonlesional epilepsy can localize pathologic seizure foci [147] and provide information about the functional integrity of cortex outside the field of resection [148]. PET has been used to select Sturge-Weber syndrome patients for surgery [79].

The contribution of single photon emission computerized tomography (SPECT) to pediatric epilepsy surgery case selection is relatively unexplored. In a single published series of 100 children with epilepsy, there were 16 abnormal SPECT scans in patients with normal anatomic findings [149]. Xenon regional cerebral blood flow (rCBF) measurement of cerebral

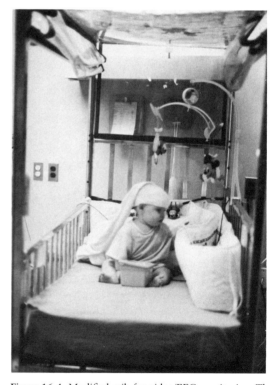

Figure 16-4. Modified crib for video/EEG monitoring. The foot end has been replaced by a sheet of clear Persplex. Video images through Persplex are indistinguishable from unobstructed images.

blood flow and regional differences in the local cerebral metabolic rate of glucose have been performed in the human neonate [150], but no data are available in children with epilepsy.

Intracranial Recording

The majority of pediatric patients have extratemporal seizure foci and require intracranial EEG monitoring for purposes of localization [151]. Epidural grid electrodes were first introduced by Goldring to localize seizures extraoperatively in unrestrained children [152,153]. This technique was an important advance over awake intraoperative studies in adults. Since the dura was left intact, complications of epidural implantation were rare [153].

More recently, flexible, small epidural peg electrodes have been substituted for large epidural grids [154]. Peg electrodes are semi-invasive and result in low morbidity since placement is made through a burr hole.

Most pediatric centers now use subdural strips or grids of electrodes to monitor infants and young children intracranially. Subdural electrodes yield accurate localizing data and facilitate mapping of eloquent cortex extraoperatively [155–157]. Compared with adults, children with chronically implanted subdural electrodes demonstrate equal success with seizure localization and cortical mapping [156]. Outcome with respect to seizure control in subdurally monitored children and adults is also comparable.

There are few published reports of depth electrode recording in children. Chronically implanted depth electrodes successfully localized seizures from the right cingulate gyrus in an 11-year-old girl [158]. Intraoperative depth electrode recording in children has also been accomplished under direct visualization using real-time ultrasound [159].

The morbidity and mortality of depth electrode placement are acceptably low. The higher proportion of extratemporal epilepsy probably contributes to their underutilization, but in mesial temporal cases, preoperative depth electrode studies would be expected to yield valuable information in children as well as in adults. Intraoperative depth studies of children have been used to provide information that is complementary to subdural EEG data [157].

Functional Mapping

The standard electrical stimulation paradigm developed to map eloquent cortex in adults is of diminished usefulness in children [160,161]. Young children consistently exhibit higher thresholds for both afterdischarges and functional responses, with thresholds showing an inverse relationship to age [160]. The refractoriness of immature cortex is probably due to incomplete myelination. The decrease in threshold with age parallels myelin production.

Functional mapping can be performed in infants and young children if stimulation is delivered at higher energy levels using stepwise increases in both intensity and duration [162]. Using this dual stimulation paradigm, infants under 1 year of age are now recognized to have well-defined hand and face regions and generate reliable electrical afterdischarges [163].

Pharmacokinetics

Proving that childhood epilepsy is medically resistant is often challenging. Children show wide variability in their pharmacokinetic profiles [164] and rapid drug clearances, and may even demonstrate total AED malabsorption [165].

Drug toxicity is also prominently related to age. Valproate-induced idiosyncratic hepatotoxicity primarily affects very young patients [166], and barbiturate-induced hyperactivity and learning disorders and phenytoin-induced gingival hyperplasia are particularly prevalent in childhood. Cases of anticonvulsant-induced Stevens-Johnson syndrome are particularly frequent in the first two decades of life.

Pharmacokinetic factors thus modify pediatric surgical referrals in contradictory ways. While the increased frequency of drug side effects and toxicity restricts the number of therapeutic options in childhood and favors earlier surgical consideration, fluctuations in serum drug concentration and the higher incidence of pediatric drug reactions make medical resistance difficult to prove and therefore mandate caution.

Neuropsychiatric Issues

Preparation for Hospitalization and Surgery

Proper emotional support should be given to all children being evaluated for epilepsy surgery. Young patients cannot interpret the nature or significance of the presurgical work-up or the surgery, cannot seek information, and are likely to misperceive the hospital experience. Too often, their parents are also unable to provide satisfactory explanations of the procedures, and the children's separation anxieties intensify. Children are therefore at high risk for serious emotional consequences of the surgery experience.

Several techniques can help prepare children for the emotional challenges of surgery. Models are the most widely employed technique to introduce the hospital routine and medical procedures. Filmed modeling requires few personnel and little equipment over and above a projector and screen. Puppet models help transmit information and alleviate anxiety in young children (Fig. 16-5). Modeling sessions also help parents cope with the stresses of their child's hospitalization and surgery.

Pediatric nursing intervention is also essential for proper emotional support of the child and parents [167]. If administered at difficult junctures during the hospitalization, nursing support increases cooperation and reduces rates of postoperative complication [168].

Family Assessment

Chronic childhood handicapping illnesses often lead to pervasive family dysfunction. Marital and parent-

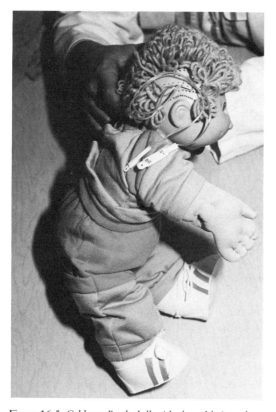

Figure 16-5. Cabbage Patch doll with shaved hair and "subdural grid." The doll helps to prepare young children for monitoring.

child conflicts intensify under the strain of chronic illness and render families vulnerable to external sources of stress. Thus, even though the burden of chronic epilepsy leads to early surgical consideration, families may find it hard to cope with intensive and prolonged hospitalizations or the psychological consequences of unsuccessful or complicated surgery.

The preoperative evaluation of the epileptic child must therefore include clear explanations of the surgical procedure and in-depth assessment of family functioning. A professional trained in developmental and/or family therapy should interview the family and document patterns of family interaction. Significant disturbances in family dynamics and individual patterns of psychiatric disability must be identified, along with unrealistic fears or expectations regarding the outcome of the surgery. These issues need to be weighed carefully prior to any surgical decision-making.

Neuropsychological Testing

Neuropsychological assessment is a standard part of the preoperative evaluation of adults for epilepsy surgery. Theoretical and methodologic considerations in children modify test scores, and since the cognitive sequelae of brain damage in early life are less predictable, neuropsychological test scores may be more difficult to interpret. Furthermore, tests standardized in normal children may not apply to the handicapped child with epilepsy. Since brain-damaged children often show short attention spans and problems initiating and maintaining set, testing may yield unrealistically low estimates of higher cortical function.

Despite these limitations, neuropsychological assessment is still indicated to document brain behavior relationships and assess preoperative levels of cognitive function [169]. Since a principal goal of early surgery is to alleviate psychosocial disability, as much baseline data as possible should be acquired. Neuropsychological testing should therefore be performed in children over the age of 6 years and in younger cooperative children of normal or near-normal intelligence. At a minimum, IQ, language skills, attention, and verbal and figural memory functions should be assessed in children of all ages.

Outcome

Focal Resection

The outcome of excisional surgery for partial epilepsy in children was first reported in 20 patients with intractable complex partial seizures of temporal lobe origin [170] and later expanded to 40 children under the age 15 years, 50% of whom were followed at least 6 years [55]. Postoperatively, 23 became seizure-free, 8 were almost seizure-free, and 5 improved significantly. This initial experience confirmed the benefit of operating early in life and has been confirmed at other centers [1,52,65,171–176]. Remission rates among centers tend to vary, but freedom or near-freedom from seizures is usually reported in 60–80% of patients. Variability probably reflects differences in the definitions of medical intractability and willingness to take on nonlesional cases.

The neuropathologic underpinnings of chronic childhood epilepsy are often antenatally acquired [176,177]. Acquired tumors (astrocytoma, ganglioglioma, ganglioneuroma) are far less common, and mesial temporal sclerosis is more typical of the adolescent [178–180].

The outcome of extratemporal resection in childhood is less favorable than that of temporal lobe surgery but similar to that reported in adults [181]. Complete remission or unambiguous improvement in the quality of life can be expected in nearly two thirds of children undergoing extratemporal resections.

Excisional surgery in children also improves neurobehavioral status [55,65,171–173]. Rage attacks, impulsivity, hyperactivity, and antisocial patterns including sexual promiscuity and juvenile delinquency have all been reported to diminish postoperatively. Whittle et al. [171] and Vaernet [172] found improved family relations and interpersonal socialization skills coincident to a reduction in seizure frequency, and the Mayo Clinic reported almost universally improved family social function [174]. Attitude toward schooling and academic performance improved as well despite absence of change in IQ scores [172].

The effect of surgery on the intellectual status of children is less convincing. Meyer et al. noted no change in the scores of children rendered seizure-free, although improved verbal and performance IQ scores correlated with shorter periods of preoperative seizures [174]. Harbord and Manson [175] and Whittle et al. [171] also noted no change in intellectual status following surgery. Adams et al. [178] reported a decline in verbal memory following left temporal lobectomy, whereas nonverbal recall was unchanged. Cavazutti et al. [182] noted improvement of functions in the nonoperative hemisphere in tumor cases but not in focal atrophy, a finding of unclear significance.

Psychotic thought disturbances in adults with complex partial seizures rarely remit after surgery. It remains unknown, however, whether psychosis is preventable by earlier intervention.

Rates of surgical complications in children are also comparable to those in adults. Superior quadrantanopic visual field defects and transient dysphasia are the most commonly reported consequences of temporal lobectomy [171–175]. Approximately 5% of children undergoing temporal and extratemporal resections suffer transient third-nerve palsies or hemipareses. Less commonly reported complications include infected bone flaps, transient rhinorrhea, subdural fluid collections, intraventricular hemorrhage, and meningitis [174].

Future studies of excisional surgery in childhood need to address behavioral, rehabilitative, and neuropsychological issues. The rationale for early surgical intervention would be strengthened considerably if it could be shown that psychosocial benefit can occur independent of seizure control.

Hemispherectomy

Removal of one cerebral hemisphere to treat epilepsy was initially developed and performed as a pediatric procedure. In the first published study, all children were rendered seizure-free, and their behavioral and psychosocial status also improved dramatically [183]. Spasticity increased in the immediate postoperative period but resolved with time, and long-term motor function ultimately improved. No children were cognitively impaired.

Subsequent hemispherectomy series reveal that 85% of patients become seizure-free or nearly so and improve with respect to rage attacks, hyperactivity, and attentional problems [184]. Surgery does not alter the behavior of children who are behaviorally normal.

Studies of long-term outcome after early hemispherectomy are also available. Of 17 patients undergoing surgery at a mean age of 11.5 years and followed for up to 36 years, 16 became seizure-free or nearly so [185]. Most were hemiplegic before age 5 years and had behavioral problems and cognitive deficits causing exclusion from normal schools. The single failure occurred in the most severely handicapped child.

Verity et al. [186] showed that neuropsychological performance improves after either right or left hemispherectomy but spatial abilities remain delayed. No children became aphasic, yet despite their seemingly impressive behavioral and intellectual gains, most patients remain handicapped due to underlying brain damage. The long-term prognosis for psychosocial function thus still remains poor.

Corpus Callosotomy

Corpus callosotomy was also developed as a pediatric procedure for treatment of lateralized seizures and cerebral hemiatrophy. Three of four children in the original series obtained a significant reduction in seizure frequency, and there were no residual sequelae although formal neuropsychological testing was not obtained [187].

More recently, commissural surgery has been advocated for a variety of childhood seizure disorders [188]. Improved outcome has been reported in the focal epilepsies and correlates with improved neuropsychological scores but not with the postoperative EEG. Callosotomy is particularly effective in children with atonic seizures, with at least 75% remitting or at diminished risk for self-injury [189,190]. Tonic seizures also respond favorably [191], but myoclonic seizures rarely improve, especially if they are the predominant seizure type [191]. Callosotomy has been advocated for simple and complex partial seizures and secondarily generalized grand mal [192], but partial seizures rarely remit after callosotomy, and focal resection remains the procedure of choice.

It has been suggested that children with mental retardation experience the poorest outcome after callosotomy [193]. However, mental retardation is multifactorial, and cognitive level is probably not a reliable contraindication for surgery. In one study, callosotomy was shown to be equally effective in retarded patients compared with patients of normal or near-normal intelligence [191].

The neuropsychological consequences of disconnecting the cerebral hemispheres in early life are even less well understood. Early acquired lesions limited to the corpus callosum are virtually unknown in childhood, and although children with congenital absence of the corpus callosum are more common, data from this population should not be extrapolated to patients whose hemispheres have been disconnected surgically [194–196]. Studies of tactile and tactuomotor integration after early and late callosotomy indicate that younger children are considerably less affected by the interruption of callosal fibers [197]. Neuropsychological outcome after early callosotomy has also been shown to reflect neurologic status, with higher intelligence predicting better outcome with respect to seizure control [198].

The indications, outcome, and effects of early callosotomy await further study. Earlier rather than later intervention appears advantageous but requires better documentation. Patients with Lennox-Gastaut syndrome may be an important group for further study since functional studies indicate the existence of at least two distinct subtypes. It is therefore possible that careful EEG and imaging may identify selected Lennox-Gastaut patients who might benefit from excisional procedures [199,200].

References

1. Jensen I. Temporal lobe epilepsy. Types of seizures, age, and surgical results. *Acta Neurol Scand* 1976; 53:335–57.
2. Rutter M, Graham P, Yule W. A neuropsychiatric study in childhood. In: *Clinics in Developmental Medicine 35/36*. London: Spastics International Medical Publications, 1970.
3. Nelson KB, Ellenberg JH. Antecedents of seizure disorders in early childhood. *Am J Dis Child* 1986; 140:1053–61.
4. Tharp BR. An overview of pediatric seizure disorders and epileptic syndromes. *Epilepsia* 1987;28 (Suppl): S36–45.
5. Ogunyemi AO, Dreifuss FE. Syndromes of epilepsy in childhood and adolescence. *J Child Neurol* 1988; 3:214–24.
6. Otahara S. Seizure disorders in infancy and childhood. *Brain Dev* (Tokyo) 1984;6:509–19.
7. De Negri M. Generalized epilepsy in childhood: some notes from a developmental perspective. *Brain Dev* 1988;10:285–8.
8. Duchowny MS. Intensive monitoring of the epileptic child. *J Clin Neurophysiol* 1985;2:203–20.
9. Sheridan PH, Sato S. Applications of intensive monitoring in epilepsy. *J Clin Neurophysiol* 1985; 2(3):221–9.
10. Jayakar P, Duchowny MS. Complex partial seizures of temporal lobe origin in early childhood. In: Duchowny MS, Resnick TJ, Alvarez LA, eds. *Pediatric epilepsy surgery*. New York: Demos. 1990.
11. Drury I. Epileptiform patterns of children. *J Clin Neurophysiol* 1989;6(1):1–39.
12. Kennard MA. Reorganization of motor function in the cerebral cortex of monkeys deprived of motor and premotor areas in infancy. *J Neurophysiol* 1983; 1:477–96.
13. Wada JA, Clarke R, Hamm A. Cerebral hemispheric asymmetry in humans. *Arch Neurol* 1975;32:239–46.
14. Chi JG, Dooling EC, Gilles FH. Left-right asymmetries of the temporal speech areas of the human fetus. *Arch Neurol* 1977;34:346–8.
15. Annett M. Laterality of childhood hemiplegia and the growth of speech and intelligence. *Cortex* 1973;9:4–39.
16. Woods BT, Teuber HL. Changing patterns of childhood aphasia. *Ann Neurol* 1978;3:273–80.
17. Woods BT, Teuber HL. Early onset of complementary specialization of cerebral hemispheres in man. *Trans Am Neurol Assoc* 1973;98:113–7.
18. Wasterlain CG. Effect of epileptic seizures on brain ribosomes: mechanisms and relationship to cerebral energy metabolism. *J Neurochem* 1977;29:707–16.
19. Dwyer BE, Wasterlain CG. Electroconvulsive seizures selectively impair myelin accumulation in the immature rat. *Exp Neurol* 1982;78:616–28.
20. Jorgensen OS, Dwyer BE, Wasterlain CG. Synaptic proteins after electroconvulsive seizures in immature rats. *J Neurochem* 1980;35:123–37.

21. Wasterlain CG, Plum F. Vulnerability of developing rat brain to electroconvulsive seizures. *Arch Neurol* 1973;20:38–45.
22. Moshe SL, Albala BJ. Kindling in developing rats: persistence of seizures in adulthood. *Dev Brain Res* 1983;4:67–71.
23. Holmes GL. Effect of serial seizures on subsequent kindling in the immature brain. *Dev Brain Res* 1983;6:190–2.
24. Olney JW, Collins RC, Sloviter RS. Excitotoxic mechanisms of epileptic brain damage. In: Delgado-Escueta AV, ed. *Advances in neurology,* vol 44. New York: Raven Press, 1986.
25. Meldrum B. Amino acid neurotransmitters and new approaches to anticonvulsant drug action. *Epilepsia* 1984;2(Suppl):S140–9.
26. Chandry MR, Pond DA. Mental deterioration in epileptic children. *J Neurol Neurosurg Psychiatry* 1961; 24:213–9.
27. Seidenberg M, O'Lery DS, Berent S, Boll T. Changes in seizure frequency and test-retest scores on the Wechsler Adult Intelligence Scale. *Epilepsia* 1981; 22:75–83.
28. Farwell JR, Dodrill CB, Batzel LW. Neuropsychological abilities of children with epilepsy. *Epilepsia* 1985;26(5):395–400.
29. Holmes GL. Do seizures cause brain damage? *Int Pediatr* 1988;3:158–64.
30. Holmes GL, Moshe SL. Consequences of seizures in the developing brain. In: Duchowny MS, Resnick TJ, Alvarez LA, eds. *Pediatric epilepsy surgery.* New York: Demos, 1990.
31. Taylor DC. Child behavioral problems and temporal lobe epilepsy. In: Parsonage M, et al, eds. *Advances in epileptology: XIVth epilepsy international symposium.* New York: Raven Press, 1983.
32. Bradley C. Behavior disturbances in epileptic children. *JAMA* 1951;146:436–41.
33. Pond DA, Bidwell B. Management of behaviour disorders in epileptic children. *Br Med J* 1954;2:1520–3.
34. Keating LE. Epilepsy and behavior in school children. *Mental Sciences* 1961;107:161–80.
35. Mulhearn RK, Kounar EH, Kun LE, Crisco JJ, Williams JM. Psychologic and neurologic function following treatment for childhood temporal lobe astrocytoma. *J Child Neurol* 1988;3:47–52.
36. Green JB. Association of behavior disorder with an electroencephalographic focus in children without seizures. *Neurology* 1961;11:337–44.
37. Shukla GD, Scivastava ON, Katiyar BC, Joshi V, Mohan PK. Psychiatric manifestations in temporal lobe epilepsy: a controlled study. *Br J Psychiatry* 1979; 135:411–7.
38. Pritchard PB, Lombroso CT, McIntyre M. Psychosocial complications of temporal lobe epilepsy. *Neurology* 1980;30:227–32.
39. Bray PF. Temporal lobe syndrome in children. A longitudinal review. *Pediatrics* 1962;617–28.
40. Lindsay J, Ounsted C, Richards P. Long-term outcome in children with temporal lobe seizures. III. Psychiatric aspects in children and adult life. *Dev Med Child Neurol* 1979;21:630–6.
41. Dinner DS, Luders H, Rothner AD, Erenberg G. Complex partial seizures of childhood onset: a clinical and electrographic study. *Cleve Clin Q* 1984; 51:287–91.
42. Hermann BP, Schwartz MS, Karnes WE, Vahdat P. Psychopathology in epilepsy: relationship of seizure type to age of onset. *Epilepsia* 1980;21:15–23.
43. McIntyre M, Pritchard PB, Lombroso CT. Left and right temporal lobe epileptics: a controlled investigation of some psychological differences. *Epilepsia* 1976;17:377–86.
44. Flor-Henry P. Psychosis and temporal lobe epilepsy. A controlled investigation. *Epilepsia* 1969;10:363–95.
45. Bourgeois BFD, Prensky AL, Palkes HS, Talent BK, Busch SG. Intelligence in epilepsy: a prospective study in children. *Ann Neurol* 1983;14:438–44.
46. O'Leary DS, Seidenberg M, Berent S, Boll TJ. Effects of age of onset of tonic-clonic seizures on neuropsychological performance in children. *Epilepsia* 1981;22:197–204.
47. Dikmen S, Matthews CG, Harley JP. Effect of early versus late onset of major motor epilepsy on cognitive-intellectual performance: further considerations. *Epilepsia* 1977;18(1):31–6.
48. Ellenberg JH, Hirtz DG, Nelson KB. Do seizures in children cause intellectual deterioration? *N Engl J Med* 1986;314:1085–8.
49. Durwen HF, Elger CE, Helmstaedter C, Penin H. Circumscribed improvement of cognitive performance in temporal lobe epilepsy patients with intractable seizures following reduction of anticonvulsant medication. *J Epilepsy* 1982;2:147–53.
50. Loiseau P, Strube E, Brouslet D, Batterlochi S, Gomeni C, Morselli PI. Learning impairment in epileptic patients. *Epilepsia* 1983;24:183–92.
51. Ounsted C, Lindsay J, Norman R. *Biological factors in temporal lobe epilepsy.* In: *Clinics in Developmental Medicine.* London: Heinemann, 1966.
52. Lindsay J, Ounsted C, Richards P. Long-term outcome in children with temporal lobe seizures. V. Indications and contra-indications for neurosurgery. *Dev Med Child Neurol* 1984;26:25–32.
53. Lindsay J, Ounsted C, Richards P. Long-term outcome in children with temporal lobe seizures. I. Social outcome and childhood factors. *Dev Med Child Neurol* 1979;21:285–98.
54. Lindsay J, Ounsted C, Richards P. Long-term outcome in children with temporal lobe seizures. II. Marriage, parenthood and sexual indifference. *Dev Med Child Neurol* 1979;21:433–40.
55. Davidson S, Falconer MA. Outcome of surgery in 40 children with temporal-lobe epilepsy. *Lancet* 1975; 1:1260–3.
56. Ward F, Bower BD. A study of certain social aspects of epilepsy in childhood. *Dev Med Child Neurol Suppl* 1978;39(20):1–63.
57. Hoare P. Does illness foster dependency? A study of epileptic and diabetic children. *Dev Med Child Neurol* 1984;26:20–4.

58. Austin JK. Childhood epilepsy: child adaption and family resources. *Child Adolesc Psychiat Ment Health Nurs* 1988;1(1):18–24.

59. Mittan RJ. Patients' fears of death and brain damage from seizures. *Merritt Putnam Quarterly* 1989; 5(6): 3–14.

60. Aicardi J. Status epilepticus in infants and children: consequences and prognosis. *Int Pediatr* 1987;2:189–95.

61. Aicardi J, Chevrie JJ. Convulsive status epilepticus in infants and children: a study of 239 cases. *Epilepsia* 1970;11:187–97.

62. Lesstma JE, Walczad T, Hughes JR, Kalelkar MB, Teas SS. A prospective study on sudden unexpected death in epilepsy. *Ann Neurol* 1989;26:195–203.

63. Hirsch CR, Martin DL. Unexpected death in young epileptics. *Neurology* 1971;21:682–90.

64. Terrence CF, Wisotzkey HM, Perper JA. Unexpected, unexplained death in epileptic patients. *Neurology* 1975;25:594–8.

65. Jensen I, Vaernet K. Temporal lobe epilepsy. Follow-up investigation of 74 temporal lobe resected patients. *Acta Neurochir* 1977;37:173–200.

66. Falconer MA, Serafetinides EA. A follow-up study of surgery in temporal lobe epilepsy. *J Neurol Neurosurg* 1963;26:154–65.

67. Stepien L, Bidzinski J, Mazurowsky W. The results of surgical treatment of temporal lobe epilepsy. *Pol Med J* 1969;8:1184–90.

68. Bebin EB, Gomez MR. Prognosis in Sturge-Weber disease: comparison of unihemispheric and bihemispheric involvement. *J Child Neurol* 1988;3:181–4.

69. Crosley CJ, Binet EF. Sturge-Weber syndrome. Presentation as a focal seizure disorder without nevus flammeus. *Skin and Allergy* 1978;17(8):606–9.

70. Taly AB, Nagaraja D, Das S, Shankar SK, Pratibha NG. Sturge-Weber-Dimitri disease without facial nevus. *Neurology* 1987;37:1063–4.

71. Peterman AF, Hayles AB, Dockerty MD, Love JG: Encephalotrigeminal angiomatosis (Sturge-Weber disease): clinical study of thirty-five cases. *JAMA* 1958; 167:2169–76.

72. Alexander GL, Norman RM. *The Sturge-Weber syndrome*. Bristol: John Wright & Sons, 1960.

73. Polani PE: Encephalotrigeminal angiomatosis (Sturge-Weber syndrome) treated by removal of affected cerebral hemisphere. *Proc R Soc Med* 1952;42:860–2.

74. Falconer MA, Rushworth RG. Treatment of encephalotrigeminal angiomatosis (Sturge-Weber disease) by hemispherectomy. *Arch Dis Child* 1960;35:433–7.

75. Hoffman HJ, Hendrick EB, Dennis M, Armstrong D. Hemispherectomy for Sturge-Weber syndrome. *Childs Brain* 1979;233–48.

76. Ogunmekan AL, Hwang PA, Hoffman HG. Sturge-Weber-Dmitri disease: role of hemispherectomy in prognosis. *Can J Neurol Sci* 1989;16:78–80.

77. Beaulieu MA, Andermann F, Rasmussen T, Olivier A, Villemure JG, Montes J. The Sturge-Weber syndrome and intractable epilepsy: surgical strategy depends on the localization and type of epileptic process. *Neurology* 1988;38(Suppl 1):280.

78. Brenner RP, Sharbrough FW. Electroencephalographic evaluation in Sturge-Weber syndrome. *Neurology* 1976;26:629–32.

79. Chugani HT, Mazziotta JC, Phelps ME. Sturge-Weber syndrome: a study of cerebral glucose utilization with positron emission tomography. *J Pediatr* 1989;114: 244–53.

80. Rosen I, Salford L, Starck L. Sturge-Weber disease—neurophysiological evaluation of a case with secondary epileptogenesis, successfully treated with lobectomy. *Neuropediatrics* 1984;5:95–8.

81. George RE, Hoffman HJ, Hwang PA, Becker LE, Chuang SH. Management of intractable seizures in unilateral megalencephaly. In: Duchowny MS, Resnick TJ, Alvarez LA, eds. *Pediatric epilepsy surgery*. New York: Demos, 1990.

82. Gomez MR. Criteria for diagnosis. In: Gomez MR, ed. *Tuberous sclerosis (2nd ed)*. New York: Raven Press, 1988.

83. Abo K, Marikawa T, Fujiwara T, Ishida S, Serno M, Wada T. Tuberous sclerosis and epilepsy. In: Parsonage M, et al., eds. *Advances in epileptology: XIVth epilepsy international symposium*. New York: Raven Press, 1983.

84. Monaghan HP, Krafchik BR, MacGregor DL, Fitz CR. Tuberous sclerosis complex in children. *Am J Dis Child* 1981;135:912–7.

85. Perot P, Weir B, Rasmussen T. Tuberous sclerosis. Surgical therapy for seizures. *Arch Neurol* 1966; 15:498–506.

86. Erba G, Duchowny MS: Partial epilepsy and tuberous sclerosis—indications for surgery in disseminated disease. In: Duchowny MS, Resnick TJ, Alvarez LA, eds. *Pediatric epilepsy surgery*. New York: Demos, 1990.

87. Dobyns WB, Stratton RF, Parke J, Greenberg F, Nussbaum RL, Ledbetter DH. Miller-Dieker syndrome: lissencephaly and monosomy 17 p. *J Pediatr* 1983; 102:552–8.

88. Aicardie J. Lissencephalic syndromes. *Int Pediatr* 1989;4(2):118–26.

89. Cameron DA, Wada JA, Farrel K, Slodmark O, Li D. Macrogyria in intractable partial seizures. *Epilepsia* 1986;27(5):594.

90. Andermann F, Olivier A, Melanson D, Robitaille Y. Epilepsy due to focal cortical dysplasia with macrogyria and the forme fruste of tuberous sclerosis: a study of 15 patients. In: Wolf P, Dam M, Janz D, Dreifuss FE, eds. *Advances in epileptology*. New York: Raven Press, 1987.

91. Kuzniecky R, Andermann F, Tampieri D, Melanson D, Olivier A, Leppek I. Bilateral central macrogyria: epilepsy, pseudobulbar palsy, and mental retardation—a recognizable neuronal migration disorder. *Ann Neurol* 1989;25:547–54.

92. Chin-Chen M, Coull BM, Golper LAC, Rau MT. Anterior operculum syndrome. *Neurology* 1989;39: 1169–72.

93. Graff-Radford NR, Bosch EP, Stears JC, Tranel D. Developmental Foix-Chaveny-Marie syndrome in identical twins. *Ann Neurol* 1986;20:632–5.

94. Taylor DC, Falconer MA, Brutton CJ, Corsellis JAN. Focal dysplasia of the cerebral cortex in epilepsy. *J Neurol Neurosurg Psychiatry* 1971;34:369–87.

95. Nordborg C, Sourander P, Sylvenius H, Blom S, Zetterlund B. Mild cortical dysplasia in patients with intractable seizures: a histological study. In: Wolf P, Dam M, Janz D, Dreifuss FE, eds. *Advances in epileptology,* vol 16. New York: Raven Press, 1987.

96. Kuzniecky R, Berkovic S, Andermann A, Melancon D, Olivier A, Robitaille Y. Focal cortical myoclonus and rolandic cortical dysplasia: clarification by magnetic resonance imaging. *Ann Neurol* 1988;23:317–25.

97. Marchal G, Andermann F, Tampieri D, Robitaille Y, Melanson D, Sinclair B, Olivier A, et al. Generalized cortical dysplasia manifested by diffusely thick cerebral cortex. *Arch Neurol* 1989;46:430–4.

98. Layton DD. Heterotopic cerebral gray matter as an epileptogenic focus. *J Neuropathol Exp Neurol* 1962; 21:244–9.

99. Potolicchio SJ, Miles R. Intractable epilepsy due to gray matter heterotopias. *Neurology* 1989;39(Suppl 1):150.

100. Sarnat HB. Disturbances of late neuronal migration in the perinatal period. *Am J Dis Child* 1987;141:969–80.

101. Hardiman O, Burket T, Phillips J, Murphy S, O'Moore B, Staunton H, Farrell MA. Microdysgenesis in resected temporal neocortex: incidence and clinical significance in focal epilepsy. *Neurology* 1988;38:1041–7.

102. Meencke HJ. Neuron density in the molecular layer of the frontal cortex with heterotopia of the gray matter. *J Comput Assist Tomogr* 1978;2:291–6.

103. Galaburda AM, Sherman GF, Roseng D, Aboitiz F, Geschwind N. Developmental dyslexia: four consecutive patients with cortical abnormalities. *Ann Neurol* 1985;18:222–33.

104. Kaufmann WE, Galaburda AM. Cerebrocortical microdysgenesis in neurologically normal subjects: a histopathologic study. *Neurology* 1989;39:238–44.

105. Robain O, Floquet CH, Heldt N. Hemimegalencephaly: a clinicopathological study of four cases. *Neuropathol Appl Neurobiol* 1988;14:125–35.

106. Tijiam AT, Stefanko S, Schenk VWD, de Vlieger M. Infantile spasms associated with hemihypsarrhythmia and hemimegalencephaly. *Dev Med Child Neurol* 1978;20:779–98.

107. King M, Stephenson JPB, Ziervogel M, Doyle D, Galbraith S. Hemimegalencephaly: a case for hemispherectomy? *Neuropediatrics* 1985;16:46–55.

108. Fitz CR, Harwood-Nash DC, Boldt DW. The radiographic features of unilateral megalencephaly. *Neuroradiology* 1978;15:145–8.

109. Mikhael MA, Mattar AG: Malformation of the cerebral cortex with heterotopia of the gray matter. *J Comput Assist Tomogr* 1978;2:291–6.

110. George RE, Hoffman HJ, Hwang PA, Becker LE, Chuang SH. Management of intractable seizures in unilateral megalencephaly. In: Duchowny MS, Resnick TJ, Alvarez LA, eds. *Pediatric epilepsy surgery.* New York: Demos, 1990.

111. Vigevano F, Bertini E, Boldrini R, Bosman C, Claps D, di Capua M, di Rocco C, et al. Hemimegalencephaly and intractable epilepsy: benefits of hemispherectomy. *Epilepsia* 1989;30(6):833–43.

112. Duchowny MS, Resnick TJ, Alvarez L. Dysplastic gangliocytoma and intractable partial seizures in childhood. *Neurology* 1989;39:601–4.

113. Leech RW, Christoferson LA, Gilbertson RL. Dysplastic gangliocytoma (L'hermitte-Duclos disease) of the cerebellum. *J Neurosurg* 1977;47:609–12.

114. Pritchett PS, King TI: Dysplastic gangliocytoma of the cerebellum—an ultrasound study. *Acta Neuropathol* (Berl) 1978;41:1–5.

115. Ambler M, Pogacar S, Sidman R. L'hermitte-Duclos disease (granule cell hypertrophy of the cerebellum). Pathological analysis of the first familial case. *J Neuropathol Exp Neurol* 1969;28:622–47.

116. Kernohan JW, Learmouth JR, Doyle JB. Neuroblastomas and gangliocytomas of the central nervous system. *Brain* 1932;55:287–310.

117. Dom R, Brucher JM. Hamartoblastome (gangliocytome diffus) unilateral de l'ecorce cerebrale: associe a une degenerescence soudanophile de la substance blanche du cote oppose. *Rev Neurol* (Paris) 1969; 44:703–8.

118. Altman N. MR and CT characteristics of gangliocytoma: a rare cause of epilepsy in children. *AJNR* 1988;9:917–21.

119. Rasmussen T, Olszewski J, Lloyd-Smith D. Focal seizures due to chronic localized encephalitis. *Neurology* 1958;8:435–45.

120. Rasmussen T, McCann W. Clinical studies of patients with focal epilepsy due to "chronic encephalitis." *Trans Am Neurol Assoc* 1968;93:89–94.

121. Gupta PC, Roy S, Tandon PN. Progressive epilepsy due to chronic persistent encephalitis. Report of four cases. *J Neurol Sci* 1974;22:105–20.

122. Dalos N, Vining EPG, Carson B, Freeman JM. Rasmussen's encephalitis: clinical recognition and surgical management. *Epilepsia* 1986;27:594.

123. Gray F, Serdaru M, Baron H, Baumas-Duport C, Loron P, Savron B, Porier J. Chronic localized encephalitis (Rasmussen's) in an adult with epilepsia partialis continua. *J Neurol Neurosurg Psychiatry* 1987; 50:747–51.

124. Piatt JH, Hwang PA, Armstrong DC, Becker LE, Hoffman HJ. Chronic focal encephalitis (Rasmussen's syndrome): six cases. *Epilepsia* 1988;29(3):268–79.

125. Rasmussen T. Further observations on the syndrome of chronic encephalitis and epilepsy. *Appl Neurophysiol* 1978;41:1–12.

126. Rasmussen T, Villemure JG. Cerebral hemispherectomy for seizures with hemiplegia. *Cleve Clin Med* 1988;56(Suppl 1):S62–8.

127. Duchowny MS. Complex partial seizures of infancy. *Arch Neurol* 1987;44:911–4.
128. Duchowny MS, Resnick TJ, Alvarez LA, Morrison G. Focal resection for malignant partial seizures in infancy. *Neurology* 40:980–4, 1990.
129. Heigbel J, Blom J, Bergfors P. Benign epilepsy of children with centrotemporal EEG foci: a study of incidence rate in out-patient care. *Epilepsia* 1975; 16:657–64.
130. Bladin PF, Papworth G. Chuckling and glugging seizures at night—sylvian spike epilepsy. *Proc Aust Assoc Neurol* 1974;11:171–6.
131. Blom S, Heijbel J. Benign epilepsy of children with central temporal EEG foci: a follow-up study in adulthood of patients initially studied as children. *Epilepsia* 1982;23:629–32.
132. Panayiotopoulos CP. Benign childhood epilepsy with occipital paroxysms: a 15 year prospective study. *Ann Neurol* 1989;26:51–6.
133. Niedermeyer E, Riggio S, Santiago M. Benign occipital lobe epilepsy. *J Epilepsy* 1988;1:3–11.
134. Gastaut H. A new type of epilepsy: benign partial epilepsy of childhoood with occipital spike-waves. *Clin Electroencephalogr* 1982;13:13–22.
135. Landau WM, Kleffner F. Syndrome of acquired aphasia with convulsive disorder in children. *Neurology* 1957;7:523–30.
136. Lou HC, Brandt S, Bruhn P. Progressive aphasia and epilepsy with a self-limited course. In: Penry JK, ed. *Epilepsy: the eighth international symposium.* New York: Raven Press, 1977.
137. Bishop DVM. Age of onset and outcome in "acquired aphasia with convulsive disorders" (Landau-Kleffner syndrome). *Dev Med Child Neurol* 1985;27:705–12.
138. Sawhney IMS, Suresh N, Dhand UK, Chopra JS. Acquired aphasia with epilepsy—Landau-Kleffner syndrome. *Epilepsia* 1988;29(3)283–7.
139. Beaumanior A. The Landau-Kleffner syndrome. In: Roger J, Dravet C, Bureau M, Dreifuss FE, Wolf P, eds. *Epileptic syndromes in infancy, childhood and adolescence.* London: Eurotext, 1985.
140. Dalla BB, Chiamenti C, Capovilla G, Trevisan E, Tassineri C. Benign partial epilepsies with affective symptoms (benign psychomotor epilepsy). In: Roger J, Dravet D, Bureau M, Dreifuss F, Wolf P, eds. *Epileptic syndromes in infancy, childhood and adolescence.* London: Eurotext, 1985.
141. Andermann F. Selection and investigation of candidates for surgical treatment of temporal lobe epilepsy in childhood and adolescence. In: Blaw ME, Rapin I, Kinsbourne M, eds. *Topics in child neurology.* New York: Spectrum, 1977.
142. Polkey CE. Selection of patients with intractable epilepsy for resective surgery. *Arch Dis Child* 1980; 55:841–4.
143. Green RC, Adler JR, Erba G. Epilepsy surgery in children. *J Child Neurol* 1988;3:155–66.
144. Resnick TJ. Evaluation of children for epilepsy surgery. *Int Pediatr* 1988;3(2):136–7.
145. Resnick TJ, Duchowny MS, Deray MJ, Alfonso I. Computerized EEG topography in children with seizures. In: *Proceedings of the sixteenth national meeting of the child neurology society.* San Diego, 1987;231.
146. Nuwer MR. Quantitative EEG: II. Frequency analysis and topographic mapping in clinical settings. *J Clin Neurophysiol* 1988;5(1):45–85.
147. Chugani HT, Shewmon DA, Shields WD, Peacock WJ, Phelps ME. Pediatric epilepsy surgery: pre- and postoperative evaluation with PET. In: Duchowny MS, Resnick TJ, Alvarez LA, eds. *Pediatric epilepsy surgery.* New York: Demos, 1990.
148. Chugani HT, Shewmon DA, Peacock WJ, Shields WD, Mazziotta JC. Surgical treatment of intractable neonatal-onset seizures: the role of positron emission tomography. *Neurology* 1988;38:1178–88.
149. Flamini JR, Konkol RJ, Wells RG, Sty JR. Cerebral iophetamine-single photon emission computed tomographic scan: analysis of 100 cases. *Ann Neurol* 1989;26:454A.
150. Younkin D, Delivoria-Papadopoulos M, Reivich M, Jaggi J, Obrist W. Regional variations in human newborn cerebral blood flow. *J Pediatr* 1988;112:104–8.
151. Luders H, Dinner DS, Morris HH, Wyllie E, Godoy J. EEG evaluation for epilepsy surgery in children. *Cleve Clin J Med* 1988;56(Suppl):S53–61.
152. Goldring S. A method of surgical management of focal epilepsy, especially as it relates to children. *J Neurosurg* 1978;49:344–56.
153. Goldring S, Gregorie E. Surgical management of epilepsy using epidural recordings to localize the seizure focus. *J Neurosurg* 1984;60:457–66.
154. Wyllie E, Burgess R, Awad I, Barnett G, Luders H. Flexible epidural peg electrodes for chronic electroencephalographic recording. *Ann Neurol* 1989; 26:471.
155. Resnick TJ, Duchowny M, Deray MJ, Alfonso I. Subdural electrode recording in the preoperative evaluation of partial seizures in children. *Ann Neurol* 1987;22(3):415.
156. Wyllie E, Luders H, Morris HH, Lesser RP, Dinner DS, et al. Subdural electrodes in the evaluation for epilepsy surgery in children and adults. *Neuropediatrics* 1988;19:80–6.
157. Resnick TJ, Duchowny M, Alvarez LA, Jayapar P, Haller JS. Comparison of depth and subdural electrodes in recording interictal activity of children being evaluated for surgery. *Epilepsia* 1989;30(5):659.
158. Levin B, Duchowny M. Childhood obsessive-compulsive disorder and cingulate epilepsy. *Biol Psychiatry* 1991;30:1049–55.
159. Altman NR, Duchowny M, Jayakar P, Resnick TJ, Alvarez LA, Morrison G. Placement of intracerebral depth electrodes during excisional surgery for epilepsy: value of intraoperative ultrasound. *AJNR* 1992;13:254–6.
160. Alvarez LA, Jayakar P. Cortical stimulation with subdural electrodes: special considerations in infancy and childhood. *J Epilepsy* 1990;3(Suppl):125–30.

161. Nespeca M, Wyllie E, Luders H, Rothner D, Kahn J, Awad I, Dinner D, Morris H, Cruse R, Erenberg G, Kotogal P, Kanner A, Estes M. EEG recording and functional localization studies with subdural electrodes in infants and young children. *J Epilepsy* 3(Suppl):107–24.

162. Jayakar P, Alvarez LA, Duchowny MS, Resnick TR. A safe and effective paradigm for functional mapping in children. *J Clin Neurophysiol* 9:288–93, 1992.

163. Duchowny M, Jayakar P. Functional cortical mapping in children. In: Devinsky O, Beric A, Dogali M, eds. *Electrical and magnetic stimulation of the brain.* (Advances in neurology,) New York: Raven, in Press.

164. Dodson WE. Special pharmacokinetic considerations in children. *Epilepsia* 1987;28(Suppl 1):556–70.

165. Gilman JT, Duchowny M, Resnick TJ: Carbamazepine malabsorption: a case report, *Pediatrics* 1988; 82:518–9.

166. Dreifuss FE, Langer DH, Moline KA, Maxwell JE: Valproic acid hepatic fatalities. II: US experience since 1984. *Neurology* 1989;39:201–7.

167. Skipper JK, Leonard RC. Children, stress and hospitalization: a field experiment. *J Health Soc Behavior* 1968;9:275–87.

168. Wolfer JA, Visintainer MA. Pediatric surgical patients' and parents' stress responses and adjustment. *Nurs Res* 1975;24:244–55.

169. Levin B, Feldman E, Duchowny M, Brown M. Neuropsychological assessment of children with epilepsy. *Int Pediatr* 6:214–9.

170. Falconer MA. Temporal lobe epilepsy in children and its surgical treatment. *Med J Aust* 1972;1:1117–21.

171. Whittle IR, Ellis HJ, Simpson DA. The surgical treatment of intractable childhood and adolescent epilepsy. *Aust NZ J Surg* 1981;51:109–96.

172. Vaernet K. Temporal lobectomy in children and young adults. In: Parsonage M, et al, eds. *Advances in epileptology: XIVth epilepsy international symposium.* New York: Raven Press, 1983.

173. Lindsay J, Glaser G, Richards P, Ounsted C. Developmental aspects of focal epilepsies of childhood treated by neurosurgery. *Dev Med Child Neurol* 1984; 26:574–87.

174. Meyer FB, Marsh WR, Laws ER, Sharbrough FW. Temporal lobectomy in children with epilepsy. *J Neurosurg* 1986;64:371–6.

175. Harbord HB, Manson JL. Temporal lobe epilepsy in childhood: reappraisal of etiology and outcome. *Pediatr Neurol* 1987;3:263–8.

176. Duchowny M, Jayakar P, Resnick TJ, Alvarez LA, Levin B, Morrison G. The outcome of very early temporal lobe epilepsy. *Cleve Clin J Med* 1990 (in press).

177. Alvarez LA, Jayakar P, Gadia C, Duchowny M, Resnick TJ: Intractable focal seizures in childhood: histopathological analysis. *Neurology* 1990;40(Suppl 1):187.

178. Adams CBT, Beardsworth ED, Oxbury SM, Oxbury JM, Fenwick PBC. Temporal lobectomy in 44 children: outcome and neuropsychological follow up. In: Duchowny M, Resnick TJ, Alvarez LA, eds. *Pediatric epilepsy surgery.* New York: Demos, 1990.

179. Falconer MA. Mesial temporal (Ammon's horn) sclerosis as a common cause of epilepsy. Aetiology, treatment and prevention. *Lancet* 1974;2:767–70.

180. Lindsay J, Ounsted C, Richards P. Long-term outcome in children with temporal lobe seizures. *Dev Med Child Neurol* 1980;22:429–39.

181. Goldring S. Surgical management of epilepsy in children. In: Engle J Jr, ed. *Surgical treatment of the epilepsies.* New York: Raven Press, 1987.

182. Cavazzuti V, Winston K, Baker R, Welch K. Psychological changes following surgery for tumors in the temporal lobe. *J Neurosurg* 1980;53:618–26.

183. Krynauw RA. Infantile hemiplegia treated by removing one cerebral hemisphere. *J Neurol Neurosurg Psychiatry* 1950;13:243–67.

184. Rasmussen T, Milner B. The role of early left-brain injury in determining lateralization of cerebral speech function. *Ann NY Acad Sci* 1977;299:328–54.

185. Lindsay J, Ounsted C, Richards P. Hemispherectomy for childhood epilepsy: a 36 year study. *Dev Med Child Neurol* 1987;29:592–600.

186. Verity CM, Strauss EH, Moyes PD, Wada JA, Dunn HG, Lapointe JS. Long-term follow up after cerebral hemispherectomy: neurophysiologic, radiologic and psychological findings. *Neurology* 1982;32:629–39.

187. Luessenhop AJ, De La Cruz TC, Fenichel GM. Surgical disconnection of the cerebral hemispheres for intractable seizures. *JAMA* 1970;213:1630–6.

188. Geoffrey G, Lassonde M, Delisle F, Decarie M. Corpus callosotomy for control of intractable epilepsy in children. *Neurology* 1983;33:891–7.

189. Amacher AL. Midline commissurotomy for the treatment of some cases of intractable epilepsy. *Childs Brain* 1946;2:54–8.

190. Gates JR, Rosenfeld WE, Maxwell RE, Lyons RE. Response of multiple seizure types to corpus callosum section. *Epilepsia* 1987;28:28–34.

191. Gates JR, Ritter FJ, Ragazzo PC, Reeves AG. Corpus callosum section in children: seizure response. In: Duchowny M, Resnick TJ, Alvarez LA, eds. *Pediatric epilepsy surgery.* New York: Demos, 1990.

192. Spencer SS, Spencer DD, Willliamson PD, et al. Corpus callosotomy for epilepsy. I. Seizure effects. *Neurology* 1988;38:19–24.

193. Spencer DS, Spencer SS. Corpus callosotomy in the treatment of medically intractable secondarily generalized seizures of children. *Cleve Clin J Med* 1989;56(Supple Part 1): S69–78.

194. Slage UT, Kely AB, Wagner JA. Congenital absence of the corpus callosum. Report of a case and review of the literature. *N Engl J Med* 1957;256:1171–6.

195. Loeser JD, Alvord EC. Agenesis of the corpus callosum. *Brain* 1968;91:523–70.

196. Ettlinger G, Blakeworth CB, Milner AB, Wilson J. Agenesis of the corpus callosum: a further behavioral investigation. *Brain* 1974;97:225–34.

197. Lassonde M, Sauerwein H, Geoffroy G, Decarie M. Effects of early and late transection of the corpus

callosum in children. A study of tactile and tactuomotor transfer and integration. *Brain* 1986;109:953–67.

198. Lassonde M, Sauerwein H, Geoffroy G, Decarie M. Long-term neuropsychological effects of corpus callotomy in children. In: Duchowny M, Resnick TJ, Alvarez LA, eds. *Pediatric epilepsy surgery.* New York: Demos, 1990.

199. Chugani HT, Mazziotta JC, Engle J, Phelps ME. The Lennox-Gastaut syndrome: metabolic subtypes determined by 2-deoxy-2(18F)fluro-d-glucose positron emission tomography. *Ann Neurol* 1987;21:4–13.

200. Theodore WH, Rose D, Patronas N, Sato S, et al. Cerebral glucose metabolism in the Lennox-Gastaut syndrome. *Ann Neurol* 1987;21:14–21.

Chapter 17

Intraoperative Electrocorticography and Functional Mapping

GEORGE A. OJEMANN

The indications for electrocorticography (ECoG) and functional mapping during resective surgery for medically intractable epilepsy depend on two aspects of a surgical epileptologist's approach to these patients. One aspect is the significance placed on variability. When the extent of the epileptogenic zone and the location of functionally important areas are considered to be anatomically uniform among patients who are candidates for resections, the resections are anatomically standardized. Examples include "measured" anterior temporal lobectomies 4–4.5 cm in the dominant hemisphere and 5–5.5 cm in the non-dominant hemisphere [1], amygdalohippocampectomy [2], and radical hippocampectomy [3]. Preoperative evaluation of patients who are to undergo one of these procedures is usually quite extensive, establishing that the epileptogenic zone is in the area of anatomic excision through ictal recording, often with intracranial electrodes. Intraoperative recording plays no role in defining the extent of the epileptogenic zone in these procedures. The location of functionally important areas is considered to be so uniform anatomically that they are spared in these standardized removals, and thus there is no need for individual identification of eloquent areas by a technique such as intraoperative functional mapping. Although seizure control has been reported in a substantial proportion of patients managed with these types of resections with generally low morbidity, language and memory disturbances after dominant-hemisphere standard anterior temporal resections have been a concern [4,5].

However, not all epileptogenic zones fall within the anatomic limits of these standardized resections. Moreover, other surgical epileptologists have viewed temporal lobe epilepsy as having variable epileptogen-ic zones, indicating resections of somewhat different extent and tailored to removal of the individual patient's focus. For example, Rasmussen reported 100 cases of temporal lobe resections, seizure-free after operation, with epileptogenic zones predominantly in lateral cortex in 46%, predominantly in medial structures in 28%, and in both in 27% [6]. In addition, the location of eloquent areas of cortex, especially those essential for language, has shown considerable variability in some studies [7]. This includes location of essential temporal lobe language areas anterior to the level of rolandic cortex, or the vein of Labbe, within the limits of anatomically standardized operations, in from one of five or six patients with dominant-hemisphere resections (Fig. 17-1). These indications of variability in location of epileptogenic zones and eloquent areas even in the temporal lobe provide the reason for recording and mapping in the individual patient.

The second aspect of the approach to resective epilepsy surgery bearing on the use of recording and stimulation is whether those techniques are to be used intraoperatively or extraoperatively. Techniques for extraoperative recording and stimulation, using chronic subdural electrodes, are described by Lüders in Chapter 7. The major advantages of extraoperative recording are the ability to record ictal onsets and interictal activity, the extra time available for stimulation mapping, and the ability to map language without the cooperation needed for a craniotomy under local anesthesia. Thus, this technique is useful in young children [8]. Major disadvantages include the need for two craniotomies, an increased risk of infection with the percutaneous leads from the chronic electrodes, the substantial extra costs associated with

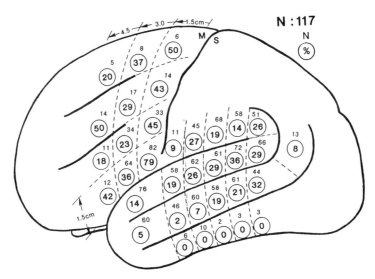

Figure 17-1. Variability in location of essential areas for language as assessed by electrical stimulation mapping during object naming in 117 patients, all left brain dominant for language. Individual patient maps are aligned by the rolandic cortex and the end of the sylvian fissure. Sites of stimulation are then assigned to the appropriate zone, indicated by the dashed lines. Numbers above in each zone indicate the number of patients with one or more sites of stimulation at that zone. Numbers in circles indicate the percent of patients with an essential site for naming in that zone, based on repeated evoked disturbances of naming. Note the marked variability in location of essential areas. (Reprinted by permission of the publisher from Ojemann G. et al. Cortical language localization in left dominant hemisphere. *J Neurosurg* 1989;71:316–26.)

the hospitalization for recording and mapping, and the somewhat less precise functional localization of stimulation through fixed chronic subdural electrodes, sometimes with problematic relation to the cortical surface. I see little justification for the additional risks and costs of chronic electrodes in patients with clear interictal epileptic foci on preoperative evaluation who can cooperate with local anesthesia. In these patients, assessment of predictors of successful outcome from surgery suggest that ictal recording contributes little if any additional certainty in localizing the epileptogenic zone over that obtained from interictal recordings [9]. Indeed, in patients with clear interictal foci, ictal recordings may erroneously lead to a decision to withhold operation [10]. Functionally important areas can be readily localized in those patients by intraoperative stimulation mapping, including language localization when the craniotomy is done while the patient is awake with local anesthesia [7,11]. Thus, intraoperative recording and stimulation are part of the approach to resective surgery indicated for these patients, who represent a large part of most series of resective epilepsy surgery. Compared with approaches using anatomically standardized resections, this approach, tailoring resection to the intraoperative findings, seems to yield at least as many seizure-free patients, with slightly lower mor-

bidity and substantially lower cost. However, the two approaches have never been compared in matched series of patients.

Intraoperative Electrocorticography

The extent of the epileptogenic zone is identified intraoperatively by the location of interictal epileptiform discharges. There is clearly a relation between the site of interictal discharges, the site of ictal onset, and the tissue that must be removed to control seizures. Interictal discharge location is an excellent predictor of where a resection is likely to control seizures [9,12]. Patients with no interictal discharges on post-resection recordings are more likely to be seizure-free than those with persisting discharges, but the relationship is by no means absolute: in one series, the probability of seizure control was about 70% without residual discharges but 30% when they were present [13]. Interictal discharges that are present in a patient with therapeutic levels of antiepileptic drugs, before any resection or other brain injury such as insertion of a depth electrode, and present in an alert patient (or during rapid eye movement sleep) may be particularly good indicators of tissue whose removal is likely to control seizures. Interictal discharges evoked by pharmacologic activation, such as a rapid intravenous bolus of methohexital (Brevital) may be a less certain indicator of the tissue needing removal. The significance of interictal discharges that appear after a resection but were not present in that location previously, Penfield's "activation by excision," is controversial. Penfield recommended resection of tissue with this change, whereas others have not [14]. Interictal spikes in insular cortex need not be excised to achieve seizure control in temporal lobe foci [15], and residual interictal activity in posterior parahippocampal gyrus is not an indication for further resection [16].

Resection is directed at removing all tissue with interictal discharges, limited by the above considerations, and sparing any area essential for motor or language functions, regardless of abnormal ECoG activity. In temporal lobe epilepsy, those resections usually differ some from the anatomically standard resections, with more extensive removal of inferior temporal cortex and less of lateral superior cortex in the "average" tailored resection, compared with a measured anterior temporal lobectomy. Even in patients with "classical" mesial temporal sclerosis, interictal epileptiform activity is usually present in anterior and inferior neocortex as well as in limbic areas, although the amplitude of this abnormal activity is often higher medially (Chatrian et al., unpublished observations). In my experience, the posterior limit of the medial resection is established in part on criteria other than the ECoG. That resection includes the anterior 1 cm of hippocampus and parahippocampal gyrus, even if recording of ECoG directly from hippocampus does not demonstrate epileptiform activity, a not uncommon finding. This is based on the observation that failure to extend the resection posteriorly to the tip of the temporal horn is associated with only a moderate number of seizure-free patients, whereas extending it to include the anterior 1 cm of hippocampal formation (including the remainder of posterior uncus) substantially increases that number [16]. Larger hippocampal removals were not associated with a higher seizure-free rate than those including just the anterior portion.

The early experience with ECoG identification of interictal epileptiform discharges as a guide for resective epilepsy surgery used local anesthesia for most cases [14]. Subsequently, resections have been reported that were tailored to ECoG recordings obtained under general anesthesia [17]. A recent comparison of results of resections guided by ECoG recorded under general or local anesthesia found no difference in effectiveness in seizure control [18].

There is some evidence that nitrous oxide is more likely to interfere with epileptiform activity than other anesthetic agents (Artru et al., unpublished observations). If general anesthesia is used, I prefer the use of systemic paralysis, with progressive lightening of anesthesia using a volatile halogenated agent until ECoG epileptiform events appear. When extensive recording is undertaken, very few patients fail to show interictal discharges. In the rare events when none are present, a rapid intravenous bolus of Brevital, 1 mg/kg, is used to "activate" epileptiform discharges. These are especially evident as the drug effects wear off. However, ideally I prefer ECoG recorded without general anesthesia or pharmacologic activation.

The ECoG recording should sample from all accessible areas, with a goal of establishing the full extent of the abnormal electrical activity. In cases of temporal lobe epilepsy, I place subdural multicontact strips under anterior and mid temporal lobes, with the most medial contacts on the uncus. Often a strip is placed under the posterior temporal lobe as well, to establish the posterior extent of inferior and medial abnormal electrical activity. A strip is also often placed on orbital frontal cortex, although in the presence of the typical picture of temporal lobe epilepsy obtained by scalp EEG, resection of the frontal cortex is seldom necessary. Usually any epileptiform events from the orbital frontal cortex disappear after the temporal resection. ECoG recording from lateral cortex is obtained through carbon electrodes placed in rows on exposed gyri. Recordings are obtained in a referential manner to a linked neck reference. The initial recording is used to plan the resection, but I repeat the ECoG recording after the lateral temporal removal is complete and the ventricle open, with recording electrodes placed directly on the hippocampus and the amygdala, as well as strip electrodes placed along the parahippocampal gyrus and the posterior margins of the resection. Recording is then repeated at the end of the resection. Acute use of depth electrodes is avoided, both because of the difficulty in identifying their location and the risk of inducing injury discharges that may provide misleading information.

Functional Mapping

Intraoperative identification of the essential areas for motor, language, and memory functions is done with electrical stimulation mapping. The goal of functional mapping is to identify those cortical areas that must be spared in a resection because of their essential functional role. These include areas essential for motor and sensory function, language, and, under certain circumstances, neocortical representation of recent verbal memory. Identification of motor cortex provides a useful landmark in temporal lobe resections and is indicated in any resection in posterior frontal or parietal lobes. Identification of subcortical motor pathways may be useful in those resections or temporal resections extending superiorly to the choroidal fissure. Identification of language cortex is indicated in any dominant-hemisphere resection in perisylvian cortex and probably in the posterior superior frontal lobe. Dominance for language is established by a preoperative intracarotid amobarbital perfusion study, the Wada test [19]. Based on studies of Ojemann and Dodrill [20,21], discussed later in this chapter, identification of the neocortical areas essential for recent verbal memory may be indicated in selected dominant-hemisphere temporal resections at high risk for a postoperative memory deficit, such as patients with evidence of bitemporal disease, patients with facile preoperative memories, or patients with memory loss when the side of the proposed resection is inactivated on the Wada test.

Sensorimotor Cortex

Sensorimotor cortex is identified by sites of evoked movements or sensation. Movements may be evoked under local or general anesthesia (without paralysis), although movements evoked under general anesthesia are less localized to one body part and have a higher threshold than those evoked under local anesthesia. In addition, the large representation of tongue is difficult to recognize under general anesthesia. Cortical localization is equally focal with general or local anesthesia, however, rarely extending more than 1–1.5 cm anterior to the central sulcus.

Stimulation identification of sensorimotor cortex uses brief trains of biphasic square-wave pulses, 1 msec in duration per phase, at 60 Hz, delivered across bipolar electrodes separated by 5 mm. Under local anesthesia the initial current level is 2 mA, measured between pulse peaks. Sensation or movements will be evoked in most awake patients at this current; rarely slightly larger currents up to 6 mA may be needed. Much larger currents are needed under general anesthesia. Then stimulation usually begins at 4 or 6 mA, and is increased at 2-mA increments until movements are evoked or 16 mA reached.

Motor or sensory responses will be evoked in most awake adolescent or adult patients with intact motor function. Occasionally the lowest sensorimotor representation will be several centimeters above the sylvian fissure and thus not included in a temporal exposure. Tumors may substantially displace motor cortex or occasionally directly invade it without producing paresis. In the presence of paresis, cortical motor representation of the involved part is usually absent. Motor and sensory responses are evoked with some difficulty from young children [22]. Subcortical motor pathways can also be identified with stimulation, using a current at or just above the threshold for cortical motor responses. Sensory cortex can also be identified by recording of somatosensory evoked potentials [23]. This technique is limited by the difficulty of evoking responses from the face. I have found it to be a much less practical way to identify rolandic cortex than motor stimulation, but recording of evoked potentials to median nerve stimulation has been of value in localizing motor cortex in some young children.

Language

Language localization makes use of a different effect of applying a current to cortex than that used to identify sensorimotor cortex. A surface current both excites and blocks function in both neurons and fibers; activity can be changed in either excitatory or inhibitory elements [24]. In motor cortex, excitatory effects predominate. Such predominantly excitatory effects seem to occur only in primary motor and sensory systems at both cortical and subcortical levels. Language is almost never evoked by stimulation. Instead, applying a current to some cortical sites where nothing was evoked in the quiet patient will block ongoing language, most likely through a predominance of depolarization. This method of identifying language cortex was developed by Penfield [11].

Penfield used object naming as the measure of language. Naming deficits are characteristic of all types of aphasias, so this measure would seem to provide a good screening test for language cortex. As with lesions, a site was related to language when that behavior failed during stimulation. Thus the relation was made only if the cortical area was essential for the language measure. In this respect, both stimulation mapping and lesions differ from blood flow or other metabolic measures [25] or physiologic measures such as neuronal recording [26] or ECoG [27]. These latter matters indicate where cortex is participating in language but not whether it is essential for it.

Penfield inferred that sites where stimulation disrupted object naming, with an arrest of speech or anomia, identified language cortex because of the congruency of the sites of these evoked responses to traditional language cortex [11]. Ojemann and Dodrill examined the relation between lesions and stimulation more directly in anterior temporal lobe resections. They found that when those resections were close to sites of stimulation-evoked disturbances of naming there was a subtle but definite postoperative deficit on a sensitive aphasia battery administered 1 month after operation that was not present when the resection did not come close to such sites; this deficit could not be accounted for by size of resection, degree of seizure control, or preoperative verbal ability [28]. Subsequently, on several occasions clinical considerations have required resection of small portions of frontal or temporal areas with repeated evoked disruption of naming, and on each occasion there has been a significant postoperative language disturbance lasting more than several weeks, although it eventually resolved (Ojemann, unpublished observations). Thus the sites where stimulation repeatedly disrupts naming seem to be areas that must be intact for normal postoperative language.

In an individual patient, the essential areas for language as assessed by stimulation-evoked disruption of object naming are usually localized to one or more "mosaics" of 1–2 cm^2 in extent, often with sharp boundaries (Fig. 17-2). Usually there is at least one frontal mosaic and one or more temporoparietal ones, but about 20% of one large series of dominant-hemisphere perisylvian cortex mapping had *only* frontal or temporoparietal language representation [7]. When the location of the essential language areas in a large series of patients, all known to be left

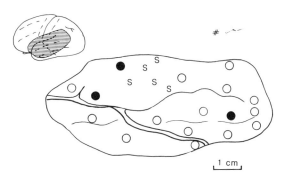

Figure 17-2. Sites essential for language as assessed by electrical stimulation mapping during object naming in left language dominant hemisphere of a 35-year-old female, verbal IQ 114. Circles are sites of stimulation; filled circles are sites with repeated evoked naming errors. Open circles are sites where patient made no error. *S* indicates sites of evoked face sensation. Mapping during naming was done at a current of 5 mA. Note the highly localized temporal site essential for naming.

dominant for language, are compared by aligning the individual maps to location of rolandic cortex and the end of the sylvian fissure, a high degree of variability is evident (see Fig. 17-1). Aside from a small area just in front of the face motor cortex, no zone of perisylvian cortex had essential language areas in more than 36% of subjects with sites sampled in that zone. Variability was evident even when larger anatomic areas were considered: only 65% of one series had essential language areas identified anywhere in the superior temporal gyrus of the dominant hemisphere [7]. Essential language areas were identified in portions of the temporal lobe considered "safe" for resection based on anatomic criteria in about one sixth of that series. The importance of this variation in individual location of essential language areas is evident in comparisons of language disturbances in dominant-hemisphere temporal lobe resections with language mapping with those based on only "safe" anatomic measurements without individual language mapping. More language deficits were noted after resections under general anesthesia based on anatomic criteria [18].

Several concepts guide the technique of identification of language by stimulation mapping. The technique requires the use of local anesthesia, with the patient quite alert during testing, because few errors must occur in the absence of stimulation. Only then can errors on the small number of stimulation-evoked responses at any given cortical site be distinguished from chance errors. Safe resection of areas without evoked language changes requires that areas with language changes also be identified; a completely negative language-mapping study does not provide assurance that a resection anywhere will not lead to an aphasia. The choice of current intensity is also crucial: too low a current may not block cortical function, whereas too large a current is likely to evoke seizures.

The exposure is designed to include both the area of proposed resection and regions where language is likely to be located. Anesthesia for an awake craniotomy with language mapping uses a scalp field block of ½% lidocaine and ¼% bupivacaine, supplemented by intravenous fentanyl and droperidol shortly before placing the block. The block should include deep infiltration around the root of the zygoma and the temporal muscle insertion. No pain sensation is elicited directly from bone, but pain fibers are present in the dura adjacent to blood vessels, especially the main trunk of the middle meningeal artery and adjacent to the transverse (but usually not sagittal) sinus. As a result, in a temporal exposure, the initial burr hole is placed over the middle meningeal trunk, and pain fibers are blocked with an intradural injection of a small amount of local anesthesia adjacent to the artery. The brain is generally insensitive to any sensation.

The current level for stimulation is selected with the aid of ECoG as the largest current that does not evoke afterdischarges in the area of cortex to be sampled. Other stimulation parameters are identical to those used for motor mapping. Once ECoG recording is completed, stimulation at 2 mA (between pulse peaks) for a 4-s train is applied to one of the recording electrodes located over the area of association cortex where language is to be mapped. Stimulation is repeated at that electrode at increasing currents in 2-mA increments until an afterdischarge is evoked. This threshold is often the same on repeated stimulations but varies widely among patients, from less than 2 mA, the threshold for responses from motor cortex, to over 10 mA, five times or more the motor threshold. Stimulation is then repeated at other electrodes covering the area of exposed cortex. Usually the afterdischarge threshold will be a few milliamperes lower in the anterior temporal or frontal lobes than in the posterior temporal lobe. The lower current level is used for mapping throughout the exposure. The marked differences in afterdischarge thresholds between adjacent electrodes described with chronic subdural arrays have been rarely encountered with direct cortical stimulation. On the few occasions when afterdischarge thresholds vary greatly over the exposure, mapping is carried out at different current levels for different groups of electrodes.

Object naming has usually been used as the measure of language. Once the current level is established, 10–20 sites of stimulation are arbitrarily selected to cover the exposed cortex. Each site is identified by a sterile numbered ticket. In my technique, the objects to be named are shown as line drawings on slides and at a rate, usually one every 3 or 4 s, that makes naming an easy task for the patient. The objects are selected as those with common names, and the patient is shown them the night before the operation. Any objects named with difficulty are deleted from those shown during mapping. After the patient has begun naming, a randomly selected site is stimulated just before a slide appears, and the current is continued until the next slide. At the end of stimulation, the number of that site is called aloud by the surgeon. After two or three more objects are named correctly, another site is stimulated, continuing until all sites have been stimulated once. The process is then repeated, stimulating sites in a different order until three samples of stimulation at each site have been

obtained. The accuracy of the patient's naming of each slide is determined as the test proceeds. Sites with repeated failures to correctly name during stimulation are considered essential for language. Errors include an arrest of all speech, or anomia, the inability to name with retained ability to speak. I have not considered hesitations alone as errors because of the difficulty in determining the level of hesitation on control slides. Conducted in this way, language mapping of perisylvian cortex requires about 20 min. If the resection is to be immediately adjacent to a site with repeated naming errors, it is wise to test naming while doing that part of the resection as well.

Although object naming has most often been used to assess language with stimulation mapping and for most purposes identifies those areas that must be preserved to avoid a postoperative aphasia, there is some evidence that naming does not identify all cortical areas essential for all aspects of language. In bilingual patients, sites essential for naming in one language are subtly different from those essential for naming the same object pictures in another language [28,29]. This separation extends to naming in oral compared with manual communication systems such as finger spelling or American sign language [30, Ojemann et al., unpublished observations]. Areas essential for reading of simple sentences also are somewhat separate from those essential for naming [28,31]. Thus, in a resection in posterior frontal or temporal lobes, additional mapping during measures of these other language functions is desirable if complete preservation of one of these language functions is particularly important.

Memory

Recent verbal memory deficits remain a major concern after dominant-hemisphere temporal lobe resections [5]. The usual approach to this concern utilizes the intracarotid amobarbital perfusion test to identify patients at risk for memory deficits (see Chapter 10). The response to a major memory loss with perfusion of the side of the proposed resection has been to either forgo surgery or limit the removal of medial temporal structures [32]. However, memory loss has been identified in patients who "passed" the intracarotid perfusion test [33] and when the extent of medial resection was modified in response to it [20]. In order to identify factors contributing to this memory loss, Ojemann and Dodrill evaluated verbal memory in 20 consecutive patients who had the medial extent of the resection reduced because the intracarotid perfusion study demonstrated memory deterioration, and who had been subjects of a research investigation of effects of lateral temporal neocortical stimulation on a recent verbal memory measure [20,21]. Ten of those patients had a deterioration in verbal memory 1 month after operation. These patients were distinguished from the 10 patients without memory deficits by several factors: those with deficits had *better* preoperative verbal memories and larger *lateral*, but not medial, resections, and their resections encroached on neocortical sites related to recent verbal memory by stimulation mapping. Based on these findings, it was proposed that sparing lateral cortical sites essential for memory as well as minimizing the medial resection would avoid a postoperative verbal memory deficit, and this was shown in two cases completely dependent on the left hemisphere for verbal memory based on intracarotid amobarbital perfusion assessment [20]. Subsequently neuronal activity related to recent verbal memory was identified in lateral temporal cortex [26]. These studies provide the basis for considering stimulation-mapping identification of essential areas for memory. Because the mapping is quite demanding on the patient and surgeon, and requires 1–1.5 hours, it is reserved for cases at risk for memory deficits: patients with good preoperative memories, patients whose livelihood depends on facile memory, and patients identified by the intracarotid perfusion study as "at risk" for a memory deficit.

Stimulation mapping during memory measures has identified several features of verbal memory representation in lateral temporal cortex. Sites essential for recent verbal memory are adjacent to, but rarely overlap with, sites essential for language [34]. Rather, the memory sites tend to surround language areas, with the memory sites in more anterior frontal, anterior temporal, and posterior parietal cortex than language sites.

Memory sites showed as much variation in location among patients, as was evident for language sites [20]. When the memory measure is designed to separate memory into three phases—the entry of information into memory (input), a phase when it is stored, and a retrieval phase—memory disturbance with stimulation of temporoparietal sites was most likely when the current was applied during the input and storage phases, whereas at frontal sites, memory disturbances most often occurred with stimulation during the retrieval phase [28,34]. Inclusion of sites where stimulation during the input or storage phases had disturbed memory in a resection was particularly likely to be associated with a postoperative memory deficit [20].

Thus, the memory measure used with stimulation is designed to separate the input, storage, and retrieval phases of memory. That measure, too, is presented as slides. Each trial has three slides. The first slide is an object picture that the patient names. This is the information that is to be retained in memory. The second slide cues a distracting task during which the memory must be stored. I use sentence reading as the distraction. The third slide is a cue for retrieval. In my paradigm, the word "recall" on a slide is used for this cue. Input and retrieval slides are usually shown for 4 s, and distraction slides for 6–8 s. Stimulation occurs on the input slide during some trials, on the distracting slide during others, and on the retrieval slide during still others, and trials without stimulation on any slide are interspersed to provide control performance measures. The patient is trained on this task prior to operation. As with language mapping, three samples of each stimulation condition are obtained for each site; a site is related to a phase of memory if the disturbance of memory with stimulation at that site during that phase has less than a 5% probability of occurring on a chance basis, based on performance on the control trials. If the control memory error rate exceeds about 40%, more than three stimulation trials for each condition at each site will be needed to establish any statistically significant changes. Because of the large number of stimulation conditions, the need for few errors with control performance, and the tendency of control errors to increase with patient fatigue, it is rarely possible to map more than 6 to 10 sites for memory. These are selected in and on the margins of the planned resection. Stimulation parameters for memory mapping are the same for language mapping. Sites with significant errors during stimulation in the input or storage phases of memory are spared in a resection designed to minimize the risk of postoperative memory deficit.

References

1. Falconer M. Anterior temporal lobectomy for epilepsy. In: Logue V, ed. *Operative surgery,* vol 14: *Neurosurgery.* London: Butterworths, 1971.
2. Wieser HG, Yasargil M. Selective amygdalohippocampectomy as a surgical treatment of mesiobasal limbic epilepsy. *Surg Neurol* 1982;17:445–57.
3. Spencer D, Spencer S, Mattson R, Williamson P, Novelly R. Access to the posterior medial temporal lobe

structures in the surgical treatment of temporal lobe epilepsy. *Neurosurgery* 1984;15:667–71.

4. Heilman KM, Wilder BJ, Malzone WF. Anomic aphasia following anterior temporal lobectomy. *Trans Am Neurol Assoc* 1972;97:291–3.

5. Delgado-Escueta AV, Treiman DM, Walsh GO. The treatable epilepsies (second of two parts). *N Engl J Med* 1983;308:1576–84.

6. Rasmussen T. Localizational aspects of epileptic seizure phenomena. In: Thompson R, Green J, eds. *New perspectives in cerebral localization.* New York: Raven Press, 1982.

7. Ojemann G, Ojemann J, Lettich E, Berger M. Cortical language localization in left dominant hemisphere. *J Neurosurg* 1989;71:316–26.

8. Ojemann G, Berger M, Lettich E. Resective surgery in young children: method for foci near eloquent areas. *Epilepsia* 1989;30:642.

9. Dodrill C, Wilkus R, Ojemann G, Ward A Jr, Wyler A, van Belle G, Tamas L. Multidisciplinary prediction of seizure relief from cortical resection surgery. *Ann Neurol* 1986;20:2–12.

10. Ojemann G, Engel J Jr. Acute and chronic intracranial recording and stimulation in the surgical treatment of epilepsy. In: Engel J Jr, ed. *Surgical treatment of epilepsy.* New York: Raven Press, 1987.

11. Penfield W, Roberts L. *Speech and brain mechanisms.* Princeton: Princeton University Press, 1959.

12. Morris H, Kanner A, Lüders H, Murphy D, Dinner D, Wyllie E, Kofagal P. Can sharp waves localized at the sphenoidal electrode accurately identify a mesiotemporal epileptogenic focus? *Epilepsia* 1989;30:532–9.

13. Bengzon A, Rasmussen T, Gloor P, Dassault J, Stephens M. Prognostic factors in the surgical treatment of temporal lobe epileptics. *Neurology* 1968;18:717–31.

14. Penfield W, Jasper H. *Epilepsy and the functional anatomy of the human brain.* Boston: Little, Brown, 1954.

15. Rasmussen T. Surgical treatment of patients with complex partial seizures. *Adv Neurol* 1975;11:415–49.

16. Ojemann L, Ojemann G, Baugh-Bookman C. What is the optional extent of the medial resection in anterior temporal lobe epilepsy? *Epilepsia* 1986;27:636.

17. Walker A. Temporal lobectomy. *J Neurosurg* 1967; 26:641–9.

18. Hermann B, Wyler A. Comparative effects of dominant temporal lobectomy under general or local anesthesia: language outcome. *Epilepsia* 1988;29:668.

19. Wada J, Rasmussen T. Intracarotid injection of sodium Amytal for the lateralization of cerebral speech dominance: experimental and clinical observation. *J Neurosurg* 1960;17:266–82.

20. Ojemann G, Dodrill C. Verbal memory deficits after left temporal lobectomy for epilepsy: mechanisms and intraoperative prediction. *J Neurosurg* 1985;62:101–7.

21. Ojemann G, Dodrill C. Intraoperative techniques for reducing language and memory deficits with left temporal lobectomy. *Adv Epileptol* 1987;16:327–30.

22. Goldring S. Epilepsy surgery. *Clin Neurosurg* 1984; 31:369–88.

23. Wood C, Spencer D, Allison T, McCarthy G, Williamson P, Goff W. Localization of human sensorimotor cortex during surgery by cortical surface recording of somatosensory evoked potentials. *J Neurophysiol* 1988;68:99–111.

24. Ranck JB Jr. Which elements are excited in electrical stimulation of mammalian central nervous system: a review. *Brain Res* 1975;98:417–40.

25. Raichle M. Circulatory and metabolic correlates of brain function in normal humans. In: Mountcastle V, Plum F, Geiger S, eds. *Handbook of physiology,* Sec I: *The Nervous System,* Vol V: *Higher functions of the brain.* Bethesda: American Physiological Society, 1987.

26. Ojemann GA, Creutzfeldt O, Lettich E, et al. Neuronal activity in human lateral temporal cortex related to short-term verbal memory, naming and reading. *Brain* 1988;111:1383–1403.

27. Ojemann GA, Fried I, Lettich E. Electrocorticographic (ECoG) correlates of language: I. Desynchronization in temporal language cortex during object naming. *EEG Clin Neurophysiol* 1989;73:453–63.

28. Ojemann G. Brain organization for language from the perspective of electrical stimulation mapping. *Behav Brain Sci* 1983;6:189–230.

29. Ojemann GA, Whitaker HA. The bilingual brain. *Arch Neurol* 1978;35:409–12.

30. Mateer C, Palen S, Ojemann G. Cortical localization of finger spelling and oral language: a case study. *Brain Lang* 1982;17:46–57.

31. Ojemann GA. Some brain mechanisms for reading. In: von Euler C, ed. *Brain and reading.* New York: Macmillan, 1989.

32. Blume W, Grabow J, Darley F, et al. Intracarotid amobarbital test of language and memory before temporal lobectomy for seizure control. *Neurology* 1973;23:812–9.

33. Rausch R, Crandall P. Psychological status related to surgical control of temporal lobe seizures. *Epilepsia* 1982;23:191–202.

34. Ojemann G. Organization of short-term verbal memory in language areas of human cortex: evidence from electrical stimulation. *Brain Lang* 1978;5:331–48.

PART FOUR
OUTCOME

Chapter 18
Outcome with Respect to Seizure Frequency

DON W. KING
JOSEPH R. SMITH
BRIAN B. GALLAGHER
ANTHONY M. MURRO
HERMAN F. FLANIGIN

This chapter reviews outcome with respect to seizure frequency of four major types of surgical procedures: anterior temporal lobectomy, extratemporal resection, hemispherectomy, and corpus callosum section. Neuropsychological outcome, psychosocial outcome, and neurologic complications of these procedures are dealt with in other chapters.

In his book, *Surgical Treatment of the Epilepsies,* Engel discussed a number of problems that must be considered in determining outcome with respect to seizure frequency [1]. First, postoperative seizure frequency is obtained from patients and families, and they may not be able to give accurate information. Many patients are unaware of the occurrence of their seizures, especially those that occur during sleep, and family members may not witness each seizure. Second, seizures that occur during the first few weeks following surgery may be different from preoperative seizures and may have little long-term prognostic significance. It has not been established how these seizures should be considered. Third, some patients have clusters of seizures, either preoperatively or postoperatively. Multiple nocturnal seizures clustered in one night have a much different effect on function than multiple daytime seizures scattered throughout the year. Fourth, it has been well documented that the frequency and pattern of seizures in an individual patient may be quite different in different postoperative years, that is, patients who are initially rendered seizure-free may have a recurrence of seizures, and those who initially continue to have seizures may later become seizure-free. As a result, an individual patient may move from one postoperative classification to another over time. Finally, seizures may occur when medications are inadvertently missed or being withdrawn. It has not been established if these seizures should be counted in the same way as those that occur during medication treatment [1].

In addition to problems in determining outcome in an individual patient, there are major difficulties in comparing outcome among centers. Each center that performs epilepsy surgery has different referral patterns, different methods of preoperative evaluation, and different criteria for patient selection. Surgical procedures and techniques also vary from one center to another, as do follow-up protocol and methods for measuring outcome. As a result of these variations, it is often difficult to compare outcome among different centers [1].

In an attempt to achieve some degree of standardization, Engel has proposed the following classification for reporting outcome with respect to seizure frequency [1]:

Class I: Seizure-free
Class II: Rare seizures (almost seizure-free)
Class III: Worthwhile improvement
Class IV: No worthwhile improvement

Each category is further subdivided in an attempt to account for some of the factors discussed above [1]. In this chapter, we use this basic information as we evaluate some of the previous studies of surgical outcome. Because most patients who undergo corpus callosotomy have multiple seizure types, it seems reasonable to report outcome with respect to each individual seizure type. This has been done in a number of recent studies and is discussed more fully in the following sections.

Temporal Lobectomy

Anterior temporal lobectomy refers to resection of the anterior 5–7 cm of the temporal lobe, including the amygdala, the uncus, and, in most patients, the anterior hippocampus. It is the most common surgical procedure used in the treatment of epilepsy. It is indicated in patients with medically intractable complex-partial seizures in whom evidence suggests that seizures arise in one of the temporal lobes. Non-invasive evidence of temporal lobe origin may include the characteristic behavioral phenomena of temporal lobe seizures, neuroimaging evidence of a temporal lobe lesion, neuropsychological evidence of temporal lobe dysfunction, interictal epileptiform discharges from the anterior/medial temporal region, and localized electrographic seizure onset from the temporal region recorded with scalp or sphenoidal electrodes. Intracranial electrodes may be used in patients whose seizures are not well localized during noninvasive investigation. The primary evidence for localization during invasive investigation is an electroencephalographic (EEG) recording of seizure onset localized to the temporal region, which precedes clinical onset.

Penfield and Flanigin in 1950 [2] and Bailey and Gibbs in 1951 [3] were the first to report the value of anterior temporal lobectomy in the treatment of complex-partial seizures. Penfield and Flanigin reported 51 patients at the Montreal Neurological Institute (MNI) followed for 1–10 years postoperatively. Using Engel's proposed classification, 27.4% were Class I, 25.5% Class II, 25.5% Class III, and 21.6% Class IV [2]. Van Buren et al. reported a series of 124 patients followed for 5–16 years postoperatively at the National Institutes of Health [4]. Of these, 21% were Class I, 46% were Class II or III, and 33% were Class IV. In a recent publication, Walczak et al. reported 100 cases undergoing temporal lobectomy at Duke University [5]. During the second postoperative year, 63% were Class I, 16% were Class II or III, and 21% were Class IV. The largest series of patients undergoing temporal lobectomy is that of the MNI. In 1983, Rasmussen reported 894 patients with follow-up of 2–44 years (median 12 years) [6]. In Rasmussen's study, 63% were seizure-free or had rare attacks (37% Class I and 26% Class II), and another 15% had marked reduction in seizure frequency (Class III).

Two major centers have used the *en bloc* resection in which the anterior temporal lobe, including medial structures, is resected in one piece [7–9]. In 1963, Falconer and Serafetinides reported 100 cases undergoing *en bloc* resection at the Maudsley Hospital who were followed for 2–10 years postoperatively [8]. They reported that 39% were Class I, 14% Class II, 30% Class III, and 17% Class IV. Cahan et al. reported results from UCLA series in 1984 [9]. Prior to 1977, all patients evaluated at UCLA were studied with depth electrodes. Of 59 patients undergoing temporal lobectomy, 44% were seizure-free (Class I), and 83% demonstrated worthwhile improvement (Class I, II, or III). After 1977, patients who met strict criteria on noninvasive evaluation underwent surgery without depth electrodes. Of 12 patients who had surgery based on non-invasive evaluation, 75% were Class I, and 100% had worthwhile improvement (Class I, II, III). Of the 35 patients who required depth electrodes, 62% were Class I, and 97% showed worthwhile improvement [9]. Their data suggest that with newer methods of evaluation, very strict criteria for surgery may lead to significantly improved results.

In 1984, Spencer et al. reported outcome following limited anterior temporal tip resection plus extensive medial temporal resection that included the entire hippocampus [10]. At 1 year postoperatively all of their patients were Class I, II, or III. Wieser and Yasargil reported results of amygdalohippocampectomy in 27 patients with seizures arising in the medial temporal region followed for 0.5–6 years after surgery [11]. Eighty-one percent (81%) were seizure-free (Class I), and an additional 7% were improved (Class II or III). A follow-up report in 1988 described outcome in 181 patients who underwent selective amygdalohippocampectomy. Of these, 87% had received worthwhile improvement [12].

Excellent results of anterior temporal lobectomy have also been reported in children and older adults. Using an *en bloc* technique, Davidson and Falconer reported that of 40 children followed postoperatively for 1–24 years, 57.5% were Class I, 20% were Class II, and 12.5% were Class III [13]. Recently, Meyer et al. reported 50 children operated on at the Mayo Clinic. At 0.5–10 years postoperatively, 78% were Class I, and an additional 10% showed worthwhile improvement [14]. Similar results have been noted in patients less than 10 years of age [15,16] and over 50 years of age [17,18].

Numerous additional reports from centers with fewer patients have confirmed that anterior temporal lobectomy is effective in both adults and children [19–27]. Summarizing these reports, at 1–2 years postoperatively, 35–75% of patients were seizure-free or nearly seizure-free (Class I or II), and 60–90% achieved worthwhile improvement (Class I, II, and

III). At the 1986 International Conference on the Surgical Treatment of Epilepsy, 40 centers responded to a survey concerning the results of anterior temporal lobectomy [1]. Of 2,338 patients reported, 56% were seizure-free (Class I), and an additional 27.7% were improved (Class II and III). Thus, despite the difficulty in determining outcome in individual cases and in comparing results among centers, there is a large body of evidence that, in selected cases, temporal lobectomy offers an excellent chance for a significant reduction in seizure frequency [1].

A number of investigators have studied the relationship between various preoperative and operative factors and outcome with respect to seizure frequency [4,8,28–41]. Results have often been conflicting, and a summary of these results was published by Dodrill et al. in 1986 [32]. We will limit this discussion to two factors that have consistently correlated with outcome—extent of resection and pathology of resected tissue—and recent data suggesting that ictal EEG data recorded from implanted electrodes may also have prognostic significance.

Numerous studies have suggested that surgical outcome is related to the extent of resection. Bengzon et al. at the MNI compared 50 patients who had worthwhile improvement (Class I, II, and III) with 54 patients who did not respond (Class IV) [29]. Of the 50 responders, 56% had complete hippocampal resection, 38% had partial hippocampal resection, and 6% had no hippocampal resection. On the other hand, of the 54 nonresponders, only 10% had complete hippocampal resection, 57% had partial resection, and 33% had no hippocampal resection [29]. In the 1975 study of Van Buren et al., there was also evidence that complete resection is more effective [4]. They divided their patients into those who had total resection, which included the amygdala and anterior hippocampus, and those who had partial resection, in which mesial temporal structures were not resected. Of the 48 patients with partial resection, only 4% were Class I, 43% were Class II or III, and 54% were Class IV. Of the 76 patients with total resection, 32% were Class I, 44% were Class II or III, and only 20% were Class IV [4]. Wyllie et al. [35] and Awad et al. [36] at the Cleveland Clinic have found similar results. Wyllie et al. defined complete resection as removal of all cortical areas with interictal and ictal epileptiform discharges. Of 19 patients with complete resection, 90% were Class I. This compared with 55% of 31 patients who became Class I following partial resection [35]. Using postoperative magnetic resonance imaging (MRI) to determine extent of resection, Awad et al. found that there was a direct correlation between extent of resection and surgical outcome. This was especially true for the extent of resection of mesial temporal structures [36] and has been further supported by two subsequent reports [39,40].

The results of reoperation in patients whose initial surgery was unsuccessful also support the notion that completeness of resection is an important factor in predicting outcome. Of the 121 patients at the MNI who underwent reoperation following unsuccessful epilepsy surgery, 45% were seizure-free or nearly seizure-free [42]. These data include temporal lobectomies and extratemporal resections. Wyler et al. reported that in their series of 16 patients undergoing additional temporal lobe resection following an initial unsuccessful temporal lobectomy, 63% were seizure-free and an additional 25% received worthwhile improvement [43].

Falconer and Serafetinides were the first to show the relationship between outcome and pathology of resected tissue [8]. Patients were followed for 2–10 years following an *en bloc* anterior temporal lobectomy. Of 71 patients with pathologic changes of mesial temporal sclerosis, tumor, or angioma, 59% were Class I or II and only 9% were Class IV. Of 22 patients with equivocal pathologic changes, only 36% were Class I or II, and 36% were Class IV [9]. In a more recent study, Duncan and Sagar reported that 63–84% of patients with Ammon's horn sclerosis, nonspecific hippocampal sclerosis, or glioma were Class I or II, but only 14% of patients with nonspecific changes were Class I or II [34]. These data plus similar results reported by others [20,29] suggest that there is a positive correlation between the finding of specific pathologic changes and good outcome.

Recent studies have suggested that ictal EEG data recorded from implanted electrodes may also have prognostic significance [33,37,38]. Lieb et al. at UCLA studied the EEG seizure propagation time from one hippocampus to the contralateral hippocampus. They found that patients with longer interhemispheric propagation times have better outcome than patients with shorter propagation times [33]. Similar data were found by Weiser and Siegel using foramen ovale electrodes [41]. Reviewing the Montreal series, So et al. reported that patients who had unilateral or unilaterally predominant depth-recorded temporal seizure onset had better outcome than patients with bitemporal independent seizure onset [37]. Similarly, Spencer et al. reported that of 18 patients whose EEG seizure onsets were limited to the hippocampal region, 89% were Class I, and an additional 6% were Class II or III [38]. None of the four patients with variable or neocortical seizure onset were seizure-free, and only 50% showed worthwhile improvement. These data suggest that various parameters of depth-recorded seizure onset may correlate well with seizure outcome. On the other hand, Hirsch et al. from the Yale group have recently reported quite good results in patients with bilateral independent seizure onset [44].

Table 18-1 summarizes results of anterior temporal lobectomy at the Medical College of Georgia during the first five years of our program. Of the 68 patients who underwent anterior temporal lobectomy, 60% were Class I, 13% were Class II, 4% were Class III, and 22% were Class IV. All nine patients with structural abnormalities were Class I or II postoperatively. Although the numbers were small, patients who met strict EEG criteria for temporal lobectomy (i.e., those with unilateral temporal interictal epileptiform discharges, localized EEG seizure onset from the ipsilateral temporal region, and no evidence suggesting contralateral temporal lobe dysfunction) tended to have better results than patients who did not meet strict criteria. Patients who did not have structural abnormalities and who did not meet strict EEG criteria underwent implantation of depth electrodes [45]. The results were similar to those of So et al. previously discussed [37]; patients who had all seizures originating in one temporal lobe had better outcomes than patients with bilateral independent seizure onset or poorly localized onset.

Extratemporal Resection

Extratemporal resection refers to the removal of cortical epileptogenic tissue plus an associated structural abnormality, if present, in the frontal, parietal, or occipital region. Posterior or lateral temporal resections that do not include the anterior/medial temporal lobe are also included in this group. Extratemporal resections are indicated in patients with partial seizures of extratemporal origin in whom adequate localization can be made. As with anterior temporal lobectomy, localization is based on a number of factors, including the clinical phenomena of the patient's seizures, evidence of structural abnormality on imag-

ing studies, neuropsychological evidence of focal dysfunction, and EEG documentation of localized interictal epileptiform activity or electrographic seizure onset. Because clinical and electrographic localization is often difficult outside the anterior/medial temporal lobe, structural abnormalities assume much greater importance in patients with extratemporal seizure origin. If a structural lesion is not present on imaging studies, patients usually require intracranial electrodes, often in multiple extratemporal sites. In addition, extratemporal seizures may arise in functionally important areas, limiting the extent of the epileptogenic tissue that can be removed. As a result of these factors, outcome following extratemporal resection is generally not as good as that following anterior temporal lobectomy.

There are fewer data concerning outcome of extratemporal resection than of anterior temporal lobectomy. In 1975, Rasmussen reported surgical outcome of patients undergoing extratemporal resections at the MNI [46,47]. Of 212 patients undergoing frontal lobe excision with follow-up of 2–39 years, 23% were seizure-free or became seizure-free after early attacks (Class I), and 32% had a marked reduction in seizure tendency compatible with Class II [36]. The results were not significantly different for patients who underwent central or sensory/motor resections (31% Class I and 26% Class II); parietal resections (31% Class I and 28% Class II); or occipital resections (26% Class I and 42% Class II) [47]. As noted previously, of 121 patients who underwent reoperation for removal of additional tissue after an initial unsuccessful procedure, 21% were seizure-free (Class I), and 24% had rare seizures (Class II) [42].

Goldring and Gregorie in 1984 reported outcome in 100 patients undergoing epidural recordings to localize the seizure focus, 80 of whom had seizures arising extratemporally [48]. Of 57 patients who underwent resection and were followed for 1–12 years, 63% achieved a good result (Class I, II, or III), and 37% were Class IV. Wyllie et al. at the Cleveland Clinic reported their results in 11 patients with extratemporal resection [35]. Forty-five percent had

Table 18-1. Outcome of Anterior Temporal Lobectomy (1–5 Year Follow-Up)

	Class I	Class II	Class III	Class IV
A. Noninvasive evaluation (28 patients)	20	3	0	5
1. Structural abnormality	(7)	(2)	(0)	(0)
2. Strict EEG criteria for temporal lobectomy	(12)	(1)	(0)	(3)
3. Other	(1)	(0)	(0)	(2)
B. Depth electrode evaluation (40 patients)	21	6	3	10
1. Unilateral temporal seizure onset	(20)	(6)	(2)	(4)
2. Bilateral independent temporal seizure onset	(0)	(0)	(0)	(2)
3. Poorly localized seizure onset	(1)	(0)	(1)	(4)

good outcome (Class I, II, or III), and 55% were Class IV. This compared with good outcome in 68% of patients undergoing anterior temporal lobectomy [35].

Hajek and Wieser recently reported their results in 30 patients who underwent extratemporal resections [49]. Their series included the following types of resection: rolandic or perirolandic resections, eight patients; premotor resections, seven patients; subtotal frontal resections, six patients; frontal basal resections, two patients; subtotal hemispherectomy, two patients; occipital with partial temporal or parietal resections, three patients; and others, two patients. At mean postoperative follow-up of 11 years, 20% were Class I, and an additional 60% were markedly improved (Class II, III). Hajek and Wieser found a correlation between outcome and completeness of resection of the "primarily epileptogenic area" [49].

Thirty-two centers reported extratemporal resections at the International Conference on the Surgical Treatment of Epilepsy. Of the 825 patients undergoing extratemporal resections, 43.2% were seizure-free (Class I), and another 27.8% were significantly improved (Class II and III) [1]. Thus, despite the fact that localization is more difficult extratemporally, and the results are not quite as good as with temporal lobe epilepsy, these data suggest that extratemporal resection is an effective procedure in well-selected patients.

Table 18-2 summarizes results of extratemporal resection during the first five years of the program at the Medical College of Georgia. In this small group of patients, patients with extratemporal structural abnormalities tended to have better outcomes than those whose extratemporal seizures were localized with implanted electrodes.

Hemispherectomy

Hemispherectomy refers to the resection of all cortical and a variable amount of subcortical tissue of one hemisphere for the control of seizures. It is indicated in patients who have extensive unilateral hemisphere damage, uncontrolled focal seizures originating in the damaged hemisphere, and a severe contralateral hemiparesis with minimal hand function. The two major categories of patients are those with static lesions causing infantile hemiplegia and those with chronic

progressive hemiparesis and seizures thought most likely to be secondary to chronic encephalitis. A number of modifications of "complete hemispherectomy" have been developed and will be discussed below.

The first report of a series of patients undergoing hemispherectomy was by Krynauw in 1950 [50]. He reported results of hemispherectomy in 12 patients with infantile hemiplegia, 10 of whom had seizures. Postoperatively, all 10 patients became seizure-free. In 1953, McKissock reported 18 patients with infantile hemiplegia who underwent complete hemispherectomy [51]. Of the 18 patients, one died perioperatively, 12 became seizure-free, four had marked improvement, and one patient was unchanged. Rasmussen et al. in 1958 reported three patients with chronic progressive encephalitis, two of whom underwent hemicorticectomy [52]. Both were seizure-free postoperatively. Subsequently Wilson reported 50 cases who underwent hemispherectomy at the National Hospital, Queen Square, because of intractable epilepsy and behavioral disturbance associated with early-onset spastic hemiparesis [53]. One patient died early in the postoperative period. Of the remainder, 68% were seizure-free, 14% had worthwhile improvement, 4% were unimproved, and 12% had inadequate follow-up [53].

Although complete hemispherectomy was shown to be very successful in controlling seizures, up to one third of patients who underwent complete hemispherectomy developed "superficial hemosiderosis" [54–56]. This condition is thought to be secondary to minor trauma causing the gradual seepage of red blood cells from granulation tissue into the hemispherectomy cavity. Superficial hemosiderosis may result in hydrocephalus, gradual neurologic deterioration, and even death.

Because of the complications associated with complete hemispherectomy, Rasmussen and his associates began performing "subtotal hemispherectomy," a procedure in which most of the hemisphere was resected but a portion of the frontal and/or occipital lobes was left in place [56]. The rationale was to prevent excessive movement of the remaining brain, thus preventing superficial hemosiderosis. In 1983, they reported results in 57 patients who underwent subtotal hemispherectomy followed for 2–31 years postoperatively. Forty-five percent were seizure-free,

Table 18-2. Outcome of Extratemporal Resection (1–5 Year Follow-Up)

	Class I	Class II	Class III	Class IV
A. Structural abnormality (5 patients)	3	0	2	0
B. EEG criteria (5 patients)	0	1	1	3
1. Localized seizure onset		(1)	(1)	(2)
2. Others		(0)	(0)	(1)

and 23% had rare seizures. Although the results were not as good as with complete hemispherectomy, chronic hemosiderosis did not develop [56].

In an attempt to obtain better seizure control, Rasmussen and colleagues further modified the procedure, performing an anatomically partial but functionally complete hemispherectomy [57]. This consists of resection of most of the hemisphere, leaving the frontal pole and occipital lobes with their blood supply intact, and isolation of the remaining frontal pole and occipital lobe from the corpus callosum and brainstem. Of 14 patients operated on at the MNI and followed for 4–13 years, 10 were seizure-free, one had rare seizures, and three showed worthwhile improvement. No patients developed chronic superficial hemosiderosis [57]. A follow-up report of 25 patients described similar outcomes [58].

Adams has proposed another procedure to prevent the development of chronic hemosiderosis [59]. Following complete hemispherectomy with "immaculate hemostasis," the superficial dura is separated from the skull and sutured to the falx, tentorium, and dura lying in the floor of the middle and anterior cranial fossa. This decreases the subdural space and increases the epidural space. Muscle is placed in the ipsilateral foramen of Monro to isolate the subdural cavity from the ventricular system. Of four patients who underwent this procedure, all were seizure-free, and no patients developed chronic hemosiderosis [59].

At the International Conference on the Surgical Treatment of Epilepsy, 17 centers reported results with hemispherectomy. Of 88 patients undergoing complete or subtotal hemispherectomy, 77.3% were seizure-free, and an additional 18.2% had achieved worthwhile improvement [1]. Thus, the data strongly suggest that hemispherectomy is an excellent procedure in appropriate cases, and with the modified techniques now used, the complication rate is relatively low.

Corpus Callosum Section

Corpus callosum section refers to the separation of the two hemispheres by dividing the corpus callosum. The rationale for this procedure in the control of seizures is that separation of the two hemispheres will inhibit the spread of a seizure from one hemisphere to the other, thus decreasing the severity of the seizure. Since the site of origin is not removed, it is unlikely that section of the corpus callosum would completely abolish seizures. Section of the corpus callosum has been combined with section of the anterior commissure, hippocampal commissure, and one fornix to provide a complete "forebrain commissurotomy." Because of the unacceptable side effects, including intraventricular infection and death, most surgeons now use microsurgical techniques and limit the procedure to the corpus callosum and hippocampal commissure, using either a one- or two-stage procedure. As with the other procedures for epilepsy, variations in patient selection criteria, surgical procedure, and methods for determining outcome make comparison of outcome among centers difficult. In addition, since most patients who undergo corpus callosotomy have multiple types of seizures, measurement of outcome following this procedure is especially complex.

Corpus callosum section was originally described by Van Wagenen and Herren in 1940 [60]. Although their results were mixed, subsequent investigators reported good results [61,62]. During the 1970s, a group of investigators at Dartmouth reported their results with corpus callosum section in a series of publications [63–67]. The first three patients underwent "complete forebrain commissurotomy"; the next five patients underwent a frontal commissurotomy including the rostral half of the corpus callosum, the anterior commissure, and one fornix; subsequent patients underwent "central commissurotomy," which included section of the corpus callosum and underlying hippocampal commissure in one or two stages. Summarizing their results in 1983, they reported that of 19 patients with good follow-up, five had three or fewer seizures per year, 11 showed reduction of seizures of greater than 50%, and three had minimal or no change in their seizures [63].

Recent reports have emphasized the effect of corpus callosum section on specific seizure types. Gates et al. reported 24 patients followed for 23–79 months after corpus callosotomy at the University of Minnesota [68]. They found a significant decrease in frequency of atonic/tonic seizures, tonic-clonic seizures, and complex-partial seizures. Seven patients became seizure-free for atonic/tonic seizures, and 12 patients became seizure-free for tonic-clonic seizures. On the other hand, six patients had an increase in complex-partial seizures following surgery, and three patients developed partial seizures that were not present prior to surgery. Three patients became totally seizure-free postoperatively [68].

In 1988, Spencer et al. reported 22 patients who underwent corpus callosum section (nine partial and 13 complete) [69]. Postoperative follow-up at two years revealed the following. One patient was totally seizure-free, and eight patients had simple partial seizures only. Seven additional patients had no postoperative generalized seizures but continued to have simple and complex partial seizures. Four of these had more intense partial seizures than prior to surgery. Six patients had no appreciable change. A complete corpus callosum section was effective in controlling secondarily generalized seizures in over 75% of patients and was twice as likely as a partial section to abolish generalized seizures. Patients with focal lesions on computed tomography (CT) were more likely to have an excellent outcome than patients without structural lesions. Patients with an intelligence quotient (IQ) of less than 45 were more likely to have a poor outcome [69].

Murro et al. reported 25 patients followed for 12–67 months after anterior two thirds corpus callosotomy [70]. Of the 18 patients with generalized tonic-clonic seizures, 6% had no further generalized tonic-clonic seizures, 17% had rare generalized tonic-clonic seizures, and an additional 22% showed worthwhile improvement. The one patient with atonic seizures became free of atonic seizures. There was also a statistically significant reduction in complex-partial seizures at 12–67 months. As noted in previous studies, 10 patients had more severe partial seizures postoperatively than preoperatively [59]. In a subsequent study of anterior two thirds corpus callosotomy in 20 children followed for at least 12 months, Makari et al. from the same center reported the following results. Two patients became seizure-free, two patients had rare seizures, and four patients had worthwhile reduction of seizures [71]. There was no relationship between outcome and various preoperative factors studied.

Purves et al. in 1988 reported 24 patients followed for 3–11 years postoperatively for anterior two thirds corpus callosotomy [72]. Eighteen patients had greater than 80% reduction in seizure frequency, and three additional patients were improved. Results were best for patients who had "unilateral" seizure onset versus multifocal independent or diffuse-onset seizures [72].

At the International Conference on the Surgical Treatment of Epilepsy, 16 centers reported results of corpus callosotomy. Of 197 patients, only 5% were seizure-free, but 71% achieved worthwhile improvement [1]. These plus the preceding data suggest that a one- or two-stage corpus callosotomy, including section of the hippocampal commissure, is helpful in patients with severely uncontrolled seizures. However, it rarely achieves complete seizure control.

Conclusion

The surgical treatment of epilepsy is effective in selected patients with intractable epilepsy. Resective procedures in patients with localized seizure onset offer the possibility of excellent seizure control. Definite pathologic abnormality and extent of resection correlate with improved outcome. Corpus callosotomy offers the possibility for improved seizure control in selected patients. Additional data concerning outcome from multiple centers should improve our understanding of epilepsy and our methods for selecting patients for epilepsy surgery.

References

1. Engel J. Outcome with respect to epileptic seizures. In: Engel J, ed. *Surgical treatment of the epilepsies.* New York: Raven Press, 1987:553–71.
2. Penfield W, Flanigin H. Surgical therapy of temporal lobe seizures. *Arch Neurol* 1950;64:491–500.
3. Bailey P, Gibbs FA. The surgical treatment of psychomotor epilepsy. *JAMA* 1951;145:365–70.
4. Van Buren JM, Ajmone-Marsan C, Mutsuga N, Sadowsky D. Surgery of temporal lobe epilepsy. In: Purpura DP, Penry JK, Walter RD, eds. *Advances in neurology,* Vol 8. New York: Raven Press, 1975:155–96.
5. Walczak TS, Radtke RA, McNamara JO, Lewis DV, Luther JS, Thompson E, Wilson WP, Friedman AH, Nashold BS. Anterior temporal lobectomy for complex partial seizures: evaluation, results, and long term follow up in 100 cases. *Neurology* 1990;40:413–8.
6. Rasmussen TB. Surgical treatment of complex partial seizures: results, lessons, and problems. *Epilepsia* 1983;24(Suppl 1):65–76.
7. Crandall PH. Cortical resections. In: Engel J, ed. *Surgical treatment of the epilepsies.* New York: Raven Press, 1987:377–404.
8. Falconer MA, Serafetinides EA. A follow-up study of surgery in temporal lobe epilepsy. *J Neurol Neurosurg Psychiatry* 1963;26:154–65.
9. Cahan LD, Sutherling W, McCullough MA, Rausch R, Engel J, Crandall PH. Review of the 20-year UCLA experience with surgery for epilepsy. *Cleve Clin Q* 1984;51:313–8.
10. Spencer DD, Spencer SS, Mattson RH, Wilkinson PD, Novelly RA. Access to the posterior medial temporal lobe structures in the surgical treatment of temporal lobe epilepsy. *Neurosurgery* 1984;15:667–71.
11. Wieser HG, Yasargil MG. Selective amygdalohippocampectomy as a surgical treatment of mesio-basal limbic epilepsy. *Surg Neurol* 1982;17:445–57.
12. Wieser HG. Selective amygdalo-hippocampectomy for temporal lobe epilepsy. *Epilepsia* 1988;29(Suppl 2):S100–13.
13. Davidson S, Falconer MA. Outcome of surgery in 40 children with temporal lobe epilepsy. *Lancet* 1975;1:1260–9.
14. Meyer FB, Marsh F, Laws ER, Sharbrough FR. Temporal lobectomy in children with epilepsy. *J Neurosurg* 1986;64:371–6.

15. Hopkin IJ, Klug GL. Temporal lobectomy for the treatment of intractable complex partial seizures of temporal lobe origin in early childhood. *Dev Med Child Neurol* 1991;33:26–31.

16. Duchowny M, Levin B, Jayakar P, Resnick T, Alvarez L, Morrison G, Dean P. Temporal lobectomy in early childhood. *Epilepsia* 1992;33:298–303.

17. Cascino GD, Sharbrough FW, Hirschorn KA, Marsh WR. Surgery for focal epilepsy in the older patient. *Neurology* 1991;41:1415–7.

18. McLachlan RS, Chavaz CJ, Blume WT, Girvin JP. Temporal lobectomy for intractable epilepsy in patients over age 45 years. *Neurology* 1992;42:662–5.

19. Greenwood J, Kellaway P. Surgical treatment for epilepsy. *Tex Med* 1969;65:64–71.

20. Jensen I, Klinken L. Temporal lobe epilepsy and neuropathology. *Acta Neurol Scand* 1976;54:391–414.

21. Green JR. Surgical treatment of epilepsy during childhood and adolescence. *Surg Neurol* 1977;8:71–80.

22. Jensen I, Vaernet K. Temporal lobe epilepsy. Follow up investigation of 74 temporal lobe resected patients. *Acta Neurochir* 1977;37:173–200.

23. Rapport RL, Ojemann GA, Wyler AR, Ward AA. Surgical management of epilepsy. *West J Med* 1977;127:185–9.

24. Olivier A. Surgical management of complex partial seizures. *Prog Clin Biol Res* 1983;124:309–24.

25. King DW, Flanigin HF, Gallagher BB, So EL, Murvin AJ, Smith DB, Oommen KJ, Feldman DS, Power J. Temporal lobectomy for partial complex seizures: evaluation, results and 1-year follow-up. *Neurology* 1986; 36:334–9.

26. Mizrahi EM, Kellaway P, Grossman RG, Rutecki PA, Armstrong D, Rettig G, Loewe A. Anterior temporal lobectomy and medically refractory temporal lobe epilepsy of childhood. *Epilepsia* 1990;31:302–12.

27. Sperling MR, O'Connor MJ, Saykin AJ, Philips CA, Morrell MJ, Bridgman PA, French JA, Gonatas N. A noninvasive protocol for anterior temporal lobectomy. *Neurology* 1992;42:416–22.

28. Bloom D, Jasper H, Rasmussen T. Surgical therapy in patients with temporal lobe seizures and bilateral EEG abnormality. *Epilepsia* 1959/1960;1:351–65.

29. Bengzon ARA, Rasmussen T, Gloor P, Dussault J, Stephens M. Prognostic factors in the surgical treatment of temporal lobe epileptics. *Neurology* 1968;18:717–31.

30. Engel J, Driver MV, Falconer MA. Electrophysiological correlates of pathology and surgical results in temporal lobe surgery. *Brain* 1975;98:129–56.

31. Lieb JP, Engel J, Gevins A, Crandall PH. Surface and deep EEG correlates of surgical outcome in temporal lobe epilepsy. *Epilepsia* 1981;22:515–38.

32. Dodrill CB, Wilkus RJ, Ojemann GA, Ward AA, Wyler AR, van Belle G, Tamas L. Multidisciplinary prediction of seizure relief from cortical resection surgery. *Ann Neurol* 1986;20:2–12.

33. Lieb JP, Engel J, Babb TL. Interhemispheric propagation time of human hippocampal seizures. I. Relationship to surgical outcome. *Epilepsia* 1986;27:286–93.

34. Duncan JS, Sagar HJ. Seizure characteristics, pathology, and outcome after temporal lobectomy. *Neurology* 1987;37:405–9.

35. Wyllie E, Lüders H, Morris HH, Lesser RP, Dinner DS, Hahn J, Estes ML, Rothner AD, Erenberg G, Cruse R, Friedman D. Clinical outcome after complete or partial cortical resection for intractable epilepsy. *Neurology* 1987;37:1634–41.

36. Awad IA, Katz A, Hahn JF, Kong AK, Ahl J, Lüders H. Extent of resection in temporal lobectomy for epilepsy. I. Interobserver analysis and correlation with seizure outcome. *Epilepsia* 1989;30:756–62.

37. So N, Olivier A, Andermann F, Gloor P, Quesney LF. Results of surgical treatment in patients with bitemporal epileptiform abnormalities. *Ann Neurol* 1989; 25:432–9.

38. Spencer SS, Spencer DD, Williamson PD, Mattson R. Combined depth and subdural electrode investigation in uncontrolled epilepsy. *Neurology* 1990;40:74–9.

39. Siegal AM, Wieser HG, Wichmann W, Yasargil GM. Relationships between MR-imaged total amount of tissue removed, resection scores of specific mediobasal limbic subcompartments and clinical outcome following selective amygdalohippocampectomy. *Epilepsy Res* 1990;6:56–65.

40. Nayel MH, Awad IA, Lüders H. Extent of mesiobasal resection determines outcome after temporal lobectomy for intractable complex partial seizures. *Neurosurgery* 1991;29:55–61.

41. Wieser HG, Siegal AM. Analysis of foramen ovale electrode-recorded seizures and correlation with outcome following amygdalohippocampectomy. *Epilepsia* 1991;32:838–50.

42. Rasmussen T. Cortical resection for medically refractory focal epilepsy: results, lessons and questions. In: Rasmussen T, Marino R, eds. *Functional neurosurgery.* New York: Raven Press, 1979:253–69.

43. Wyler AR, Hermann BP, Richey ET. Results of reoperation for failed epilepsy surgery. *J Neurosurg* 1989; 71:815–9.

44. Hirsch LJ, Spencer SS, Spencer DD, Williamson PD, Mattson RH. Temporal lobectomy in patients with bitemporal epilepsy defined by depth electroencephalography. *Ann Neurol* 1991;30:347–56.

45. Flanigin HF, Smith JR. Depth electrode implantation at the Medical College of Georgia. In: Engel J, ed. *Surgical treatment of the epilepsies.* New York: Raven Press, 1987:609–12.

46. Rasmussen T. Surgery of frontal lobe epilepsy. In: Purpura DP, Penry JK, Walter RD, eds. *Advances in neurology,* Vol 8. New York: Raven Press, 1975:197–205.

47. Rasmussen T. Surgery for epilepsy arising in regions other than the temporal and frontal lobes. In: Purpura DP, Penry JK, Walter RD, eds. *Advances in neurology,* Vol 8. New York: Raven Press, 1975:207–26.

48. Goldring S, Gregorie EM. Surgical management of epilepsy using epidural recordings to localize the seizure focus. Review of 100 cases. *J Neurosurg* 1984;60:457–66.

49. Hajek M, Wieser HG. Extratemporal, mainly frontal epilepsies: surgical results. *J Epilepsy* 1988;1:103–19.

50. Krynauw RA. Infantile hemiplegia treated by removing one cerebral hemisphere. *J Neurol Neurosurg Psychiatry* 1950;13:243–67.

51. McKissock W. Infantile hemiplegia. *Proc R Soc Med* 1953;46:431–4.

52. Rasmussen T, Olszewski J, Lloyd-Smith D. Focal seizures due to chronic encephalitis. *Neurology* 1958; 8:435–45.

53. Wilson PJE. Cerebral hemispherectomy for infantile hemiplegia. A report of 50 cases. *Brain* 1970;93:147–80.

54. Oppenheimer DR, Griffith HB. Persistent intracranial bleeding as a complication of hemispherectomy. *J Neurol Neurosurg Psychiatry* 1966;29:229–40.

55. Rasmussen T. Postoperative superficial hemosiderosis of the brain, its diagnosis, treatment and prevention. *Trans Am Neurol Assoc* 1973;98:133–7.

56. Rasmussen T. Hemispherectomy for seizures revisited. *Can J Neurol Sci* 1983;10:71–8.

57. Tinuper P, Andermann F, Villemure JG, Rasmussen TB, Quesney LF. Functional hemispherectomy for treatment of epilepsy associated with hemiplegia: rationale, indications, results and comparison with callosotomy. *Ann Neurol* 1988;24:27–34.

58. Smith SJM, Andermann F, Villemure JG, Rasmussen TB, Quesney LF. Functional hemispherectomy: EEG findings, spiking from isolated brain postoperatively, and prediction of outcome. *Neurology* 1991; 41: 1790–4.

59. Adams CBT. Hemispherectomy—a modification. *J Neurol Neurosurg Psychiatry* 1983;46:617–9.

60. Van Wagenen WP, Herren RY. Surgical division of commissural pathways in the corpus callosum. Relation to spread of an epileptic attack. *Arch Neurol Psychiatry* 1940;44:740–59.

61. Amacher AL. Midline commissurotomy for the treatment of some cases of intractable epilepsy. *Childs Brain* 1976;2:54–8.

62. Luessenhop AJ. Interhemispheric commissurotomy: (the split brain operation) as an alternate to hemispherectomy for control of intractable seizures. *Am Surg* 1970;36:265–8.

63. Harbaugh RE, Wilson DH, Reeves AG, Gazzaniga MS. Forebrain commissurotomy for epilepsy: review of 20 consecutive cases. *Acta Neurochir* 1983;68:263–75.

64. Wilson DH, Culver C, Waddington M, Gazzaniga M. Disconnection of the cerebral hemispheres. An alternative to hemispherectomy for the control of intractable seizures. *Neurology* 1975;25:1149–53.

65. Wilson DH, Reeves A, Gazzaniga M. Division of the corpus callosum for uncontrollable epilepsy. *Neurology* 1978;28:649–53.

66. Wilson DH, Reeves AG, Gazzaniga MS. "Central" commissurotomy for intractable generalized epilepsy: series two. *Neurology* 1982;32:687–97.

67. Wilson DH, Reeves A, Gazzaniga M, Culver C. Cerebral commissurotomy for control of intractable seizures. *Neurology* 1977;27:708–15.

68. Gates JR, Rosenfield WE, Maxwell RE, Lyons RE. Response of multiple seizure types to corpus callosum section. *Epilepsia* 1987;28:28–34.

69. Spencer SS, Spencer DD, Williamson PD, Sass K, Novelly RA, Mattson RH. Corpus callosotomy for epilepsy. I. Seizure effects. *Neurology* 1988;38:19–24.

70. Murro AM, Flanigin HF, Gallagher BB, King DW, Smith JR. Corpus callosotomy for the treatment of intractable epilepsy. *Epilepsy Res* 1988;2:44–50.

71. Makari GS, Holmes GL, Murro AM, Smith JR, Flanigin HF, Cohen MJ, Huh K, Gallagher BB, Ackell AB, Campbell R, King DW. Corpus callosotomy for the treatment of intractable epilepsy in children. *J Epilepsy* 1989; 2:1–7.

72. Purves SJ, Wada JA, Woodhurst WB, Moyes PD, Strauss E, Kosaka B, Li D. Results of anterior corpus callosum section in 24 patients with medically intractable seizures. *Neurology* 1988;38:1194–201.

Chapter 19

Language Function, Temporal Lobe Epilepsy, and Anterior Temporal Lobectomy

BRUCE P. HERMANN
ALLEN R. WYLER

The purpose of this chapter is to review the literature pertaining to the adequacy of interictal language function among patients with partial seizures of temporal lobe origin, and the effects of anterior temporal lobectomy (ATL) on subsequent language ability. In general, there has been little interest in the status of preoperative interictal language function, but there has been considerable interest in protecting eloquent cortex during focal cortical resection. Functional mapping of language and memory areas is a time-honored procedure conducted by many (but not all) surgical epilepsy centers, using either acute intraoperative or chronic extraoperative functional mapping techniques [1–5]. Given the time, effort, and expense inherent in functional mapping, the cumulative number of cases that have undergone such procedures, and the fundamental controversies regarding the necessity of mapping and the comparative efficacy of intraoperative versus extraoperative mapping, one might expect to find a considerable amount of literature addressing the issue of post-ATL language function. However, that is not the case. Only a small number of language-outcome studies have been published.

In the following material, the literature is reviewed. Our own group has published several preoperative versus postoperative evaluations of language function, as well as a study of the adequacy of interictal language function among patients with temporal lobe epilepsy (TLE). Because these investigations have all relied on one particular aphasia battery, a brief review of the procedures is presented first. This is followed by a discussion of the adequacy of interictal

language function, concluding with a review of language function following ATL.

The Multilingual Aphasia Examination

Language function can be evaluated by any number of specialized tests or batteries. One particular language battery, the Multilingual Aphasia Examination (MAE) [6], has been administered at the Epi-Care Center* since 1985. Details of the battery are presented so that its strengths and weaknesses will become evident. Table 19-1 provides a brief narrative of the individual subtests, and Figures 19-1 to 19-3 provide examples of some of the stimulus materials.

Obvious advantages of the MAE include (a) the ability to assess a variety of core language functions in a standardized fashion in an efficient timeframe; (b) the ability to correct scores for patient age and education, an important clinical advantage; and (c) the availability of norms for both nonaphasic and aphasic populations. Disadvantages include (a) the relatively easy nature of a few subtests, resulting in subsequent ceiling effects; (b) several interesting as well as important aspects of language function are not assessed (e.g., prosodic elements of language); and (c) the MAE has not been utilized as often and is not as familiar to researchers and clinicians as some classic aphasia batteries (e.g., Boston Diagnostic Aphasia Examination).

*Baptist Memorial Hospital/University of Tennessee, Memphis/Semmes-Murphey Clinic.

Table 19-1. Multilingual Aphasia Battery

Subtest	Description
Visual Naming	The stimulus material consists of 10 pictures calling for 30 naming responses.
Sentence Repetition	This test consists of 14 sentences of progressively increasing length, ranging from 3–18 words.
Controlled Oral Word Association	The subject is required to make verbal associations with a letter of the alphabet by saying all the words that he or she can think of beginning with that letter. Three letters of increasing associative difficulty are presented.
Oral Spelling	The subject is asked to spell 11 different words orally.
Token Test	Twenty large and small circles and squares in five colors are employed to assess the patient's ability to comprehend and carry out simple commands.
Aural Comprehension	This is a multiple-choice test of aural comprehension. A variety of visual stimuli (six pages, each with four possible choices) assess comprehension of 11 single words and seven short phrases.
Reading Comprehension	This test is the reading counterpart of the multiple-choice aural comprehension test. Stimulus materials consist of 18 single words or short phrases calling for pointing responses to the same stimulus material as the aural comprehension test.

Source: Benton AL, Hamsher K: *Multilingual aphasia examination.* Iowa City: AJA Associates, 1989, with permission.)

Nevertheless, use of the MAE has facilitated a systemic approach to the assessment of core language functions, and comparisons of language outcomes in the context of varying surgical approaches have allowed systematic hypotheses to be developed.

Prior to examining the issue of language outcome following ATL, a brief review of the relatively neglected issue of preoperative (interictal) language function is presented.

Adequacy of Preoperative Interictal Language Function

An extensive neuropsychological literature exists that examines the effects of epilepsy on a diversity of higher cognitive functions [7–11]. Interestingly, as reviewed by Perrine et al. [11] only a preliminary understanding of the adequacy of interictal language function is known.

Mayeux et al. [12] examined the performance of left ($n = 14$) and right ($n = 7$) TLE patients, as well as a generalized epilepsy group ($n = 8$), on measures of visual confrontation memory (Boston Naming Test) and associative verbal fluency (Controlled Oral Word Association Test). They found that the left TLE group exhibited significantly poorer performance on the Boston Naming Test than did the right TLE and generalized epilepsy groups. These differences remained significant when the influence of education

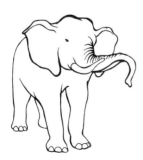

Figure 19-1. Stimulus item from visual naming test. The patient is asked to name the animal, and the examiner points to the animal's ear, tusk, and trunk and asks the patient to provide the correct names for these. (From Benton AL, Hamsher K: *Multilingual aphasia examination.* Iowa City: AJA Associates, 1989, with permission.)

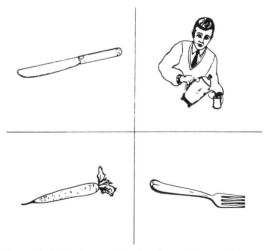

Figure 19-2. Aural comprehension items. The examiner asks the patient to point to the picture depicting the word "edible." (From Benton AL, Hamsher K: *Multilingual aphasia examination.* Iowa City: AJA Associates, 1989, with permission.)

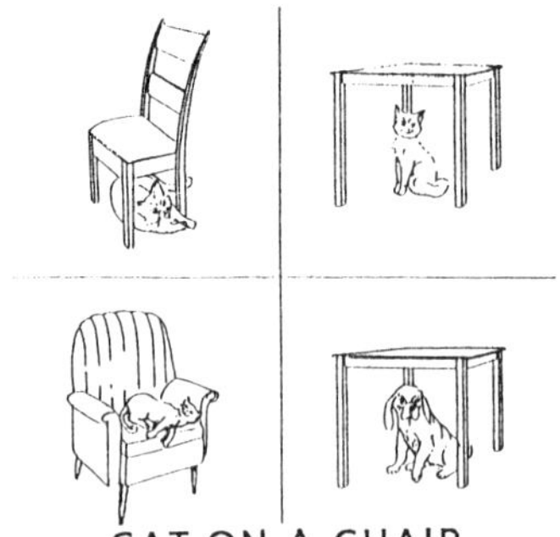

CAT ON A CHAIR

Figure 19-3. Reading comprehension item. Pictorial stimuli and the printed phrase are placed before the patient and he or she is asked to point to the correct picture. (From Benton AL, Hamsher K: *Multilingual aphasia examination*. Iowa City: AJA Associates, 1989, with permission.)

and the WAIS Vocabulary scores were controlled. No differences were found on the test of verbal fluency.

Our center recently examined preoperative interictal language function in 99 patients who were candidates for ATL. Patients were not mentally retarded (full-scale intelligence quotient [IQ] > 69), were left hemisphere dominant for speech as determined by intracarotid sodium amobarbital (Amytal) testing, did not have lesions on magnetic resonance imaging (excluding mesial temporal sclerosis), and had unilateral temporal lobe origin of their seizures as documented by invasive electroencephalographic (EEG) monitoring of spontaneous seizures (left temporal = 47, right temporal = 52) [13]. Table 19-2 shows the MAE results.

Table 19-2. Preoperative Language Function in Unilateral Temporal Lobe Epilepsy*

Subtest	Left Temporal (n = 47)	Right Temporal (n = 52)
Visual Naming	20.7 (24.5)	39.0 (30.4)†
Sentence Repetition	29.4 (26.95)	41.1 (27.1)‡
Controlled Oral Word Association	34.2 (30.9)	40.1 (29.4)
Oral Spelling	38.6 (28.1)	39.6 (26.6)
Token Test	42.9 (31.5)	56.0 (26.6)‡
Aural Comprehension	38.5 (29.3)	47.7 (25.1)‡
Reading Comprehension	33.9 (25.5)	47.0 (21.9)†

*Percentile scores are reported with standard deviations in parentheses.
†$p < .01$
‡$p < .05$
(From Hermann BP, Seidenberg M, Haltiner A, Wyler AR: Adequacy of language function and verbal memory performance in unilateral temporal lobe epilepsy. *Cortex* 1992;28:423–33, with permission.)

Several findings are noteworthy. First, the left TLE group performed significantly worse than the right TLE group on five of the seven MAE subtests: Visual Naming, Sentence Repetition, Token Test, Reading Comprehension, and Aural Comprehension. These results suggest that even in a clinically nonaphasic TLE population, the adequacy of interictal language function is adversely affected by left TLE. These results replicated the findings of Mayeux et al. [12] that visual confrontation naming was significantly worse in left TLE compared with right TLE but also suggested that the effects were not merely limited to naming ability. Multiple aspects of language ability, both expressive and receptive, were affected. The etiology underlying this abnormality could be due to any number of factors (alone or in combination) and includes propagation of interictal discharges to lateral temporal cortex, ipsilateral cortical hypometabolism, and other factors.

Second, the standard deviations for all subtests, for both the left and right TLE groups, were quite large. There appears to be significant variability in the adequacy of language function within both the left and right TLE groups, and to date the factors responsible for this variability remain to be identified.

Third, the right TLE group scored below the 50th percentile on six of the seven subtests, raising the possibility that even their language capabilities had been compromised. There are several possible explanations for such performance. It may merely be consistent with expectations, given their overall level of intellectual ability (full-scale IQ = 88, approximately the 21th percentile). It may also be possible that their language function had been adversely affected by a variety of seizure-related factors (e.g., secondarily generalized seizures, head injuries secondary to seizure-related injuries) that influenced dominant-hemisphere function.

Nevertheless, it should be evident that if left and right TLE patients were assessed *only* following ATL, and if the pattern of results depicted above were obtained, some might infer that surgery had pernicious effects on language ability when in fact these differences preexisted preoperatively. Clearly, both preoperative and postoperative assessment is needed.

Effects of Anterior Temporal Lobectomy on Language Function

Postoperative Testing Only

A small number of articles examined selected aspects of postoperative language function. Heilman, Wilder, and Malzone [14] provided a very brief report on 10 patients who underwent ATL and were available for postoperative testing. The patients underwent non-standardized evaluation of spontaneous speech, comprehension of spoken and written language, repetition, writing, praxis, constructional ability, elements of Gerstmann's syndrome, and naming. Four of the 10 patients were said to have a nontransient anomic aphasia, and all had undergone left ATL. It is not clear how many patients in all had left ATL, and few details were presented regarding the surgery, including whether or not the patients had undergone preoperative functional mapping.

Lifrak and Novelly [15] examined a total of 30 left and right ATL patients who had undergone either total or partial hippocampectomy. They were assessed no sooner than 4 months and up to 7 years postoperatively. Patients were administered two tests of object naming (Boston Naming Test, Lifrak Naming Test), a measure of auditory language comprehension (Revised Token Test), and two tests of associative verbal fluency (letter and category). Patients were tested postoperatively only and had not undergone functional mapping. The dominant ATL patients had lower scores on both naming tests postoperatively compared with the nondominant ATL group. There was no effect of partial versus total hippocampectomy on nominal speech, and latencies to word finding did not differ between dominant and nondominant ATL groups. There were also no differences between the dominant and nondominant groups on measures of fluency or comprehension. Finally, the patients were compared with a control group of 18 healthy individuals, the latter of whom scored significantly better than the ATL patients on all measures except unrestricted verbal fluency.

Cherlow and Serafetinides [16] examined selected aspects of language function in 36 patients (21 right ATL, 9 left ATL, 6 with diagnostic implantation of depth electrodes only). Patients were tested postoperatively only, from 6 months to 12.5 years after surgery. Mapping of language functions had not been carried out. Patients were administered two abbreviated tests from the Boston Diagnostic Aphasia Examination.

1. *Visual Confrontation Naming* (five categories of items depicted on cards including objects, letters, geometric forms, numbers, and actions). The examiner pointed to each of the 27 items, and the patients were asked to provide the correct name, and the number of delays before responding were noted.
2. *Reading Sentences.* Seven sentences, each of which ended with a blank word or phrase, were pre-

sented on cards. Four choices were presented below each card, only one of which would complete the sentence correctly. The results indicated that there were no significant differences among the subject groups for either measure.

Frisk and Milner [17] reported transient deficits in sentence comprehension and rapid naming following left ATL in the acute postoperative period (2 weeks postoperatively), but longer-term follow-up was not reported.

Summary

These investigations all involved postoperative testing only, and the patients did not undergo intraoperative or extraoperative functional mapping. Some investigators, but not all, reported postoperative language abnormalities in left ATL patients generally involving visual confrontation naming ability. The particular tests of visual naming ability were different in each investigation.

Preoperative-to-Postoperative Assessments

Because language differences can be found between left and right TLE groups prior to surgery, the results of preoperative-to-postoperative assessments are needed to more clearly assess the impact of surgery. Those investigations that specifically examined preoperative to postoperative language performance are reviewed below.

Bornstein et al. [18] reported neuropsychological outcomes in a very small sample of left ($n = 4$) and right ($n = 5$) ATL patients who were all left hemisphere dominant for language. It was not stated whether functional mapping had been conducted, and the mean intertest interval was over 1 year for both groups. The left ATL group showed a significant preoperative-to-postoperative *improvement* in associative verbal fluency (Controlled Oral Word Association Test), whereas the right ATL group showed no change. This is an interesting report of improvement in a discrete language ability following left ATL.

Martin et al. [19] administered the same test of verbal fluency (Controlled Oral Word Association Test), as well as a measure of category (semantic) fluency (animals and fruits and vegetables) both prior to and approximately 1 week after left ($n = 15$) or right ($n = 17$) ATL. A normal control group was also included. All patients were right-handed and left hemisphere dominant for language. Functional mapping was not reported. Performance declined significantly for *both*

ATL groups on *both* tasks. Left ATL patients did not show greater declines than right ATL patients.

It is probably reasonable to suspect that the deficits in verbal fluency noted by Martin et al. [19] are attributable to the acute postoperative timing of their assessment, particularly as Bornstein et al. [18] reported improvement on an identical test in the left ATL group and no change in the right ATL group when tested at a time more distant from surgery. However, this hypothesis needs to be confirmed directly via prospective assessment.

Multiple studies of preoperative-to-postoperative language outcome have come from two centers and are reviewed in the following, concluding with a review of language outcome in children following ATL.

Comprehensive Epilepsy Center (CEC), Graduate Hospital, Philadelphia

Stafiniak et al. [20] investigated changes in visual confrontation naming in patients following left (n = 22) or right (n = 23) ATL. Testing was carried out in the acute postoperative period (2–3 weeks after surgery). Functional mapping was not conducted either intraoperatively or extraoperatively. All patients were right-handed and were grouped by side of surgery and presence or absence of early (age 5 years or under) risk factors for epilepsy (i.e., suspected underlying etiologic insult, not necessarily age at onset of epilepsy). After left ATL, 60% of the patients *without* early risk factors exhibited what the authors considered to be a significant decline on the Boston Naming Test (25% loss or greater), whereas none of the left ATL patients *with* early risk factors showed a change in confrontation naming ability. There were no changes after right ATL. These findings suggested that early insult to the left cerebral hemisphere resulted in intrahemispheric or interhemispheric functional reorganization of language ability. This reorganization did not occur in those with a later age at seizure risk, and left ATL resulted in an increased risk of acute postoperative dysnomia. The permanence of these declines in visual confrontation naming ability is the subject of an ongoing prospective investigation by the authors, although they note that there has been appreciable improvement in some patients at one year postoperatively.

Robinson and Saykin [21] examined this issue further in an expanded series of patients (32 right ATL and 32 left ATL), along with a healthy control group (n = 32). All patients had been assessed in the acute postsurgical interval (median 18 days postoperatively), and none had undergone functional mapping. An expanded battery of language tests was administered (including confrontation naming, phonemic and semantic fluency, repetition, comprehension, and reading recognition). Robinson and Saykin [21] were able to confirm that decline in visual confrontation naming occurred primarily in left temporal ATL patients who presented with an absence of early risk factors. Declines were also noted on other language subtests for this group, but the most dramatic effect occurred for naming ability.

Epi-Care Center, Baptist Memorial Hospital/University of Tennessee, Memphis

Intraoperative Mapping and Language Outcome. The first comprehensive preoperative-to-postoperative evaluation of language outcome in patients who underwent intraoperative functional mapping with tailored resection did not appear until recently [22]. We compared patients who underwent dominant (n = 15) or nondominant ATL (n = 14), using the latter group as a control for test-retest effects. The dominant and nondominant ATL groups were comparable in age, education, age at onset, IQ, and duration of epilepsy. All had undergone intracarotid amobarbital testing to determine cerebral dominance for speech. Two patients were right hemisphere dominant for language and underwent right ATL. Thirteen of the 15 patients undergoing dominant ATL received intraoperative functional mapping. There was concern that the other two patients might not tolerate the procedure because of psychiatric difficulties and/or compromised intelligence, and they received general anesthesia without benefit of mapping. Based on the results of functional mapping and electrocorticography (ECoG), the majority of the dominant ATL group (13 of 15) underwent a tailored resection.

As shown in Table 19-3, overall group results revealed that dominant ATL patients did not show significant worsening in any area of language ability and even showed some statistically significant improvements compared with the nondominant ATL group. The dominant ATL group showed significant gains in complex receptive language comprehension (Token Test) and associative verbal fluency (Controlled Oral Word Association Test). The overall pattern of results therefore suggested that the use of intraoperative mapping of language ability helped to preserve preoperative levels of language ability.

In addition to these analyses of *group* data, several subsequent analyses were carried out to determine whether there were any significant deviations in the performances of *individuals* who underwent dominant ATL. Although there were individual differences

Table 19-3. Preoperative-to-Postoperative Language Function: Study 1*

Subtest	Dominant ATL ($n = 15$)	Nondominant ATL ($n = 14$)
Visual Naming	-0.1 (8.0)	3.1 (8.7)
Sentence Repetition	3.3 (9.9)	3.8 (12.2)
Controlled Oral Word Association	3.7 (5.5)	1.3 (8.2)†
Oral Spelling	0.3 (5.8)	-1.2 (9.2)
Token Test	6.8 (11.3)	3.4 (8.5)†
Aural Comprehension	-1.5 (4.5)	-1.3 (4.1)
Reading Comprehension	-0.8 (5.5)	1.9 (7.9)

*Scores are postoperative T-scores minus preoperative T-scores (standard deviation in parentheses). Negative scores represent postoperative performance declines, positive scores represent postoperative performance improvements.
†$p < .05$. Significantly greater preoperative-to-postoperative improvement for dominant ATL group.
(From Hermann BP, Wyler AR: Effects of anterior temporal lobectomy on language function: a controlled study. *Ann Neurol* 1988;23:585–88, with permission.)

in the pattern of language outcome, factors predictive of this variability could not be identified. We did not, however, examine the influence of age at first risk for epilepsy or the age at onset of epilepsy.

Language Outcome With Versus Without Intraoperative Mapping

One important question concerns the status of language outcome in groups of patients who do or do not undergo functional mapping. A unique comparison was undertaken in a small series of consecutive patients who underwent dominant ATL under either local anesthesia with acute intraoperative functional mapping ($n = 13$) or under general anesthesia without mapping ($n = 13$) [23]. Intraoperative functional mapping was slowly abandoned at the EpiCare Center (for nonlesional cases of mesial temporal lobe onset) because of the difficulty that some patients experienced with the procedure and, more importantly, because clinical experience suggested that surgical outcome was associated with the extent of hippocampal resection [24]. Surgery under local anesthesia limits head positioning during surgery, is painful when dissection is near the tentorium, and is not conducive to use of the operating microscope. Thus, since it was believed the outcome was improved with more complete resection of hippocampus we changed to performing all cases under general anesthesia.

The MAE was administered preoperatively and 6 months postoperatively. The two groups were comparable in age, education, gender distribution, age at onset of epilepsy, duration of epilepsy, etiology, verbal IQ, and preoperative performance on all the MAE subtests. The group that underwent dominant ATL with mapping and corticography had a more extensive lateral temporal resection compared with the patients who had dominant ATL under general anesthesia without mapping.

Preoperative and postoperative scores were converted to T-scores (mean = 50, standard deviation = 10), and Table 19-4 shows the mean postoperative minus preoperative difference scores (negative scores representing performance decline). In general, the magnitude of change for both groups was very small. More importantly, comparison of MAE performance from preoperative to postoperative assessments showed a marginally significant ($p = .05$) decline on the Visual Naming subtest for the group that did not undergo functional mapping (Fig. 19-4). This decline in word-finding ability was on the order of approximately half a standard deviation.

This study would appear to suggest that mapping does protect against mild nontransient postoperative dysnomia. It should be remembered that patients were assessed at 6 months following surgery, and it is unclear whether the alterations in naming ability resolved over time. It is interesting to note that at 6 months follow-up, 69% of patients operated on under general anesthesia were completely seizure-free compared with 46% of those undergoing ATL under local anesthesia with functional mapping. Although this length of follow-up is clearly too short to predict long-term outcome, it was consistent with expectations.

Table 19-4. Preoperative-to-Postoperative Language Function: Study 2*

Subtest	Left ATL With Mapping	Left ATL Without Mapping
Visual Naming	0.8	-4.9†
Sentence Repetition	2.5	5.6
Controlled Oral Word Association	3.0	3.4
Oral Spelling	0.9	0.5
Token Test	6.7	3.6
Aural Comprehension	-1.8	0.3
Reading Comprehension	-0.9	1.6

*Mean postoperative T-scores minus preoperative T-scores.
† t = 0.05.
(From Hermann BP, Wyler AR: Comparative results of dominant temporal lobectomy under general or local anesthesia: language outcome. *J Epilepsy* 1988:1:127–34.)

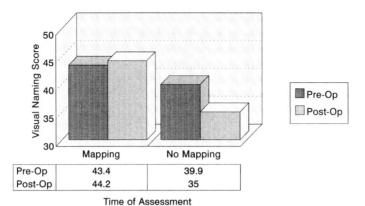

Figure 19-4. Change in confrontation naming with, versus without, use of intraoperative mapping techniques.

Language Outcome Without Functional Mapping but With Conservative Cortical Resection

In the third investigation [25], none of the patients underwent intraoperative or extraoperative mapping of language ability. All the patients (dominant [left] ATL [n = 29], nondominant [right] ATL [n = 35]) had intractable epilepsy and were without any MRI visible lesion (tumor, stroke, arterovenous malformation). All patients had undergone invasive monitoring of spontaneous seizures and had been found to have unilateral temporal lobe onset, primarily from medial structures. Therefore, a very conservative resection of dominant lateral temporal cortex was carried out. The median resection was 4.25 cm.

The MAE was administered preoperatively and 6 months postoperatively, and the groups were comparable in age, education, and IQ. The dominant ATL group had an earlier age at onset and longer duration of epilepsy. Median preoperative-to-postoperative change scores were examined in the dominant and nondominant ATL groups (Table 19-5). There were no impairments in language function following dominant ATL compared with the nondominant group. The dominant ATL group again showed a significant improvement on the Token Test compared with the nondominant controls, but in this investigation no improvement was shown on the measure of verbal fluency. Another point of interest was that with the conservative resections done in this series, there was very little overall alteration in language function. In fact, the median preoperative-to-postoperative change score was 0 for 12 of the 14 MAE comparisons. We were again largely unable to find any subject variables that were predictive of postoperative decrements or improvements in language function following ATL.

While these findings need to be confirmed in different surgical populations using alternative aphasia batteries, the results to date tentatively suggest that with *conservative* resections of dominant lateral temporal cortex in patients with epilepsy of mesial temporal lobe origin, preoperative levels of basic language function can be largely preserved. Before concluding that dominant ATL has few pernicious effects of postoperative language function, investigations are needed that assess the use of language in the service of higher cognitive abilities (e.g., reasoning, expression of ideas), evaluate the effects of different surgical procedures (e.g., *en bloc* vs. amygdalohippocampectomy) on language outcome, and utilize additional or alternative testing procedures and aphasia batteries.

Table 19-5. Preoperative-to-Postoperative Language Function: Study 3*

Subtest	Left ATL (n = 29)	Right ATL (n = 35)
Visual Naming	0 (−28–10)	0 (−10–8)
Sentence Repetition	0 (−2–50)	0 (−2–6)
Controlled Oral Word Association	−3 (−11–34)	0 (−21–12)
Oral Spelling	0 (−2–4)	0 (−2–3)
Token Test	1 (−5–8)	0 (−6–6)
Aural Comprehension	0 (−5–3)	0 (−2–2)
Reading Comprehension	0 (−2–5)	0 (−2–1)

*Median postoperative minus preoperative difference scores are depicted. There were no significant differences.
(From Hermann BP, Wyler AR, Somes G: Language function following anterior temporal lobectomy. *J Neurosurg* 1991;74:560–6, with permission.)

Language Outcome in Children Following Anterior Temporal Lobectomy

Adams et al. [26] reported the surgical and neuropsychological outcome of ATL in 44 children under the age of 16 years. Functional mapping was apparently not conducted. Measures of language function were administered to a subgroup of children preoperatively and at both acute (3–6 weeks) and chronic (6 months) follow-up. Language tests included confrontation naming (Oldfield-Wingfield Object Naming) and two tests of comprehension (Test for Recognition of Grammar [TROG], Shortened Token Test [STT]). Ten children underwent language assessment after left-sided operations, and at acute assessment (3–6 weeks) they showed a significant decline in object naming that resolved by 6 months following surgery. No changes were seen on the measures of comprehension. Sixteen children were seen after right-sided operations, and there were no language changes acutely, with significant improvement on the TROG at 6 months but still no change on the SST.

This study is particularly important because it demonstrates that the acute naming problems seen in the immediate postoperative period, which has been noted by others, tend to resolve at longer-term follow-up.

Conclusions

Based on the above review, the following observations are offered. First, given the approximately half-century history of functional mapping, there has been a remarkable lack of empirical research designed to evaluate its efficacy. Strong opinions have been voiced regarding the general necessity of such procedures, as well as of the relative superiority of one technique over the other. These opinions have been offered within the context of an almost total lack of published outcome data. In fact, several of the reviewed investigations did not perform functional mapping and reported that naming deficits (a) were seen acutely but appeared to resolve over time, (b) were not detected at 6 months after surgery, or (c) persisted in a subgroup of individuals, suggesting that mapping may be important for certain subgroups of potential left ATL patients. While this clearly requires further study, it would certainly seem fair to ask those who routinely submit their patients to intraoperative mapping to demonstrate the efficacy of their procedures.

Second, the information that is now available should be considered to be very preliminary. As is generally appreciated, surgical centers vary widely in their criteria for patient selection, surgical technique, test-retest interval and length of follow-up, language-assessment procedures, determination of speech/language dominance on intracarotid amobarbital testing, and a host of other variables that certainly influence language outcome results. While it has become a tired cliché, it is nonetheless abundantly clear that additional research is needed so that a better understanding of this important aspect of surgical outcome can be derived.

Third, there has in general been little appreciation for the adequacy of preoperative interictal language function. The available evidence suggests that abnormalities are more common in left than in right TLE, but there is considerable variability within both groups, the cause of which remains to be determined. More research and clinical interest should be devoted to this important domain of cognitive function.

References

1. Lüders H, Hahn J, Lesser RP, Dinner D, Morris H, Wyllie E, Friedman L, Friedman D, Skipper G. Basal temporal subdural electrodes in the evaluation of patients with intractable epilepsy. *Epilepsia* 1989;30:131–42.
2. Lesser RP, Lüders H, Klem G, Dinner D, Morris H, Hahn J, Wyllie E. Extraoperative cortical functional localization in patients with epilepsy. *J Clin Neurophysiol* 1987;4:27–53.
3. Ojemann G, Ojemann J, Lettich E, Berger M. Cortical language localization in left, dominant hemisphere. *J Neurosurg* 1989;71:316–26.
4. Ojemann G. Individual variability in cortical localization of language. *J Neurosurg* 1979;50:164–9.
5. Ojemann GA. Cortical organization of language. *J Neurosci* 1991;11:2281–7.
6. Benton AL, Hamsher K. *Multilingual aphasia examination.* Iowa City: AJA Associates, 1989.
7. Bennett TL, Krien LK. The neuropsychology of epilepsy: psychological and social impact. In: Reynolds CR, Fletcher-Janzen E, eds. *Handbook of clinical child neuropsychology.* New York: Plenum Press, 1989.
8. Dikmen S. Neuropsychological aspects of epilepsy. In: Hermann BP, ed. *A multidisciplinary handbook of epilepsy.* Springfield, IL: Charles C. Thomas, 1980:36–73.
9. Dodrill C. Neuropsychology. In: Laidlaw J, Richens A, Oxley J, eds. *A textbook of epilepsy.* New York: Churchill Livingstone, 1988.
10. Hermann BP. Contributions of traditional assessment procedures to an understanding of the neuropsychology of epilepsy. In: Dodson E, Kinsborne M, eds. *Computerized neuropsychological assessment in epilepsy.* New York: Demos Publications, 1991.
11. Perrine K, Gershengorn J, Brown ER. Interictal neuropsychological function in epilepsy. In: Devinsky O, Theodore W, eds. *Epilepsy and behavior.* New York: Wiley-Liss, 1991:181–93.

12. Mayeux R, Brandt J, Rosen J, Benson DF. Interictal memory and language impairment in temporal lobe epilepsy. *Neurology* 1980;30:120–5.

13. Hermann BP, Seidenberg M, Haltiner A, Wyler AR. Adequacy of language function and verbal memory performance in unilateral temporal lobe epilepsy. *Cortex* 1992;28:423–33.

14. Heilman KM, Wilder BJ, Malzone WF. Anomic aphasia following anterior temporal lobectomy. *Transactions of the American Neurological Association* 1972;97:291–3.

15. Lifrak MD, Novelly RA. Language deficits in patients with temporal lobectomy for complex partial seizures. In: Porter RJ, et al., eds. *Advances in neurology: XVth epilepsy international symposium.* New York: Raven Press, 1984:469–73.

16. Cherlow DG, Serafetinides EA. Speech and memory assessment in psychomotor epileptics. *Cortex* 1976; 12:21–6.

17. Frisk V, Milner B. The relationship of working memory to the immediate recall of stories following unilateral temporal or frontal lobectomy. *Neuropsychologia,* 1990;28:121–35.

18. Bornstein RA, McKean JDS, McLean DR. Effects of temporal lobectomy for treatment of epilepsy on hemispheric functions ipsilateral to surgery: preliminary findings. *Int J Neurosci* 1987;37:73–8.

19. Martin RC, Loring DW, Meador K, Lee GP. The effects of lateralized temporal lobe dysfunction on formal and semantic word fluency. *Neuropsychologia* 1990; 28: 823–9.

20. Stafiniak P, Saykin AJ, Sperling MR, Kester MS, Robinson LJ, O'Connor MJ, Gur RC. Acute naming deficits following dominant anterior temporal lobectomy: prediction by age at 1st risk for seizures. *Neurology* 1990;40:1509–12.

21. Robinson LJ, Saykin AJ. Psychological and psychosocial outcome of anterior temporal lobectomy. In: Bennett TL, ed. *The neuropsychology of epilepsy.* New York: Plenum Press, 1992:181–97.

22. Hermann BP, Wyler AR. Effects of anterior temporal lobectomy on language function: a controlled study. *Ann Neurol* 1988;23:585–8.

23. Hermann BP, Wyler AR. Comparative results of dominant temporal lobectomy under general or local anesthesia: language outcome. *J Epilepsy* 1988;1:127–34.

24. Wyler AR, Hermann BP. Comparative results of temporal lobectomy under local or general anesthesia: seizure outcome. *J Epilepsy* 1988;1:121–5.

25. Hermann BP, Wyler AR, Somes G. Language function following anterior temporal lobectomy. *J Neurosurg* 1991;74:560–6.

26. Adams CBT, Beardsworth ED, Oxbury SM, Oxbury JM, Fenwick PBC. Temporal lobectomy in 44 children: outcome and neuropsychological follow-up. *J Epilepsy* 1990;3(Suppl 1):157–68.

Chapter 20

Psychiatric Assessment and Temporal Lobectomy

Desirability of Psychiatric Assessment

Epileptic patients are disadvantaged not only because of their epilepsy and their seizures, but also because of the difficulties they often experience in other areas of their lives. Patients admitted to surgical programs for temporal lobectomy commonly experience difficulties in interpersonal relationships, work relationships, and sexual relationships [1–5]. Thus, an epilepsy surgery program should not aim simply to stop seizures, but also to identify these difficulties in an initial presurgical assessment and so help patients cope with the difficulties in their personal lives. Once it is known whether the fits have been controlled, the impact of surgery on the patient's whole life adjustment and situation should be assessed. Some patients may not be improved or may be disadvantaged by the operation, and they will require special care. It is also surprisingly not uncommon to find patients who are distressed by a complete remission of their seizures and who have difficulty in coping without epilepsy.

Psychiatric Illness in Patients with Temporal Lobe Epilepsy

The patient with epilepsy has recurrent, often widespread, transient disturbances of brain function. Yet despite these disturbances and the accompanying social stigmata caused by the resulting changes in behavior, non–brain-damaged patients with epilepsy as a group are relatively normal. A high prevalence of psychiatric morbidity is associated with several different factors, each of which is important and some of which are cumulative. A brief review of the preva-lence and causes of psychiatric disorders may be helpful before looking at the psychiatric outcome of the temporal lobe surgery program reported in the literature.

Prevalence of Psychiatric Morbidity in Epilepsy

Accurate estimates of psychiatric morbidity in epilepsy are hard to find. Existing estimates tend to be biased because of the selection of the populations studied.

Gudmundsson [6], in a community survey of epilepsy in Iceland, found that only half the epileptic patients sampled were psychologically normal. He found the same rate of neuroticism (10%) for men as did Helgason [7] in a community survey of the general population, but Gudmundsson reported a significantly higher rate of neuroticism (25%) in women with epilepsy. Pond and Bidwell [8] have suggested that at least 29% of people with epilepsy have psychological difficulties. In the Isle of Wight population survey of children, the overall rate of psychiatric disorder with uncomplicated epilepsy was 28.6%, four times the control rate, rising up to 58.3% in children with brain damage [9]. A follow-up study of a sample of children with epilepsy 25 years after they had entered a population survey found that two thirds of that population suffered minimal or no ill effects [10,11]. A study of the Medical Research Council National Longitudinal Survey of Health and Development of Children born in 1946 in Great Britain found that by the age of 26 years about 35% of the 46 epileptic patients studied (mainly those with definite brain damage) were graded as "complicated" and did not perform as well socially and in employment as the controls or as those patients with uncomplicated epilepsy [11]. Thus, a figure between one third and one half for the prevalence of psychiatric morbidity in people with epilepsy would seem reasonable.

Diffuse lesions with generalized brain damage lead to intellectual impairment with an increased prevalence of psychiatric morbidity, as described above, and focal lesions may lead to specific cognitive deficits. Of greater importance, however is the recent finding that temporal lobe lesions have a significant relationship to the genesis of psychiatric morbidity. Gudmundsson [6] showed that 50% of patients with temporal lobe epilepsy had psychological difficulties compared with 25% of those with other types of attacks. Pond and Bidwell's study [8] showed similar results; nearly 20% of those with temporal lobe epilepsy had been in mental hospitals compared with 7% of the group as a whole. Rodin et al. [12], in a study of patients with temporal lobe epilepsy, also found a significantly higher rate of psychiatric morbidity.

Rodin et al. [12] showed a clear relationship between temporal lobe epilepsy and psychiatric morbidity, but they also showed that patients with temporal lobe epilepsy were more difficult to control, took a greater number of drugs, and frequently had more than one seizure type—all confounding variables, which again suggests that an important underlying factor is likely to be brain damage. In a series of 100 patients with temporal lobe epilepsy followed longitudinally for a number of years, brain damage was again found to be associated with psychiatric disorder, personality difficulties, and sexual dysfunction [13]. Currie et al. [14] found a surprisingly low prevalence rate of psychiatric morbidity. Their hospital study of patients with temporal lobe epilepsy suffers from all the deficits mentioned above, but in view of the fact already mentioned that patients with temporal lobe epilepsy and psychiatric illness are more frequently referred to a hospital, a higher prevalence rate might have been expected.

Depression has been frequently mentioned in the literature as affecting patients with seizure disorders. Several recent reviews have looked at this in detail and all agree that depression is common [14a–14d]. There is, however, little consensus as to the cause of depression. There have been attempts to relate occurrence and severity of depression to features of the epilepsy. Little convincing relationship has been shown between seizure type, seizure frequency and age of onset of the epilepsy. There is some suggestion, however, [14e] that patients with left temporal lobe seizures are more prone to depression than those with

a focus on the right side. However, this finding has not been replicated in other studies. Psychosocial factors are often named but without adequate studies or control groups it is never possible to be sure which of these are important.

Locus of control is a measure of the degree to which a patient feels in control of his life. In a review of the relationship between locus of control and depression in patients with epilepsy, Benassi et al. [14f] showed that there was a small correlation of approximately 0.31. A study of 37 patients prior to temporal lobe surgery looked at the influence on depression of locus of control. It was found in this study also that this accounted for 9% of the variance of depressive symptoms [14d]. This study indicated that patients with severe drug resistant epilepsy were no more likely to be involved than patients with epilepsy who were not going forward in an epilepsy surgery program.

More recently, Trimble and Perez [15], reviewing those studies that had used questionnaire scoring of the relationship between psychopathology and type of seizure, show that there is an association between an increased prevalence of psychiatric pathology and temporal lobe epilepsy.

Factors Leading to Psychiatric Morbidity

The "epileptic personality" often described is seldom due to the epilepsy alone. Brain damage; medication; the stigma of epilepsy; difficulties with schooling, employment, and interpersonal relationships; and, in a small proportion of patients, institutionalization, all contribute [16–19].

Gibbs [20], Gastaut [21], and others have suggested that seizure discharges within the limbic system (temporal lobe epilepsy) lead to a specific temporal lobe syndrome. Waxman and Geschwind [22] and Geschwind [23] suggest that some patients with temporal lobe epilepsy showed altered sexual behavior and an altered religious view of life, and that they became compulsive writers (hypergraphia). Bear [24] and Bear and Fedio [25] describe a sensory limbic hyperconnection syndrome. They suggested that one effect of temporal lobe epilepsy is to cause the patient to add excessive meaning to his or her world, and that the hyperconnection syndrome was a reverse Klüver-Bucy [26] syndrome. Other workers have shown that if patients with psychiatric illness are removed from the epilepsy group, most of the differences between patients with temporal lobe epilepsy and other patient groups disappear [27–30]. It is thus likely that the findings of excessive emotion initially reported by Bear and Fedio [25] are related to psychiatric illness rather than specifically to temporal lobe epilepsy.

There is also a continuing controversy about whether it is the seizures themselves or the underlying brain damage that causes the suggested personality alteration. The most widely accepted view is that of Stevens and Hermann [31], who said "There are a number of factors which increase the risk of psychopathology in patients with temporal lobe epilepsy. The most powerful factors identified are clinical, EEG and radiological evidence of bilateral, deep or diffuse cerebral pathology." These points need careful consideration when looking at the composition of populations coming forward for temporal lobectomy.

Brain Damage

An association between brain damage and psychiatric morbidity has been described in many studies. The relationship between epilepsy, brain damage, and chronic illness has been shown by Rutter et al. [9] in the results of a total survey of the school children on the Isle of Wight. They found an overall rate of psychiatric morbidity of 6.8% for the control sample. The highest prevalence was found for those with brain damage and epilepsy—58.3%. The association of brain damage with epilepsy is thus an important factor. This study also found that the presence of temporal lobe seizures, emotional instability in the patient's mother, and low social class significantly influenced the occurrence of psychiatric morbidity.

Studies by Lennox [32] and Lennox and Lennox [33] showed the importance of brain damage and also found that early age of onset of the epilepsy carried a poorer prognosis for mental functioning. Reitman [34] also showed that the younger the age at which brain damage occurs, the greater will be its effects on the development of the person's intellect and personality. Personality disorders are found more frequently the earlier the seizures start and the more widespread the convulsions (generalized rather than focal) [9,35].

The level of intellectual performance is also affected by the type of epilepsy and the size of the brain lesion. Generalized diffuse brain damage tends to produce a global reduction in intelligence quotient (IQ) scores but no specific reduction in subtest scores, whereas localized lesions may produce focal cognitive deficits. Dominant (left) temporal lesions, for example, generally produce a deterioration in verbal IQ and verbal memory, whereas nondominant (right) temporal lesions may show no specific change or, sometimes, impaired verbal memory and reduced verbal IQ. A few studies show nonverbal memory impairment. However, focal epileptogenic lesions usually lead to focal cognitive deficits, and those patients with focal deficits are more at risk for psychiatric illness than those without.

Multiplicity of Factors

Taylor [36] has consistently emphasized that it is no longer sufficient to clump all patients with temporal lobe epilepsy together. He has shown that in patients undergoing temporal lobectomy, "a number of effects—pathological sinistrality, the balance of cognitive skills, complexity of the aura experience, aggression, extraversion and liability to psychosis—were partially dependent on the time of origin of the temporal lobe lesion, its left or right location, and on the patient's sex" [37]. Taylor [35] also showed that aggressiveness is more often associated with left temporal lobe lesions.

Comparing children with epilepsy with nonepileptic controls, Stores [38] found that epileptic children were significantly more socially isolated, inattentive, overactive, and anxious. They were also emotionally dependent on their mothers. His most significant finding, however, was that boys with epilepsy were more affected than were girls, and children of both sexes who had left, rather than right, temporal epileptic foci were more frequently affected. This finding was confirmed in the follow up study of children with temporal lobe epilepsy by Lindsay et al. [13], who again suggested that males with a left temporal focus were particularly at risk.

Family Factors

The family's response to and ability to cope with a disadvantaged child play an important part in the genesis of psychiatric morbidity. Rutter [9] found that disturbed home backgrounds and broken family relationships were important causes of psychiatric morbidity. It is a general finding that parents of epileptic children are often overprotective [39], so that the children tend to be emotionally immature and excessively dependent on their families, particularly on their mothers. The child's immaturity, lack of social skills, and fear of independence may lead to a stormy adolescence and difficulty in breaking away from the family. Often the result is a hostile, dependent adult, who may never succeed in leaving the parental home.

Temporal Lobe Surgery Programs

Prevalence of Psychiatric Disorder in Candidates for Surgery

Psychiatric morbidity varies widely among surgery series. Some report almost all their patients as psychologically healthy, for example Montreal Neurological Institute (personal communication), while others give very high rates of psychiatric illness. Mihara et al. (1990) found that 18 (27%) patients entering the epilepsy surgery program were rejected because of psychological problems. Amongst those rejected, the high numbers (3–15%) of patients with psychotic illnesses should be noted. The 27% represent 14% of the total patients who entered the epilepsy surgery program. Walker and Blumer [40] report that 32% of their sample required psychiatric hospital admission, whereas Jensen and Larsen [2] report that only 8% of their sample were psychiatrically normal.

Psychiatric Indications for Surgery

Surgery is indicated if there is a clear relationship between seizures and alterations in behavior. Thus, patients who have postictal confusional states or postictal psychotic episodes are likely to be helped by surgery. There may be specific psycho-syndromes, as yet not clearly defined, that would improve if surgery were successful. The Danish experience was that some patients who had had a poor life adjustment and had been out of work showed improvement and returned to work after lobectomy [2]. It would be advantageous if this group could be identified preoperatively.

The relationship between disorders of behavior and surgery is important. Experience in several centers has already shown that in some patients behavior improves following successful temporal lobectomy. It could thus be argued that temporal lobectomy was a suitable treatment for disorders of behavior. This argument could lead to the use of temporal lobe surgery as psycho-surgery, directed at altering behavior rather than at seizure control. However, behavior is better regarded as the final outcome of many different factors, some internal and some situational. It is difficult to argue that seizure discharges within the limbic system, whether directly visible on the scalp electroencephalogram (EEG) or confined to the depth EEG, are always responsible for disordered or anti-social behavior [41,42]. The primary aim of temporal lobe surgery should be directed toward seizure control rather than specifically at behavioral modification. However, Walker and Blumer [40] found that hyposexuality and aggressiveness tended to improve after temporal lobectomy, whereas temporal lobe viscosity of personality did not. Experience from the first Maudsley series, too, was that aggressiveness was reduced after temporal lobectomy [43].

In 1987, a questionnaire study was submitted to all 53 centers in the world carrying out temporal lobe surgery [44]. In answer to the question, "In your view, are there any absolute psychiatric indications to TLE surgery?" 20 units replied "no." When the questionnaire was repeated in 1989, 19 units replied, 16 of whom still felt there were no psychiatric indications for surgery. However, two centers now suggested that postictal psychosis or postictal psychopathology was sufficient reason for surgery, and one suggested ictal rage was an indication for surgery. In my view, clear stereotyped behavioral (aggressive, psychotic, etc.) changes following seizures are a clear indication for assessment for temporal lobectomy and operation if suitable.

Contraindications to Surgery

There are, however, contraindications to temporal lobe surgery. Many psychiatrically disadvantaged patients present themselves for epilepsy surgery. It is essential to detect these patients early in the assessment procedure and to decide whether facilities for rehabilitation and support are available for them during both the assessment phase and the postoperative period of the surgery program. If such facilities are not available, then this would be a contraindication to surgery. Again it must be emphasized that patients are seeking improvement of their life situation and not only seizure control. This point is an important one and has been given little attention so far in the literature, possibly because there has been insufficient evidence to support it. However, if the findings of the recent analysis of the old Maudsley series (see below) are confirmed by other units, it is possible to differentiate a group of patients whose seizures may be helped but who become psychiatrically disadvantaged. It is thus questionable whether these patients should be operated on, even though surgery might result in seizure control. The loss of seizures can be catastrophic for vulnerable patients whose personal identity is linked to seizure occurrence. Without adequate preparation and counseling before surgery, the result of successful seizure control could be more devastating than a continuation of the seizures [45].

Severe brain damage and poor memory functioning are generally recognized as strong contraindications to surgery. However, it should be recognized that any decision will be influenced by the overall severity of the seizures and the possibility of further reduction in cognitive and behavioral functioning due to continuing seizures.

Several epilepsy surgery programs are believed to reject patients with an interictal psychosis of epilepsy. There is evidence that psychosis is neither enhanced nor decreased by surgery [2,46,47]. It could be argued that there are patients with a psychosis who would be better off without seizures, even though it is recognized that the operation would not influence the course or severity of the psychotic process. Although the original suggestion from the Maudsley series was that patients with psychosis should not be operated on, reanalysis of the series (see below) indicates that left temporal lobectomies may more frequently lead to a remission in psychoses, whereas right temporal lobectomies may induce a psychosis. Further work is needed to confirm these findings.

There are only limited data on the numbers of patients who are rejected by epilepsy surgery programs before being admitted to the assessment procedure. Because of the wide variation among centers and the number of patients who have psychiatric illnesses, it must be presumed that some centers are operating on a policy of rejection, either overtly or covertly. It will not be possible to understand fully the relationship between psychiatric morbidity and outcome until information is available about the psychiatric composition of the populations involved. *There is thus a need for each center to state its policy with regard to patients with psychiatric illness and the numbers of patients who are rejected or admitted for assessment.*

In the 1987 questionnaire mentioned above [44], 20 units answered the question, "In your view are there any absolute contraindications to temporal lobe surgery?" Seven replied "yes," and 13 "no." The most common contraindications were psychosis (5), psychiatric disorder that is more disabling than the seizures (1), and severe passive-aggressive disorder (1). The questionnaire was repeated in 1989, when the answers were essentially similar. On this occasion, 18 units replied: severe psychosis (9), severe depressive illness with the likelihood of suicide (7), unrealistic attitudes to outcome (2), personality disorder (2), frequent pseudoseizures (1), and low IQ (1). Interestingly, six units on this occasion felt there were no psychiatric contraindications.

Assessment of Results of Surgery Programs

One of the major difficulties in assessing the results of a temporal lobe surgery program lies in lack of knowledge of the initial patient input. Precise descriptions of the psychiatric, psychological, and seizure state of preoperative surgical candidates are seldom available. To remedy this, it is essential that all patients should be psychiatrically assessed before detailed investigation for surgery. It is as important to report in detail the psychiatric state of those who are rejected from the program as of those who are to be included. In this way, similarity or difference in populations of those entering the surgery program in different units can be assessed.

Preliminary studies of social and personal, sexual, and work functioning and the major life variables of the operated populations have been carried out by Hill et al. [48], Green et al. [49], James [50], Taylor [51], Taylor [35], Serafetinides and Falconer [52], Taylor and Falconer [43], Taylor and Marsh [53], Polkey [4], Jensen and Varnet [1], Jensen and Larsen [2], and Walker and Blumer [40]. A recent study from Japan reports that 27% (18) patients were rejected from pretemporal lobe surgery assessment because of psychological problems. The psychological problems detailed were psychotic, character abnormalities, drug noncompliance, and uncooperative with investigatory procedures. This would suggest that considerable filtering of psychiatric patients before surgery may occur in some studies [53a]. However, behavioral and psychiatric data have not been studied in as much detail as seizure variables, and there is still a need for further detailed work.

Psychiatric Complications after Surgery

The nature of psychiatric complications and the immediate psychiatric complication rate following surgery have not yet been adequately described. Between 5% and 10% of the population operated on may have some degree of immediate postoperative psychiatric morbidity. Walker and Blumer [40] report a 4% immediate postoperative change in behavior that was disruptive to other patients in the ward. Many of these postoperative states are transient changes of mood that rapidly clear over a few days. Questionnaire surveys that I carried out (Fenwick 1987; 1989) reveal similar figures for the immediate postoperative 3 months. In the first survey, 19 units replied to the question, "How many temporal lobe epilepsy patients had significant psychiatric complications within 3 months of surgery?" There was a mean of 1.5 patients per unit (10%) with a range of 0–10 patients. In the second questionnaire, 17 units replied; the mean was 1.1 (6%) with a range of 0-4 patients (0–16%). These are overall slightly higher than the figure of 4% given by Blumer, although they are clearly in the same ballpark.

The prevalence of immediate postoperative psychotic states is probably considerably lower, but, again, little hard information is available. The general impression of members at the workshop on temporal lobe surgery held at Palm Springs [54] was that the overall postoperative complication rate is decreasing. The reasons for this are probably multifactorial. Some of the important factors are rejection for surgery of patients with psychiatric illness, presurgery identification of those who are psychiatrically vulnerable, operations on progressively younger populations, and the inclusion in some surgery programs of postoperative psychiatric support and counseling. A new factor that will require evaluation is the modification of the temporal lobe surgical resection procedure. It could be predicted, although this will have to await evaluation, that modified amygdalohippocampectomies with preservation of much of the temporal cortex will lead to fewer cases of psychiatric disturbances.

Long-Term Postoperative Psychiatric Morbidity

Social and Behavioral Variables

Milner [55,56] was one of the first to point out that significant cognitive deficits might follow temporal lobectomy. Hill et al. [48] were among the first to study in detail neuropsychiatric changes following temporal lobectomy. Their paper reported 27 cases. All except one patient were regarded as mentally abnormal before operation. Eighteen had character disorders, three hysteria, three predominantly affective disorders, and two hallucinatory psychosis, mainly paranoid. The cases were studied for 2–5 years after operation. Hill et al. reported a marked reduction in aggressiveness, which they described as "taming" (a partial Klüver-Bucy syndrome). Relatives reported that the patients were less irritable and showed

less impulsive anger. Postictal depression was reported in 12 cases, and in several patients depression was so severe that hospitalization became necessary because of the fear of suicide. Electroconvulsive therapy was given to five patients. The depressive episodes tended to recur up to 18 months after operation, but many patients made a spontaneous recovery. In some patients there was a swing to paranoid, hostile attitudes. Eight of the cases were dominant and four were nondominant lobectomies. This is about the same proportion as in the sample as a whole, and there is thus no evidence that those with right-sided lesions were more susceptible to affective illnesses. There was a change in the intensity, libido, and sexual choice of 14 of the patients. This was in the direction of increased sexual drive and potency. One patient became hypersexual postoperatively, but this resolved with treatment. Two patients lost their perverse sexual tendencies, and one lost his sexual promiscuity. Most cases showed an increase in warmth and friendliness postoperatively, although there were examples of remoteness and rudeness following operation. There was overall a relationship between improvement in psychological status and postoperative freedom from seizures.

Hill [57] felt that surgery should not be recommended for patients with lower than average intelligence, particularly if the operation was to be on the dominant hemisphere. However, Blakemore and Falconer [58] in their series of 86 patients pointed out that postoperative complications a year after surgery did not necessarily lead to a poor outcome, as the brain was plastic and could recover. It is not the purpose of this chapter to detail these cognitive deficits, since they are comprehensively dealt with elsewhere.

The foundation paper, looking at the relationship between clinical, socioeconomic, and psychological changes following temporal lobectomy, was published by Taylor and Falconer [43]. They devised their own rating scale and looked at early development, background social data, and items of social adjustment, including such features as family relationships, leisure activities, sexual performance, work performance, and mental state, together with other variables relating to their epilepsy, IQ, and so on. In the 100 patients studied, 47% showed mesial temporal sclerosis, whereas 62% were largely relieved of their fits. Taylor and Falconer pointed out that the social background of their sample was considerably disturbed. Of the patients in their study, 40% had a family history of mental illness, 27% were separated from at least one parent before the age of 15 years, 45% had experience of life in an institution, and 37% were unemployed preoperatively. The operation was, however, of some overall benefit and produced a simple reduction in seizure frequency. "At follow-up, 51% had good social adjustment, 29% had usefully improved, but 12% had deteriorated. The most consistently good effects were on working ability and interpersonal relationships, rather than on use of leisure or sexual adjustment, and 35% were considered psychiatrically normal at follow-up, compared with 13% prior to operation."

These authors comment that surgery offers the best hope to those patients whose social maladjustment is primarily due to epilepsy. Prognosis was poor in those patients in whom the major problem was not epilepsy, but rather psychosis, low IQ, or a family history of mental illness. In these latter cases seizure relief did not always correlate with social improvement, and this too had been found by Ferguson and Rayport [45].

Davidson et al. [58a] reported nine cases of temporal lobectomies which were carried out in children whose ages ranged from 9 to 16 years. Six were seizure-free and three were much improved. The behavior was much improved in three and improved in six. There was some improvement in educational achievements; one child was able to leave a special school with remedial teaching for a normal school. All the children showed a greater improvement in confidence and social ability. One child with a left-sided lesion who before operation had shown episodes of aggressive rage and murderous assaults on his mother had returned to school, with excellent reports of improved progress and social adjustment: his behavior was described as impeccable.

In a subsequent paper, Davidson and Falconer [59] give the findings on 40 children in two groups of 20. Before operation 19 of the boys were aggressive and many of them were accused of bizarre behavior. "Although none was in trouble with the law, the boys were often involved in gangs and the girls in promiscuous behavior. Many were accused of stealing. Their antisocial behavior usually involved intolerable provocation of schoolmates and teachers. Their tempers were unusually short and some reacted strongly to teasing. Many had formidable reputations as fighters. Our referring colleagues saw their future with foreboding . . ." Five boys in the first group made a good adjustment; but ten did not, and the outcome of the remaining five was between these two extremes. In the second group of 20 patients, many of whom are still adolescents, only three are unemployable and seven are working.

Rausch et al. [60], in a prospective study, looked at preoperative psychosocial functioning and personality factors and postoperative outcome. They used the same scale as Taylor and Falconer, mentioned above, together with the Minnesota Multiphasic Personality Inventory (MMPI). They found that three patients who had normal personality tests preoperatively were rated as having good psychosocial functioning following surgery. Of the seven patients who showed psychopathology preoperatively, three were rated as having good and four as having poor psychosocial functioning postoperatively.

Jensen and Vaernet [1], in a summary paper of their previous work [61–63] reported that 92% of their patients were psychiatrically abnormal preoperatively but that a further 22% became normal following surgery. The majority of these patients had either no seizures or a marked reduction in seizure frequency. Of those who were abnormal preoperatively, 27% were rated as markedly improved and 7% as improved. There was usually, though not always, a clear relationship between psychiatric improvement and a reduction in seizure frequency.

In a review paper, Fraser [64] discusses the functional rehabilitation outcome following epilepsy surgery. He points to difficulties in methodology in that rates of new employment are seldom reported and students and housewives are merged in a category of those actively competing for employment. Consequently it is difficult to assess what true outcome variables are. Augustine et al. [65] followed 32 surgical patients. They were rated 2 years before operation, 1 year postoperatively, 2 years postoperatively, and the latest year postoperatively. The number of patients employed on a full time basis increased from 14 (43%) to 23 (66%). The underemployed decreased from eight (25%) to zero. Those who were unemployed prior to operation (10–31%) remained unemployed (nine postoperatively). There was no difference in seizure reduction between the two groups, thus suggesting that the variables that lead to epilepsy patients being disadvantaged preoperatively, such as severe psychiatric disorders, substance abuse, and disability income, were not altered by the operation [66–68]. There was a significant difference in the side of the lesion among the unemployed. One was dominant, whereas eight were nondominant.

Hermann et al. [68a] studied the relationship between preoperative psychological adjustment and the degree of postoperative seizure reduction in determining both emotional and psychosocial outcome following temporal lobectomy. Ninety-seven patients were studied; 53 became seizure-free and 44 were significantly improved. They showed, on a range of measures, that there was a clear and significant relationship between preoperative and postoperative psychosocial adjustment. They also showed that becoming seizure-free was associated with a markedly improved behavioral/emotional outcome. They did, however, show that freedom from seizures and good presurgical adjustment only accounted for 36% of the variance explaining postoperatively psychosocial adjustment. Thus, 64% of the variance is accounted for by other measures as yet unidentified.

The authors point out that different results may be obtained from different tests, and thus unless centers all use the same tests the differences found between centers may simply reflect differences in their measuring instrument. As an example, they point out that the later age of onset of the epilepsy was associated with an improved psychosocial outcome after surgery on the GHQ (General Health Questionnaire) but not on the MMPI or the WPSI (Washington Psychosocial Seizure Index).

Bladin [68b] has reviewed the results of the Austin Hospital (Melbourne, Australia) Epilepsy program. The author interviewed 107 patients of an original series of 115 patients. The follow-up ranged from 12 months to ten years after operation. 27% of patients had a follow-up of over 5 years. Those patients who lost their seizures did best, and most found employment postoperatively. If seizures continued then employment outcome was bleak. An important point made by the authors relates to what they call "the burden of normality." Some patients who lost their seizures missed their epilepsy; some were resentful that they had not been operated on earlier, while a few more were unable to develop the social graces that were now required by normal psychosocial functioning. In the group that lost their seizures, 39, (46%) reported an improvement in sexual functioning postoperatively. Only 3 (4%) reported worsening sexual functioning. In the group whose seizures were either worse or unimproved there was no improvement in sexual functioning; 2 (20%) were worse.

Psychosis

A serious and major complication of temporal lobe surgery is the development of a long-term schizophreniform psychotic illness, which occurs in clear consciousness and is not related to seizure activity. It is important to know which patients are likely to develop such a psychosis and whether the psychosis is specific to the operative procedure or is part of a spontaneously developing schizophreniform illness. For example, in the Danish series [2] overall 27% suffered from psychosis: 15% were psychotic preoperatively and 12.3% developed a psychosis postoperatively. One (0.9%) patient did, however, lose the psychosis. Stevens [69], reviewing a small series of patients who had had temporal lobectomies at the

University of Oregon, reports a rate of psychosis of 26% before surgery, suggesting that she was dealing with a psychiatrically disadvantaged population, and 45% postoperatively. Three (27%) developed a disabling paranoid psychosis 2–3 years after operation. Taylor [35] reported that 12% of the patients in the first Maudsley temporal lobectomy series had interictal psychoses before surgery, whereas the rate increased to 19% postoperatively. The rate of schizophrenia in the general population is about 1 in 100; thus the mean rate for these three series of 25.3% is significantly elevated. These very high postoperative rates, if reported from other units, would raise serious questions about whether temporal lobe surgery should be continued.

Lower rates are reported by other units. Walker and Blumer [40] give an overall figure of 10%. In a retrospective study, Koch-Weser et al. [70] looked at the risk for serious psychopathology in 25 patients with treated epilepsy, compared with 25 matched presurgical patients. They found the rate of psychosis in the postoperative group to be 8%. Bladin [68b] reports short psychotic episodes in 3 (2.6%) patients [68b] in his series. These seem to have been postictal psychoses as they cleared with treatment. Both the Montreal Neurological Institute and UCLA [71] report considerably lower rates. This may be because many units do not have specialist psychiatric assessment of their patients postoperatively. However, this explanation is inadequate, as it is unlikely that florid psychoses would go undetected. Postoperative psychosis rates will also be lower if patients with psychosis are excluded preoperatively. Differences in follow-up may also be responsible for the higher rates of psychosis.

Sherwin [47] describes seven cases of schizophreniform psychosis diagnosed preoperatively, occurring in 61 patients who underwent temporal lobectomy at UCLA. Of these seven, five were left-sided and two were right-sided lobectomies. Six of the seven cases were seizure-free after more than 5 years follow-up, and the seventh patient had less than four seizures a year. Despite the reduction in seizure frequency, the psychiatric picture did not improve substantially. In two patients the psychiatric features appeared to progress despite the relief of their seizures. The interesting point of this series is the failure of any of the patients to show psychiatric improvement with temporal lobectomy. It is also surprising that over 11% of patients with psychosis should be found when the policy of the unit was deliberately to exclude those with serious mental illness. Males were over-represented among the psychotic patients.

Laterality of the lesion is another variable said to be associated with the genesis of schizophreniform psychosis. Psychosis is said to be associated with dominant-hemisphere temporal lobe foci. However, there is a wide division of opinion in the literature, ranging from the report of Jensen and Larsen [2], who found no association between side of lesion and psychosis; Taylor [35], who found a weak association with left-sided lesions and pathology (mainly alien tissue lesions—hamatomas); to those of Sherwin [47] and Sherwin et al. [72], who showed a clear relationship with left-sided lesions. Some of the possible mechanisms of psychosis have been suggested by Ferguson and Rayport [46], with clinical illustrations from their operated series. Further work is required in this area.

The current view of a number of surgical units is that many of the earlier studies that gave overall rates of postoperative schizophreniform psychosis of 10–40% do not give a true picture, first because fewer patients with psychosis are now admitted to the surgery program and second because patients do not seem to develop psychosis in the numbers previously reported. To gain some objective evidence in the questionnaires circulated to the 52 epilepsy surgical units in 1987 and 1989, referred to above, eleven centers responding to the first questionnaire and 16 responding to the second were asked to "estimate the percentage of patients operated on for TLE who subsequently develop a fixed psychosis." The mean for those units was 0.2% in the first questionnaire, with a range of from 0–3% [44], and 2.5% in the second questionnaire, with a range of 0–33%. However, if the Westmead Unit (which had operated on only three patients, one of whom developed a psychosis) is excluded from the second questionnaire, then the rate is 0.4%, a figure very similar to that of the first survey.

This is considerably below the level expected for the general population and raises the question as to whether there is indeed a close link between temporal lobectomy and the development of postoperative psychoses. This will need to be examined further by appropriate follow-up studies. However, with more rigorous screening before surgery and the limiting of operations to a psychiatrically less disadvantaged group of patients, the link between temporal lobectomy and chronic postoperative schizophreniform psychosis looks less convincing.

Depressive Illness

Depressive illnesses are said to occur commonly in patients after lobectomy, although precise figures are difficult to obtain. Most are short transient episodes that clear rapidly and do not usually last for more than the first three months, although some may go on for a year. Patients with epilepsy are known to have a higher rate of suicide, estimated by Barraclough to be

five times that of the general population: those with temporal lobe epilepsy had a rate 25 times that of the general population [73]. In Taylor's post-temporal lobectomy study [74] there were nine suicides when only 0.2 would have been expected. This showed a rate 45 times higher than would have been expected. A similarly increased figure was found by Jensen and Larsen [2].

Bladin [68b] reports that 5 patients (4.3%) in his series became depressed postoperatively. One of these patients committed suicide; of the others, one attempted suicide, and all four were helped with antidepressant medication. They do, however, report that their most common postoperative finding (in 50% of patients) was an anxiety state. This settled down in the majority of cases. There seemed to be some relationship to a left-sided lobectomy.

Fenwick [44] in two questionnaire studies asked for an estimation of the percentage of patients operated on for TLE who subsequently developed a severe depressive illness. Fourteen units responding to the first questionnaire [44] and 16 responding to the second were asked to "estimate the percentage of patients operated on for TLE who subsequently develop a severe depressive illness." The mean for the first questionnaire was 4.4% per unit, with a range of 0–25%, and 6.1% for the second questionnaire, with a range of 0–20%. It is very surprising that in one unit one fourth of the patients were reported as developing a severe postoperative depressive illness. Fifteen units in the first questionnaire and 17 in the second (with some overlap) were asked to "estimate the percentage of patients operated on for TLE who subsequently commit suicide." In both questionnaires, the mean was 0.15%, which is what might be expected in subgroups of the general population. The range was from 0–2% in the first questionnaire and 0–2.5% in the second, which again is very much lower than that found in earlier studies.

The question of the relationship between laterality and post-lobectomy depression has not been adequately addressed in the literature. It is generally stated by those units that have carried out large numbers of resections that when depressive illnesses occur following surgery they usually do so in those who have nondominant resections. It is, however, difficult to find conclusive data to support this. More work needs to be done in this area.

Reanalysis of Maudsley Data

Bruton [75] has reanalyzed the data from Falconer's 1950–1975 temporal lobectomy series from a neuropathologic standpoint. These results are worth examining in some detail, as this series gives the most detailed account so far of the relationship between pathology and psychosocial outcome. An important caveat, which should be borne in mind, is that the ratings are from the notes and not from patient interviews. In the eyes of some commentators, this significantly reduces the value of this study. Bruton rates the outcome of neurosurgery for 248 patients, measuring the number of their seizure fits and their psychiatric and social status.

Left temporal lobectomies were carried out on 80 males and 47 females, whereas right temporal lobectomies were carried out on 75 males and 46 females. The data for this reanalysis were gathered in the following way. The neuropathologic specimens for each patient were reexamined, and the specimens were allocated to different pathologic groupings. The case notes were reviewed for psychiatric data, and a composite score for social outcome was calculated. The composite contained subscores for social adjustment, sexual adjustment, work adjustment, and schooling. The case notes were also reviewed for frequency of seizures. The patients were allocated to various neuropathologic diagnostic groups. Ammon's horn sclerosis accounted for 107 cases; nonspecific Ammon's horn disease for 41 cases; alien tissue lesions for 38 cases; indefinite lesions for 25 cases; double pathology for 18 cases; inflammatory lesions for eight cases; trauma for seven cases; and developmental lesions for five cases.

Overall the results were as follows. Seizures were improved in 68% of patients and were unaltered or worse in 32% of patients. Personality and adjustment were improved in 48% of patients and unaltered in 52% of patients. There were clear differences in the way that patients with different pathologic lesions responded to surgery, both from the point of view of their fits and their psychosocial functioning. Alien tissue lesions showed the highest rate of improvement—79%. Social functioning was improved in 60%. Those with double pathology showed a 78% improvement in seizure frequency but only a 39% improvement in social outcome. Ammon's horn sclerosis showed a 74% improvement in seizures, with a 60% improvement in social outcome, a figure very similar to that of patients with alien tissue lesions. Inflammatory lesions showed a good outcome for seizures, with 63% improved. However they had a poor social outcome, only 38% being improved and 50% being worse. Where no pathology was found, the outcome was poor for both seizures and social functioning. Seizures were worse in 51% and improved in only 41%. In social functioning, 73% were worse, and there was improvement in only 20%. Those who were described as having indefinite lesions

had the worst outcome of all. Seizures were worse in 66%, and 80% were worse socially.

Thus, in summary, those who had Ammon's horn sclerosis did well, with a significant reduction in seizures and an improvement in psychosocial outcome. Those who had equivocal lesions, inflammatory lesions, lesions of post-traumatic origin, and developmental pathology, and those whose specimens showed no pathology had poor seizure control and were significantly worse psychosocially. Those with alien tissue lesions showed a mixed outcome: those with early onset showed an improvement in their seizures but were worse psychiatrically; in those who had a late onset, seizures were unchanged, and the psychosocial outcome was variable. Many of them died.

Psychoses of Epilepsy

Eighteen patients (6%) were schizophrenic before operation, and 19 patients (7%) were schizophrenic following surgery. Seven became schizophrenic during surgery, whereas six lost their psychoses. The percentage of patients in each pathologic grouping who had schizophrenia and the outcome in these cases were as follows.

Pathology	Pre-operative	Post-operative
No pathology found	10%	12%
Alien tissue	8%	8%
Indefinite	8%	8%
Ammon's horn sclerosis	6%	7%
Double pathology	0%	11%
Developmental lesions (only 5 cases)	20%	0%

Of the nine schizophrenic patients who had hamartomas, four became schizophrenic following operation even though their seizures were improved. The six schizophrenic patients whose psychoses resolved showed no clear relationship with any specific pathology. Thus, hamartomas seem to be clearly related to the onset of schizophrenia following surgery in this series. Of those patients who were unchanged after operation, seven had a left-sided lesion and five had a right-sided lesion. Of those caused by operation, three had left-sided lesions and four had right-sided lesions, whereas of those who were cured by operation, five had left-sided lesions and one had a right-sided lesion. These data would suggest that in those patients already suffering from schizophrenia, the removal of the damaged left temporal lobe in some cases ameliorated the psychosis.

Depression

Before operation, only one person (0.4%) was rated as suffering from a depressive illness. Postoperatively, 24 people (10%) became depressed. Sixteen had left-sided and eight had right-sided lobectomies. Of the 24 depressed subjects, six committed suicide. Five had left-sided lobectomies and one had a right-sided lobectomy. The following shows the percentage of patients with each pathology who developed a postoperative depression and those who committed suicide.

Pathology	Depression	Suicide
No abnormality detected	22%	2%
Double pathology	22%	6%
Indefinite	8%	4%
Ammon's horn sclerosis	7%	2%
Alien tissue	3%	3%

These figures again suggest that there is a relationship between depression, poor social outcome, and failure to control seizures. In this series, there is no clear relationship between right-sided lobectomies and depression or suicide.

The New Maudsley Series

Polkey [4] describes the postoperative results in a series of 40 patients from the Maudsley Hospital. Of his patients, 80% were either seizure-free or had fewer than 10% of their previous number of seizures, whereas 20% were the same or worse. Two patients developed a schizophreniform psychosis postoperatively, and both had nondominant temporal lobectomies. Both showed poor verbal scores, compared with performance scores, on psychometric testing. One patient died in a road traffic accident, and the other's psychosis was said to have improved. By the time the number of patients in the series had reached 125, one more patient had developed a psychosis, bringing the number of patients with psychosis to four, or 3.2% of the total. Factors associated with poor prognosis were similar to those already mentioned above: a right-sided focus with a verbal IQ that was significantly lower than performance IQ and an amobarbital test suggestive of bilateral damage.

With regard to depression, a survey of the case notes was carried out in 96 postoperative patients. Twenty-five patients (26%) had shown depressive symptoms postoperatively. Of these, 18 (72%) had right-sided lobectomies, whereas seven (28%) had left-sided lobectomies. In the nondepressed patients, 42% had right-sided lobectomies and 57% had left-sided lobectomies. There is thus a clear overrepresentation of right-sided lobectomy patients among the depressed group, together with an underrepresentation of left-sided lobectomies. There was a tendency for the depressed patients to have been operated on after the age of 20 years: nondepressed, 43%, and depressed, 67%. The age of onset of epilepsy was not significantly different: 96% in the nondepressed group and 84% in the depressed group had an age of onset younger than 20 years. Type of seizure and pathologic findings made no difference. Eight patients in the series died, all of whom had had right-sided lobectomies. Only one of the deaths was clearly related to a depressive episode; the patient committed suicide by self-poisoning.

Ffytch is carrying out a psychosocial postal questionnaire study of 100 of these postlobectomy patients with more than a 2 year follow-up (in preparation). So far 52 replies have been received. Of these patients, 84% felt the operation was successful and only 4% that it was unsuccessful; 91% were satisfied and 2% dissatisfied; 98% would choose the operation again, and 100% would recommend it to a friend; 75% said they had not been made worse in any way, and 92% said that they had been made better; 62% said that they went out more frequently postoperatively, while only 7% said they did not. Forty-one percent enjoyed their social life more postoperatively, only 4% said they enjoyed it less; 55% said they spent more time on their hobbies than previously; 49% said that their sexual interest had increased since the operation and 62% were now satisfied with their sex life. However, only 42% had a girl or boyfriend. Forty-three percent said they got along better with their family and friends after the operation; 10% got along worse.

The Oxford Series

The Oxford series consisted of 111 operated patients. All had enbloc resections, 68 of which were right-sided and 43 of which were left-sided lobectomies. The series contained a large number of young patients; 45 were under the age of 16 years [76]. This series shows a surprisingly low rate of postoperative psychoses compared with the first Maudsley series and even compared with the second. Only one patient in the Oxford series was diagnosed as suffering from schizophrenia before operation. She had a left-sided temporal lobectomy, and the diagnosis was an indolent glioma. She became seizure-free, but her psychosis remained unchanged. She committed suicide within 2 years. None developed a schizophreniform psychosis postoperatively.

The absence of psychosis requires explanation. A possible factor is the age of the children. Some of these children may yet go on to develop a psychosis when they reach late adolescence, but it is not possible to know whether they might have done so without surgery. A second factor is the referral pattern. Although these patients come from all over the country, they are mainly neurologic referrals, whereas the Maudsley series included many psychiatric patients who are possibly more at risk of developing a psychosis. (See above for the factors that influence the development of psychiatric morbidity and psychosis.)

Six patients were diagnosed preoperatively as having personality disorders. Of the two left-sided lobectomy patients, one had an indolent glioma and one had Ammon's horn sclerosis. Both became seizure-free, but their personality remained unchanged. Of the four patients with right-sided lobectomies, the pathology was Ammon's horn sclerosis in two and indolent glioma in two. Two became seizure-free and two had less than 10% of their previous seizures. Their personalities remained unchanged.

One patient with a right-sided lobectomy became psychopathic after surgery, although her seizures had been reduced to less than 10%. Her epilepsy was due to a scar on the right temporal lobe following trauma. Another patient was diagnosed preoperatively and postoperatively as suffering from acute anxiety, despite a right temporal lobectomy for a glioma that left him seizure-free. A preoperatively depressed patient remained depressed after a successful right-sided lobectomy for Ammon's horn sclerosis.

Two children were maladjusted preoperatively and postoperatively. Both had left-sided lobectomies, one for a glioma and one for Ammon's horn sclerosis. In both cases, seizures were reduced to less than 10%.

Passingham is carrying out a psychosocial postal questionnaire study of 86 of these post-lobectomy patients with more than a 2 year follow-up (in preparation). So far 61 replies (71%) have been received. 70% of patients felt the operation was successful and only 5% felt that it was unsuccessful; 87% were satisfied and 6% dissatisfied; 90% would choose the operation again, and 90% would recommend it to a friend; 67% said they had not been made worse in any way, and 95% said that they had been made better. Fifty-eight percent said that they went out more frequently post-operatively, while 20% said they did not; 58% said they spent more time on their hobbies than previously. Fifty-three percent said that their sexual interest had increased since the operation and 46% were now satisfied with their sex life; 49% had a girlfriend or boyfriend; 43% said they got along better with their family and friends after the operation; 16% got along worse.

In summary, the Oxford series shows very few psychoses but some personality disorders, which remain unchanged after operation. On balance, the results of psychosocial questionnaires in both the new Maudsley and the Oxford series indicate that the operation is highly successful and clearly brings both epileptic and psychosocial improvement.

Prevalence of Psychiatric Assessment

Fifty-two different units throughout the world are carrying out epilepsy surgery. Some are in academically isolated centers, while others have only recently begun their programs. The standard of psychiatric assessment in different units and the psychiatric facilities available for such assessment therefore vary widely. In some units each patient is assessed before entering the epilepsy program, and psychiatric assessments are carried out at varying intervals before and after surgery. In others, psychiatric assessment is used only for crisis intervention. However, in the majority, no psychiatric opinion is sought at any point.

Standardization of Assessment

Among those units where psychiatric assessment is carried out, a very wide range of protocols is used. Few units give their figures for psychiatric diagnoses using the standard international classifications. One view is that it is inappropriate to use either diagnostic systems or assessment protocols that have been developed for psychiatric patients without brain damage or epilepsy. Unless the features of an organic psychosyndrome can be quantified and reported, descriptive terminology is probably more helpful. For example, descriptive statements are much more valuable in assessing psychiatric symptomatology in children or brain-damaged patients than are the results of rating scales that have been developed for and standardized on non–brain-damaged adult populations. An alternative view is that although standardized mental state and psychiatric assessment protocols may not have been specifically developed for patients with organic psychiatric syndromes, they are the best available at present and are valuable in psychiatric assessment.

At the Palm Springs workshop [54] the conclusion was that cross-center consultation should be carried out so that some degree of standardization in psychiatric assessment could be achieved. This could probably be most easily achieved by agreeing on a standardized assessment protocol. Diagnosis should always be given in one of the international diagnostic classifications that are widely used at present. The North Americans were more in favor of the *DSM 3* whereas the Europeans tended toward the *ICD 9* (now ICD 10). Other rating instruments that could be considered were the Washington Psycho-Social Inventory of Dodrill, the MMPI, the Present State Examination (PSE), the Hamilton and Beck, Neppe's Temporal Lobe Symptom Profile, and so on. In addition, some units had developed their own protocols and symptom-rating procedures. It was clear that, ideally, one single system should eventually be adopted.

The conclusions of the psychiatric workshop at the Palm Springs meeting were as follows [44]:

1. At present, psychiatric investigation of patients in epilepsy surgery programs leaves much to be desired.
2. Ideally, every program undertaking epilepsy surgery, and especially temporal lobe surgery, should offer full psychiatric assessment for every patient both preoperatively and postoperatively.
3. This should, if possible, be carried out in a standardized form to make comparison among centers both possible and meaningful.
4. Centers with epilepsy programs should be invited to help design and use a standardized assessment.
5. Every patient coming to surgery should have a psychiatric diagnosis using one of the international, generally accepted, psychiatric diagnostic classifying systems, such as *ICD 9* (now *ICD 10*) or *DSM 3* (now *DSM3-R*).
6. There should be a rigorous definition of the psychiatric morbidity of the population who come to be accepted into a surgical epilepsy program. Differences in the initial population could significantly affect outcome in many ways.
7. Standardized assessment schedules in many cases were unsuitable to describe patients with epilepsy who also had associated brain damage. It is thus necessary to describe the abnormal behavior as well as to use standard rating scales.
8. Detailed psychiatric assessment was required after surgery so that the prevalence and nature of postoperative psychiatric morbidity could be recorded. The first postoperative assessment should be at 3 months, then at 6 months, and finally yearly.
9. There are few, if any, purely psychiatric considerations for surgery (see above).
10. Patients with postictal psychiatric episodes, or behavioral changes, would benefit from surgery.
11. Brain damage, low IQ, and memory impairment were all seen as contraindications to surgery (see above).
12. Some patients with psychiatric illness required extensive rehabilitation and supportive programs, together with counseling, before and after surgery. Such patients should not be admitted into the program until support is available.
13. Many centers have either covert or overt exclusion policies for patients with psychiatric illness. It is important that each center make its policy clear, so that outcome figures with regard to psychiatric morbidity can be accurately assessed in the light of detailed figures concerning the range and rate of psychiatric illness before operation.

There is thus a need to determine the exact rates of psychiatric morbidity in the patient populations from whom the candidates for temporal lobectomy are drawn, in those who undergo temporal lobe surgery, and in those who have had the operation.

Census of Psychiatric Availability

Two questionnaires have been circulated worldwide to all centers carrying out temporal lobe surgery in order to determine the exact range of psychiatric facilities available and the range of psychiatric morbidity. The first was circulated in 1987 (with 273 patients reported on) and the second in 1989 (with 268 patients reported on). The results were essentially the same for both series, showing little had changed between 1987 and 1989. Asked whether any patients were psychiatrically assessed before epilepsy surgery, 87% said yes. This rate is surprisingly high, but it must be remembered that most of the units that replied were from the West and were well established. Following surgery, just under half (42%) were assessed. Clearly there is a need for further psychiatric assessment after surgery.

Psychiatric diagnosis is important, and using an international classification system should be standard practice in all units. However, although 73% of the units who replied said they used a psychiatric assessment protocol, only 44% used *DSM 3* or *ICD 9* for psychiatric diagnosis. All units said that, provided psychiatric expertise was available, they would be willing to use a standardized psychiatric assessment. The Europeans tended to prefer *ICD 9* and the Americans *DSM 3*.

Suggested Psychiatric Assessment

It is clear that some units have access to psychiatric expertise, whereas some do not. Thus, two different protocols for psychiatric assessment will be required. It should be stated straight away that it is preferable for psychiatric assessment to be carried out by trained psychiatrists. Dr. Ferguson and I have put together a protocol (which has yet to be agreed on) to be used by those units without a psychiatrist. A copy can be obtained from the author. Associated with this are two questionnaires that take 10–15 minutes to rate and could be rated by neurosurgeons. The first one is the psychotic symptom questionnaire, which produces scales relating to hypomania, delusions, thought disorder and interference, and hallucinations. The second is the clinical information schedule of Goldberg, which extracts neurotic symptoms relating to depression, anxiety, phobias, obsessions and compulsions, and depersonalization. It also has scales that measure somatic symptoms: fatigue, sleep disturbance, irritability, and lack of concentration. Although these questionnaires are not standardized for patient populations with brain damage, they are nevertheless reliable.

It is essential that patients should be psychiatrically assessed preoperatively and then at regular intervals postoperatively. It was suggested at the outcome symposium held at the Palm Springs workshop [54] that assessment three times a year in the first postoperative year, and then at longer intervals in the second and subsequent years, would be appropriate.

One area of assessment that was given considerable attention in the 1950s, but much less recently, is sexual behavior and functioning. Assessment of sexuality should be detailed. Indications of sexual functioning, such as frequency of sexual thoughts and orgasms, fertility, and, in males, potency, should all be measured. Hormonal profiles and, in males, measurement of nocturnal penile tumescence give an objective measure of sexual functioning and should also be included [76–78, 40].

Conclusion

Temporal lobectomy has now been carried out for more than 50 years. The early investigators were concerned with the effect of the operation on personality and the psychiatric consequences of removing a significant volume of the temporal lobe. The concepts then used were derived from bilateral ablation of the temporal lobes in monkeys, which had led to the Klüver-Bucy syndrome. It became clear that in some cases a psychiatric penalty was exacted by the operation. High rates of psychosis occurred, together with some minor increase in personality disorders. However, there was clear evidence that both social functioning and aggressive behavior improved if sei-

zure frequency declined. Seizure frequency and improvement then became the main target of research studies, and, for a period in the 1970s, almost no research papers were published looking in detail at psychiatric variables. The recent publication of a re-analysis of the first Maudsley series [75] stresses the importance of pathology in both seizure and psychiatric outcome. The value of looking at results according to pathology rather than only according to seizure frequency has continually been stressed by the Oxford group. Evidence from the recent questionnaire study suggests that the high rates of psychiatric morbidity found by the original investigators do not occur today, although the reason for this is not yet apparent. One possibility is the difference in the psychiatric morbidity of input populations, since the operation is no longer seen as a last-resort method of treatment, and the operation itself has been modified so that less brain is removed. An additional factor is the improvement in preoperative diagnosis so that only appropriate cases are operated on.

We are now entering a new era in which the relevant variables related to psychiatric outcome have been defined. Thus there is the opportunity for further detailed studies. More information is required concerning the rates of psychiatric morbidity in patients undergoing temporal lobectomy and in its occurrence postoperatively. Until this is known, we cannot be sure whether there are special subgroups of patients with temporal lobe epilepsy who are specifically at risk for the development of psychiatric illness postoperatively. There is now growing evidence that the type of pathology affects not only seizure outcome but also psychiatric and psychosocial outcome. If the patients at risk can be identified, clearly much can be done in the preoperative and postoperative periods to support and help them.

References

1. Jensen I, Vaernet K. Temporal lobe epilepsy. Follow up investigation of 74 temporal lobe resected patients. *Acta Neurosurg* 1977;37:173–200.
2. Jensen I, Larsen K. Mental aspects of temporal lobe epilepsy. *J Neurol Neurosurg Psychiatry* 1979;42:256–65.
3. Rausch R, Crandall PH. Psychological status related to surgical control of temporal lobe seizures. *Epilepsia* 1982;23:191–202.
4. Polkey C. Effects of anterior temporal lobectomy apart from the relief of seizures: a study of 40 patients. *J R Soc Med* 1983;76:354–8.
5. Lindsay J, Ounsted C, Richards P. Long-term outcome in children with temporal lobe seizures. 5. Indications and contraindications for neurosurgery. *Dev Med Child Neurol* 1984;26:25–32.

6. Gudmundsson G. Epilepsy in Iceland: a clinical and epidemiological investigation. *Acta Neurol Scand* 1966;23(Suppl 25):100–14.

7. Helgason T. Epidemiology of mental disorders in Iceland. *Acta Psychiatr Scand* 1964;40:Suppl 173:1.

8. Pond D, Bidwell B. A survey of epilepsy in 14 general practices. II. Social and psychological aspects. *Epilepsia* 1960;1:285–99.

9. Rutter M, Graham P, Yule W. A neuropsychiatric study in childhood. *Clinics in Developmental Medicine* 1970; Nos. 35/36.

10. Britten N, Wadsworth M, Fenwick P. Stigma in patients with early epilepsy: a national longitudinal study. *J Epidemiol Community Health* 1984;38:291–5.

11. Adams C, Beardsworth E, Oxbury S, Oxbury J, Fenwick P. Temporal lobectomy in 44 children: outcome and neuropsychological follow up. *J Epilepsy* 1990; 3(Suppl):157–68.

12. Rodin EA, Katz M, Lennox K. Differences between patients with temporal lobe seizures and those with other forms of epileptic attacks. *Epilepsia* 1976; 17:313–20.

13. Lindsay J, Ounstead C, Richards P. Long-term outcome in children with temporal lobe seizures. 3. Psychiatric aspects in childhood and adult life. *Dev Med Child Neurol* 1979;21:630–6.

14. Currie S, Heathfield W, Henson R, Scott D. Clinical course and prognosis of temporal lobe epilepsy: a survey of 666 patients. *Brain* 1971;94:173–90.

14a. Robertson MM, Trimble MR. Depressive illness in patients with epilepsy: a review. *Epilepsia* 1983; 24(suppl 2):S109–16.

14b. Hermann BP, Whitman S. Behavioral and personality correlates of epilepsy: a review, methodological critique, and conceptual model. *Psychol Bull* 1984; 95:451–97.

14c. Robertson MM, Trimble MR, Townsend HRA. Phenomenology of depression in epilepsy. *Epilepsia* 1987;28:364–72.

14d. Hermann BP, Wyler AR. Depression, locus of control, and the effects of epilepsy surgery. *Epilepsia* 1989;30(3):332–38.

14e. Mendez MF, Cummings JL, Benson DF. Depression in epilepsy: significance and phenomenology. *Arch Neurol* 1986;43:766–70.

14f. Benassi VA, Sweeney PD, Dufour CL. Is there a relation between locus of control orientation and depression? *J Abnorm Psychol* 1988;97:357–67.

15. Trimble M, Perez M. The phenomenology of the chronic psychoses of epilepsy. *Advances in Biology and Psychiatry* 1980;8:98–105.

16. Betts TA, Merskey H, Pond DA. In: Laidlaw J, Richens A, eds. *A Textbook of Epilepsy*. Psychiatry. Edinburgh: Churchill Livingstone, 1976.

17. Tizard B. The personality of epileptics: a discussion of the evidence. *Psychol Bull* 1962;59:196–210.

18. Lishman WA. *Organic psychiatry*. London: Blackwell Scientific Publications, 1978.

19. Scott D. Psychiatric aspects of epilepsy. *Br J Psychiatry* 1978;132:417–30.

20. Gibbs FA. Ictal and non-ictal psychiatric disorders in temporal lobe epilepsy. *J Nerv Ment Dis* 1951; 113:522–8.

21. Gastaut H, Collomb H. Etude du comportement sexuel chez les epileptiques psychomoteurs. *Ann Med Psychol* 1954;2:657–96.

22. Waxman SG, Geschwind N. The interictal behavior syndrome of temporal lobe epilepsy. *Arch Gen Psychiatry* 1975;32:1580–6.

23. Geschwind N. Behavioral changes in temporal lobe epilepsy. *Psychol Med* 1979;9:217–9.

24. Bear D. Temporal lobe epilepsy—a syndrome of sensory-limbic hypoconnection. *Cortex* 1979;15: 357–84.

25. Bear D, Fedio P. Quantitative analysis of inter-ictal behavior in temporal lobe epilepsy. *Arch Neurol* 1977;34(8):454–67.

26. Kluver H, Bucy P. Preliminary analysis of functions of the temporal lobe in man. *Arch Neurol Psychiatry* 1939;42:979–1000.

27. Hermann BP, Riel P. Interictal personality and behavioral traits in temporal lobe and generalized epilepsy. *Cortex* 1981;17:125–8.

28. Mungus D. Interictal behavior abnormality in temporal lobe epilepsy. *Arch Gen Psychiatry* 1982;39:108–11.

29. Bear D, Levin K, Bloomer D, Chetham D, Ryder J. Interictal behavior in hospitalized temporal lobe epileptics: relationship to idiopathic psychiatric syndromes. *J Neurol Neurosurg Psychiatry* 1982;45:481–8.

30. Sensky T, Fenwick P. Religiosity, mystical experience and epilepsy. In: Rose FC, ed. *Progress in epilepsy*. London: Pitmans, 1982;214–220.

31. Stevens JR, Hermann BP. Temporal lobe epilepsy. Psychopathology and violence: the state of the evidence. *Neurology* 1981;31·1127 32.

32. Lennox W. Brain injury, drugs and environment as causes of mental decay in epilepsy. *Am J Psychiatry* 1942;99:174–80.

33. Lennox W, Lennox M. *Epilepsy and related disorders*. Vols 1 and 2. Boston: Little, Brown, 1960.

34. Reitan R. Psychological testing of epileptic patients. In: Vinken P, Bruyn G, eds. *Handbook of clinical neurology*. Amsterdam, 1976; Chapter 30.

35. Taylor DC. Mental state and temporal lobe epilepsy. *Epilepsia* 1972;13:727–65.

36. Taylor D. Brain lesions, surgery, seizures, and mental symptoms. In: Reynolds E, Trimble M, eds. *Epilepsy and Psychiatry*. Edinburgh: Churchill Livingstone, 1981: 227–41, 1981.

37. Taylor DC. Psychological aspects of chronic sickness. In: Rutter M, Herslov L, eds. *Child and adolescent psychiatry: modern approaches*.

38. Stores G. Schoolchildren with epilepsy at risk for learning and behaviour problems. *Dev Med Child Neurol* 1978;20:502–8.

39. Hartledge LD, Green JB. The relationship of parental attitudes to academic and social achievement in epileptic children. *Epilepsia* 1972;13:21–6.

40. Walker AE, Blumer D. Behavioral effects of temporal lobectomy for temporal lobe epilepsy. In: Blumer D,

ed. *Psychiatric Aspects of Epilepsy.* Washington, DC: American Psychiatry Press, 1985.

41. Ferguson SM, Rayport M, Couie W. Neuropsychiatric observations on behavioural consequences of corpus callosum section for seizure control. In: Reeves A, ed. *Epilepsy and the corpus callosum.* New York: Plenum Press, 1985;501–14.

42. Ferguson SM, Rayport M, Couie W. Brain correlates of aggressive behavior in temporal lobe epilepsy. In: Doane B, Livingstone D, eds. *The limbic system: functional organization and clinical disorder.* New York: Raven Press, 1986:183–93.

43. Taylor DC, Falconer MA. Clinical, socioeconomic and psychological changes after temporal lobectomy for epilepsy. *Br J Psychiatry* 1968;114:1247–61.

44. Fenwick PBC. Postscript: what should be included in a standard psychiatric assessment? In: Engel J, ed: *Surgical treatment of the epilepsies.* New York: Raven Press, 1987:505–10.

45. Ferguson SM, Rayport M. The adjustment to living without epilepsy. *J Nerv Ment Dis* 1965;140:26–37.

46. Ferguson SM, Rayport M. Psychosis in epilepsy. In: Blumer D, ed. *Psychiatric aspects of epilepsy.* Washington, DC: American Psychiatry Press, 1985;229–71.

47. Sherwin I. Psychosis associated with epilepsy: significance of the laterality of the epileptogenic lesion. *J Neurol Neurosurg Psychiatry* 1981;44:83–5.

48. Hill JD, Pond DA, Mitchell W, Falconer MA. Personality changes following temporal lobectomy for epilepsy. *J Ment Sci* 1957;103:18–27.

49. Green JR, Steelman HF, Duisberg RE, McGrath WB, Wick SH. Behavioral changes following radical temporal excision in the treatment of focal epilepsy. *Res Publ Assoc Nerv Ment Dis* 1958;36:295–315.

50. James IP. Temporal lobectomy for psychomotor epilepsy. *J Ment Sci* 1960;106:543–58.

51. Taylor DC. Ontogenesis of chronic epileptic psychoses: a reanalysis. *Psychol Med* 1971;1:274–53.

52. Serafetidines EA, Falconer MA. The effects of temporal lobectomy on patients with psychosis. *J Ment Sci* 1962;108:584–93.

53. Taylor DC, Marsh SM. The influence of sex and sides of operation on personality questionnaire responses after temporal lobectomy. In: Gruzelier J, Flor-Henry P, eds. *Hemisphere asymmetries of function in psychopathology.* Development and psychiatry. New York: Elsevier, 1979:391–400.

53a. Mihara T, et al. Surgical treatment of epilepsy in the comprehensive care program: advantages and considerations. *Jpn J Psychiatr Neurol* 1990 44:275–281.

54. Engel J, ed. *Surgical treatment of the epilepsies.* New York: Raven Press, 1987.

55. Milner B. Intellectual function of the temporal lobes. *Psychol Bull* 1954;51:42–62.

56. Milner B. Psychological defects produced by temporal lobe excision. *Res Publ Assoc Nerv Ment Dis* 1958; 36:244–57.

57. Hill D. Indications and contraindications to temporal lobectomy. *Proc R Soc Med* 1958;51:610–3.

58. Blakemore C, Falconer M. Long-term effects of anterior temporal lobectomy on certain cognitive functions. *J Neurol Neurosurg Psychiatry* 1967;30:364–7.

58a. Davidson S, Falconer M, Stroud C. The place of surgery in the treatment of epilepsy in childhood and adolescence. A preliminary report in 13 cases. *Dev Med Child Neurol* 1972;14:796–803.

59. Davidson S, Falconer M. Outcome of surgery in 40 children with temporal lobe epilepsy. *Lancet* 1975; 1:1260–3.

60. Rausch R, McCreary C, Crandall PH. Predictions of psychological functioning following successful surgical treatment of epilepsy. *J Psychosom Res* 1977;21: 141–6.

61. Jensen I. Temporal lobe epilepsy. Aetiological factors and surgical results. *Acta Neurol Scand* 1976;53:103–18.

62. Jensen I. Temporal lobe epilepsy. Type of seizures, age and surgical results. *Acta Neurol Scand* 1976;53: 335–57.

63. Jensen I. Temporal lobe epilepsy. Social conditions and rehabilitation after surgery. *Acta Neurol Scand* 1976; 54:22–44.

64. Fraser RT. Improving functional rehabilitation outcome following epilepsy surgery. *Acta Neurol Scand* 1988;78(Suppl 117):122–8.

65. Augustine EA et al. Occupational adjustment following neurosurgical treatment of epilepsy. *Ann Neurol* 1984;15:68–72.

66. Crandall PH. Postoperative management and criteria for evaluation. In: Purpura D et al. Eds.: *Advances in Neurology.* New York: Raven Press, 1975:265–79.

67. Hurley et al. Life events and emotional status in the first year following temporal lobe resection. Presented at the 15th International Epilepsy Symposium, Washington DC, September 27th, 1983.

68. Dennrell RD et al. *Neurological, psychological and social factors related to the employment of persons with epilepsy.* Michigan Epilepsy Center, 1965.

68a. Hermann BP, Wyler AR, Somes G. Preoperative psychological adjustment and surgical outcome and determinants of psychosocial status after anterior temporal lobectomy. *J Neurol Neurosurg and Psychiatr* 1992; 55:491–96.

68b. Bladin PF. Psychosocial difficulties and outcome after temporal lobectomy. *Epilepsia* 1991.

69. Stevens J. Biological background of psychosis in epilepsy. In: Canger R, Angeleri F, Penry JK, eds. *Advances in epileptology: XIth epilepsy international symposium.* New York: Raven Press, 1980:167–72.

70. Koch-Weser M, Garron DC, Gilley DW, Bergen D, Bleck TP, Morrell F, Ristanovic R, Whisler WW. Prevalence of psychological disorders after surgical treatment of seizures. *Arch Neurol* 1988;45:1308–11.

71. Anderman F and Engel J: Personal communication.

72. Sherwin I, Person-Magnan P, Bancaud J, et al. Prevalence of psychosis in epilepsy as a function of the laterality of the epileptogenic lesion. *Arch Neurol* 1982;39:621–5.

73. Barraclough B. Suicide and epilepsy. In: Reynolds E et al., eds. *Epilepsy and Psychiatry*. New York: Churchill Livingstone, 1980:72–6.

74. Taylor DC, Marsh SM. Implications of long-term follow-up studies in epilepsy: with a note on the cause of death. In: Penry JK, ed. *Epilepsy: the VIIIth international symposium* New York: Raven Press, 1977:27–34.

75. Bruton CJ. *The Neuropathology of Temporal Lobe Epilepsy*. New York: Oxford University Press, 1988.

76. Fenwick PBC, Toone BK, Wheeler MJ, Nanjee MN, Grant R, Brown D. Sexual behavior in a centre for epilepsy. *Acta Scand Neurol* 1985;71:428–35.

77. Fenwick P, Mercer S, Grant R, Wheeler M, Nanjee N, Toone B. The relationship of nocturnal penile tumescence and serum testosterone levels in patients with epilepsy. *Arch Sex Behav* 1986;15:13–21.

78. Toone B, Garralda M, Ron M. The psychosis of epilepsy and the functional psychoses. A clinical and phenomenological comparison. *Br J Psychiatry* 1982;141:256–61.

Chapter 21
Vocational Outcome

ROBERT T. FRASER
CARL B. DODRILL

As national interest increases in the benefits of the surgical treatment of epilepsy, a growing area of concern is whether the operation has a significant benefit on the occupational lives of patients. This chapter reviews the existing literature on vocational outcome following epilepsy surgery, overviews recent research data from a comprehensive study at the University of Washington Regional Epilepsy Center, and suggests steps toward improving vocational and other functional outcome for patients undergoing the operation.

This chapter concerns itself principally with changes in competitive vocational functioning. Explicitly, as a function of the operation, are the patients actually better able to work on a competitive remunerative basis within the labor market? It is important to maintain this perspective because this is often not the perspective that is maintained in a number of studies within existing research. It can be helpful to document subtle work-related changes, but an emphasis of our research should be focused on whether the surgery and encompassing psychosocial intervention are really making a change in patients' ability to financially support themselves within the local labor market. It is only by clarifying what actually occurs around the surgical intervention that we can better formulate rehabilitation programs and plan interventions that will better complement the increasing effectiveness of the surgical operation on a client's medical functioning (see Chapter 18).

Literature Review

A number of studies have assessed vocational relevance of epilepsy surgery using a diverse number of outcome measures [1–13]. Review of these studies indicates a number of consistent difficulties in attempting to assess whether surgery has made a significant functional difference. These issues include the following:

1. Younger patients (who are often students) are grouped with older patients, and it is difficult to assess whether vocational changes are a function of the intervention or simply occur within the course of social maturation.
2. Working criteria do not always relate to paid competitive employment and include homemaker categories, sheltered work activity, and other subjective ratings of employment functioning.

A review of these studies suggests that the work by Augustine et al. [1] may present an accurate picture of what generally occurs. This 1984 study followed 32 surgical patients at four status points: 2 years before the operation, 1 year postsurgery, 2 years postsurgery, and the latest year postsurgery follow-up available. While the number of patients employed on a full-time basis increased from 14 to 23, the number underemployed decreased from eight to zero. Unemployment, however, remained basically constant. Vocational gains were made, therefore, chiefly by the underemployed. Patients did not progress vocationally unless they had some vocational involvement prior to the surgery.

In this study, there were no significant differences in seizure-related variables (seizure reduction, use and serum levels of anticonvulsant drugs, or medication compliance) in employed or unemployed groups. As compared with the employed, however, the unemployed group appeared to have significantly more nondominant side resections (Chi-square significant,

The preparation of this chapter and a portion of the reported research was supported by grants 24823 and NS 17111 awarded by the National Institute of Neurological Disorders and Stroke, DHS/DHHS, USA.

$p < .01$). Although similar to the employed group on verbal intelligence quotient (IQ) scores, the unemployed group evidenced a "dull normal" performance IQ compared with an average performance IQ for the employed group. This unemployed group had consistent performance IQ deficits both before and after the operation. Although a relatively small sample size ($n = 9$), the unemployed group had a significantly higher number of moderate to severe psychiatric disorders, legal difficulties/substance abuse histories, and a preoperative history of disability income (all Chisquare significant, $p < .01$).

There is also a consistent trend in the literature that improvement in psychosocial functioning to include occupational activity can be limited to individuals who become essentially seizure-free [7,9]. Although not congruent with the findings of Augustine et al. [1], work at our center by Hale et al. [13] supports the value of seizure-free status on vocational functioning. This study involved 54 surgery patients (44 temporal lobe and 10 other surgical sites). Table 21-1 reviews preoperative and postoperative groups by seizure status. It is apparent that only the seizure-free group achieved a significant gain within the vocational functioning category. It is of interest, however, that 2 years postsurgery there appeared to be no significant change relative to independent living. Since these study participants averaged 28 years of age, it may be particularly difficult to alter established dependent behaviors.

Other studies at our center [4] showed basically no significant employment gains from presurgery to

postsurgery for a group of 51 temporal lobe resection patients (27 right temporal lobe and 24 left temporal lobe). This study, however, did not control for seizure status, specifically the seizure-free category. These patients were interviewed 1–4 years postsurgery.

In sum, the available research suggests that epilepsy surgery is not making a significant contribution to employment functioning except for those patients who are on the employment track prior to surgery, albeit underemployed, and those achieving a seizure-free status. It is also probable that psychiatric functioning, receipt of financial subsidy, and below-average cognitive functioning—particularly in the motoric and visual/spatial abilities areas—also influence employment outcome. Patients with fewer concerns in these areas are better able to mobilize their resources.

Horowitz and Cohen [14] and Horowitz et al. [5] indicate some of the more subtle concerns that are more difficult to document. Following dramatic seizure improvement or relief, some patients can be undergoing dramatic identity reformulations, which interfere with the ability to focus on a work transition. Other difficulties include a preexisting inadequate personality or inadequate personality secondary to the early onset of a more severe type of seizure disorder, and retarded rates of development or maturation secondary to the disability. In order to document the effects of these types of variables, we need to embark on more comprehensive and discreet evaluation prior to surgery. It is important to better clarify

Table 21-1. Comparison of Psychosocial Functioning Preoperatively and Two Years Postoperatively*

Variable	Before Surgery		After Surgery		
	Mean	SD†	Mean	SD	t
Seizure-free					
Vocational status	2.45	.80	2.73	.63	−2.10‡
Independent living	1.45	.91	1.50	.91	−1.00
Overall	3.95	1.46	4.23	1.38	−2.28‡
Significantly Improved					
Vocational status	1.43	1.28	1.14	1.29	.76
Independent living	.78	.97	.86	1.03	−1.00
Overall	2.21	2.01	1.86	1.75	.94
Not Significantly Improved					
Vocational status	1.33	1.19	1.44	1.20	−0.58
Independent living	1.28	.96	1.39	.92	−0.74
Overall	2.61	1.54	2.83	1.76	−0.96

*Coding Note:
  Vocational status: 0 = unemployed; 1 = token employment; 2 = part-time employment; 3 = full-time employment.
  Independent living: 0 = fully dependent; 1 = semi-independent; 2 = independent.
  Overall functioning score combines the vocational status and independent living scores.
†SD = standard deviation.
‡ $p < .05$.

the role played by obvious and more subtle variables in movement toward work and a greater range of functional life activity. Without careful documentation of these variables, it is more difficult to develop timely and effective interventions.

Current Research at the University of Washington Epilepsy Center

A comprehensive effort is currently being made at our center to examine the effects of epilepsy surgery at 5 and 10 years postoperation with the inclusion of matched controls. For our purposes, we review only the available vocational data. Homemakers were excluded from the study because it is difficult to assess the support that they receive within the home or their actual functional level.

Table 21-2 reviews comparative vocational data at 5-year follow-up between surgical patients and matched controls. Controls were patients with intractable partial seizures who were being medically managed on anticonvulsants. There were 39 surgical patients and 24 controls. For the surgical group, 21 patients were working before and after the surgery, whereas 11 patients were not working either presurgery or postsurgery. Fifteen of the people that were working presurgery and postsurgery indicated improved functioning on the job, whereas six indicated that their employment functioning was about the same. Among the controls, only six were working presurgery and postsurgery, and five of the six indi-

cated improved functioning during this period of time. Numbers in the other vocational categories are very small. It is of interest that in the surgical group, however, three individuals were working after surgery but not before. Ratings of employment functioning were scored as follows: 1 = decreased functioning, 2 = functioning the same, or 3 = functioning improved. These ratings were related to the consistency of their competitive employment, salary increases, more responsible job tasks, a greater range of tasks, or actual job promotions.

In Table 21-2, student transition to work was examined separately. There were only two students in the surgical group, one going to full-time work and one going to full-time subsidy. The control group, however, appeared to be doing reasonably well, with only two of the nine in a sheltered work category at 5 years after initial evaluation. The other seven students were either working or continuing within a school program.

Table 21-3 reviews findings on 17 surgical patients 10 years postsurgery and on 24 matched controls. Of four surgical patients working before and after surgery, all four indicated improved employment functioning on the job. Of seven individuals who did not work before and after the surgery, four indicated the same employment functioning, whereas three indicated reduced employment potential.

Among the 10-year controls, although seven were working before and 10 years after initial evaluation, their perception of their employment functioning was not as positive as that of the surgical group. Only two

Table 21-2. Five-year Follow-up

	Surgical Patients Work Status: Before and After Surgery				Controls Before and After Initial Evaluation			
		Vocational Functioning Level*				Vocational Functioning Level*		
	No.	1	2	3	No.	1	2	3
Working before and after	21		6	15	6		1	5
Not working before and after	11	1	9	1	5		4	1
Working before/not after	4	3		1	3	2		1
Working after/not before	3			3	1		1	
	39	4	15	20	15	2	6	7
		Student status:† One working full-time, one on government subsidy				Student status:† Four working full-time, one working part-time, two in marginal/sheltered work, two in continuing school programs		

*Coding Note:

　　Vocational functioning level: 1 = work functioning has deteriorated; 2 = work functioning is the same; 3 = work functioning has improved.

†Student status relates to follow-up of individuals who were students at the time of surgery or initial clinic evaluation.

Table 21-3. Ten-year Follow-up

| | Surgical Patients Work Status: Before and After Surgery | | | | Controls Before and After Initial Evaluation | | | |
| | Vocational Functioning Level* | | | | Vocational Functioning Level* | | | |
	No.	1	2	3	No.	1	2	3
Working before and after	4			4	7	2	3	2
Not working before and after	7	3	4		8	1	7	
Working before/not after					3	2	1	
Working after/not before					1	1		
	11	3	4	4	19	5	12	2
	Student status:† Four working full-time, one working part-time with full-time school, one on government subsidy				Student status:† One working full-time, four on government subsidy			

*Coding Note:
   Vocational functioning level: 1 = work functioning has deteriorated; 2 = work functioning is the same; 3 = work functioning has improved.
†Student status relates to follow-up of individuals who were students at the time of surgery or initial clinic evaluation.

indicated improved functioning, whereas three indicated no change in employment functioning and two indicated a decreased level of employment functioning.

Review of student performance 10 years after surgery or initial evaluation shows an interesting trend. Five of the six students who had surgery moved to full-time work or a full-time school and part-time work program, and only one student made the transition to subsidy status. Among the five students within the control group, four students were on subsidy status, and only one had found full-time work. The patients who were students at the time of surgery appeared to be adapting considerably better than the controls. This may support the early benefit of the surgery on these students' rate of development and occupational gains. It will be of interest to examine vocational differences at 10-year follow-up between surgical patients and controls as the patients evaluated increase through the duration of our study. It may require 10 years of follow-up in order to have a more accurate picture of the vocational impact of the surgery.

Steps in Creating Functional Change

For clients without significant cognitive, emotional, and personality deficits, significant intervention will still be required in order to achieve functional life changes among the adult population. Several authors [5,15] have emphasized that although patients may be relieved of seizure concerns, many have learned to live with the disability and in a number of cases have adopted the identified patient role within the family structure. Horowitz et al. [5] emphasize that this can be a critical period of time in which the counseling therapist and other team members must use their resources to assist the patient in the effort to identity reformulation, reevaluation of assets and deficits, and establishing new patterns of interaction with family, friends, and coworkers (if the person is working).

During the early phases of postoperative rehabilitation, individuals may go through a number of changes. In an earlier study at our center, Hurley et al. [4] indicated that 41% of surgery patients endure some negative emotional or cognitive difficulties in the first postoperative year. These are primarily emotional, involving depression, anxiety, apathy, and irritability. Most of these, however, appear to be reactive and related to changes in seizure status, dealing with new expectations and other such factors, and primarily seem to resolve in the initial postoperative year or years.

These data do suggest a significant subgroup of patients who go through a series of psychosocial changes. Horowitz et al. [5] suggest that these changes can be both intrapersonal and interpersonal. On an intrapersonal basis, patients may be waiting to see if improvement will be maintained, reappraising their abilities, dealing with the polarities of great expectations and the acceptance of the operation's failure if it does occur, giving up an assumed patient role, and so forth. Some individuals have difficulty adjusting and begin to substitute symptoms, become depressed, deny change, and cling to their established disabled person role.

Rehabilitation team members, family, friends, and other associates are challenged to both continue support and make some reasonable expectations for change on the part of the patient. This can be a delicate balancing interaction between the continuance of support, with the establishment of realistic goals and expectations for the patient relative to increased household and work responsibilities.

As previously reported [16], a small group of patients (four in the earlier University of Washington series) experienced a postoperative psychotic incident, primarily an atypical psychosis with paranoid ideation. These patients, although not having a prior hospitalization, had limited social support, experienced seizures of very early onset, were improved but not seizure-free, and had some history of community counseling or therapy. These patients were treated as having transient psychosis at the University of Washington Neurology or Epilepsy Center service. Following a period in which their seizures were stabilized by medication, the patient and family were educated relative to the probable transient nature of this illness. These individuals gradually returned to work, initially using a volunteer work experience with gradual transition to paid part-time and full-time work. They were coached relative to handling emotionally stressful events on the job and referred to a community support group and therapist. In all cases, these individuals stabilized and were able to maintain independent living and employment without being subject to a label of mental illness through referral to a psychiatric institution. A major effort was made to frame these incidents as acute and transient difficulties and to avoid chronic disability.

Assessment

It is very important that these patients be carefully assessed cognitively and psychosocially as a complement to effective surgical intervention. Assessment includes neuropsychological and psychiatric interviews and testing, functional academic testing, vocational interest assessment, and work values identification, and may include the use of work samples. This assessment not only identifies those patients who may have more adjustment difficulties but also enables the establishment of reasonable postoperative goals toward which progress can be made even before the surgery.

Framing Intervention

To truly bring about a successful rehabilitation, the surgery may be conceptualized to the patient and

family members as only part of the intervention that may render them more successful within their personal lives. Nonmedical team members such as the counseling psychologist, neuropsychologist, vocational counselor, recreational therapist, social worker, and recreation specialist can provide clients with a profile of their assets and areas of deficit as they approach the surgery. Patients and their significant others can be securing information about different job or work goals prior to the surgery. Based on seizure frequency, individuals can be placed on volunteer or even temporary paid work as they approach the surgical event (if they are not working at the time of surgery). They can explore reasonable living alternatives as well as community activities in which they have a greater potential for participation postsurgery. For clients with a longstanding patient role within the family and community, gains made in social interaction skills through volunteer work or involvement in organized community activities can be immensely helpful in improving employment potential. Improved socialization skills can compensate, to some degree, for even cognitive limitations within the employment market.

Based on response to the surgery, these community activities may need to proceed slowly in the immediate postoperative period. Some patients, however, can again begin to pick up on a fuller range of life activities relatively early in the postoperative period and make significant progress toward achieving new work, independent living, and social goals.

Functional Goals

It is important to emphasize that functional goals are established through review of assessment data as well as through interaction with the patient and family members, members of the interdisciplinary team (neurosurgeon, neurologist, neuropsychologist, rehabilitation counselor, social worker, etc.). Based on the client's progress, these goals may have to be reformulated, but if they are not set it is more likely that the client will not make a functional change because of established life patterns, anxiety over barriers that need to be overcome, and/or currently existing financial subsidy. If a patient has significant neuropsychological, emotional, or other deficits, these areas of concern will require more careful interdisciplinary team attention.

Utilization of the Rehabilitation Team

Surgery for epilepsy should be conducted within a team framework in order to optimize functional outcome. For many neurosurgical groups, there may be no social worker, vocational rehabilitation counselor, or other nonmedical team members. If this is the case, the activities of these professionals should be secured on a consultant basis from the community and coordinated by a nursing care coordinator or a social worker. For a majority of clients, it appears unlikely that these operations will result in substantial functional improvement (even if relief from seizures is experienced) unless a team or coordinated psychosocial intervention is made.

Maintaining Functional Gains: The Continuing Role of Psychotherapy and Education

As clients begin to make progress, it will be important that the primary therapist or counselor (psychologist, rehabilitation counselor, etc.) maintain contact with the client and family. There is often a tendency to regress to previously established roles that are not conducive to maintaining functional life progress. As more of these operations are performed, it would become valuable to establish 1- to 2-week psychoeducational programs for clients and family members that will provide more information about the patients' new medical status, the world of work, restructuring of their family interactions, emotional support as they challenge themselves with new expectations, and so on. Epilepsy associations may be of assistance in developing self-support groups for postsurgical patients. In considering the extent of change that will be required in the lives of many of these patients, however, it would behoove medical facilities conducting these operations to establish a short-term psychoeducational program as a basis for the rehabilitation effort. At times, family members can be more resistive than patients to establishing more functional rehabilitation goals within the lives of their sons or daughters. It may require a very comprehensive effort to really bring about change.

Summary

This chapter reviews a number of concerns related to vocational and, to some degree, other functional life changes following epilepsy surgery. Certain groups appear to be making postsurgical vocational and psychosocial progress, but these tend to be individuals who were already on a vocational track prior to the surgery, were students, or generally were of a higher cognitive level and better integrated psychosocially. Total relief of seizures can be a factor affecting vocational change, but findings are inconsistent and may be related to presurgical functioning. This will not be the case among the majority of individuals undergoing this operation. Consequently, the onus of bringing about successful changes in daily life functioning as a complement to seizure resolution rests on the staff of our medical facilities or the consulting teams that these facilities can draw from the community. Although further research is ongoing at our center and at others, existing data suggest that we are not yet able to effect the changes that are necessary to maximize these individuals' functional capacities as a complement to their usually improved medical status. Continuing research at our center should be helpful in further clarifying salient variables related to functional surgical outcome and the interrelationships among these variables.

References

1. Augustine EA et al. Occupational adjustment following neurosurgical treatment of epilepsy. *Ann Neurol* 1984; 15:68–72.
2. Crandall PH. Post-operative management and criteria for evaluation. In: Purpura et al. *Advances in neurology*, vol. 8. New York: Raven Press, 1975:265–79.
3. Dodrill CB. Commentary: psychological evaluation. In: Engel J Jr, ed. *Surgical treatment of the epilepsies*. New York: Raven Press, 1987:197–201.
4. Hurley P, Fraser RT, Wyler AR. Life events and emotional status in the first year following temporal lobe resection. Presented at the 15th Epilepsy International Symposium. Washington, DC, September 27, 1983.
5. Horowitz MJ, Cohen FM, Skolnikoff AZ, Saunders FA. Psychomotor epilepsy: rehabilitation after surgical treatment. *J Nerv Ment Dis* 1970;150:273–90.
6. Jensen I. Temporal lobe epilepsy. Social conditions and rehabilitation after surgery. *Acta Neurol Scand* 1976; 54:22–44.
7. Rausch R, Crandall PH. Psychological status related to surgical control of temporal lobe seizures. *Epilepsia* 1983;23:191–202.
8. Roth DL, Bachelor SD, Connell B, Faught E. Psychological changes after unilateral temporal lobe surgery. *Epilepsia* 1989;30:709.
9. Taylor DC, Falconer MA. Clinical, socio-economic, and psychological changes after temporal lobectomy. *Br J Psychiat* 1968;114:1247–61.
10. Savard RJ, Walker E. Changes in social functioning after surgical treatment for temporal lobe epilepsy. *Social Work* 1965;10:87–95.
11. Walzak TS, Radtke RA, Lewis DV. Factors predicting success in temporal lobectomy for complex partial seizures. *Epilepsia* 1987;28:610.
12. Weiss AA. Criteria of prediction of successful rehabilitation after temporal lobectomy from pre-operative psychological investigation. *Isr Ann Psych Relat Discipl* 1965;3:65–72.

13. Hale DK, Miller JK, Erickson T, Dodrill CB. Patient responses to their cortical resection surgery and their relationship to seizure control. Presented at the annual meeting of the American Epilepsy Society, Seattle, WA, November 1986.

14. Horowitz MJ, Cohen FM. Temporal lobe epilepsy: effect of lobectomy on psychosocial functioning. *Epilepsia* 1968;9:23–41.

15. Ferguson SM, Rayport M. The adjustment to living without epilepsy. *J Nerv Ment Dis* 1965;140:26–37.

16. Fraser RT. Improving outcome following epilepsy surgery. *Acta Neurol Scand* 1976;54:22–44.

Chapter 22

Reoperation for Failed Epilepsy Surgery

ALLEN R. WYLER

A certain percentage of patients who undergo epilepsy surgery do not obtain an acceptable reduction in seizure frequency. In many such cases the surgeon may consider reoperation in the hope of improving the initial surgical outcome. Reoperation is practiced in many epilepsy centers, although little has been published concerning its indications, morbidity, and outcome. The purpose of this chapter is to review the outcome of my series of 37 repeat epilepsy operations. Of these 37 cases, 31 were focal resections after initial focal resections or stereotaxic lesions, and six cases were focal resections following anterior corpus callosotomies. These data were previously published [1], but, even with a larger experience, the conclusions that were originally made still appear to be valid.

The 37 patients included in this report are from a larger series of 350 epilepsy surgery patients. Of these 37 patients, 10 (27%) originally underwent surgery elsewhere, and I initially operated on the other 27 patients (73%), two of whom were from my University of Washington series.

Data that clearly define a failure following epilepsy surgery have not been published. As a functional definition, we used these criteria: (a) at least 6 months have passed since the original surgery, (b) the person continues on optimal anticonvulsant drug therapy, and (c) seizures persist in sufficient frequency to significantly hinder development of an independent lifestyle.

Prior to reoperation, the patients underwent an evaluation that included a magnetic resonance imaging (MRI) scan to document the extent of the original resection and repeat, long-term electroencephalographic (EEG)/video monitoring with scalp (and sphenoidal) electrodes using the 10/20 International System. For patients not originally operated on by our

team, the data from the initial presurgical evaluation were obtained if possible.

In all cases the second operation was done under general anesthesia. For frontal lobe surgery, sensorimotor cortex was identified by either direct cortical stimulation or by recording somatosensory evoked cortical potentials [2]. Further frontal lobe resection was carried back to one gyrus anterior to the precentral gyrus in the nondominant hemisphere. We have not had occasion to reoperate on a dominant frontal lobe. Repeat temporal lobe resections involved opening dura over the previous resection cavity and selectively resecting additional hippocampus posteriorly, approximately to the level of the superior colliculus.

Outcomes from surgery were defined as follows:

1. *Seizure-free.* The patient was completely seizure-free from the time of discharge from hospital. Since auras are considered simple partial seizures, patients with auras only were not considered to be seizure-free.
2. *Significant Improvement.* At least a 75% reduction of seizures was maintained during the entire follow-up period. Patients with auras only were included in this group.
3. *Unchanged.* All patients who did not achieve at least a 75% reduction in total number of seizures (measured per year) were included in this group.

Results of Repeat Surgery

Focal Resections

A total of 31 patients underwent reoperation after initial focal resection. Mean age for this group was 22

241

years (range, 5–47 years). Average age of onset of epilepsy was 11.2 years. Of these 31 patients, the second resections were temporal in 23 cases, frontal in six cases, and parietal in two cases. Outcomes for the entire group of 31 cases were as follows and are shown in Table 22-1: 15 (48%) were seizure-free, eight (26%) were significantly improved, and nine (29%) showed no change. Follow-up periods for these patients ranges from 1 to 8 years. Complications from reoperation were quadrantanopsia in two patients and contralateral hemiparesis in one patient.

Of the 23 patients whose second operation involved the temporal lobe, 12 (52%) became seizure-free, five (22%) were significantly improved, and six (26%) were not helped by reoperation. Of the six not helped, four had their original resection on the frontal lobe. An additional case originally had stereotaxic lesions done by another surgeon; these were thought to be bilateral cingulotomies, but no operative report could be obtained. The remaining patient failed to benefit from repeat temporal lobectomy.

Outcomes for patients who had the second operation on a different lobe of brain than the first operation are shown in Table 22-2. It should be noted that the two patients who became seizure-free after the second operation had structural lesions. The first patient had initially undergone a right frontal lobectomy at another institution based only on interictal scalp EEG data. Four years later she was referred to our center, where an MRI scan demonstrated a tumor in the right temporal lobe. The tumor and adjacent temporal lobe were removed, and the patient has been seizure-free since surgery (greater than 2-year follow-up). In this case, it is clear that the frontal lobe was erroneously removed at the time of the surgery. The second person had developed a large right frontal-temporal infarction following severe sinusitis and probable cerebritis. The initial operation removed the frontal lobe, with a modest reduction in seizures. The second operation removed the temporal lobe, which has resulted in a seizure-free outcome. In this case, it is not clear if the focus was missed or simply incompletely resected during the first operation, since both the frontal and temporal lobes were involved in the cortical infarction.

For seven patients the first surgery involved a structural lesion that was incompletely removed. In all cases the remainder of the lesion was removed during the second operation. The outcome from reoperation and the pathology of the resected lesions are listed in Table 22-3. One patient, mentioned above, had a large cortical infarction involving two (frontal and temporal) lobes. Two pediatric patients had focal cortical dysplasia within the frontal lobe that had been incompletely removed at initial operation. Two patients had oligodendrogliomas; in one the lesion was incompletely removed at first operation; the other patient had the frontal lobe incorrectly removed initially. Six (86%) of the seven patients have been seizure-free thus far. The single patient who continues to have seizures has tuberous sclerosis with multiple cortical lesions in addition to those removed from the left frontal lobe. As a group, those patients with incompletely removed structural lesions after first operations have done well following a second surgery.

The entire patient sample was then reexamined to determine how the initial presurgical evaluation had influenced outcome of the second operation. Because we were most interested in how the method of EEG localization affected outcome, patients with structural lesions were removed from the sample, leaving 24 patients who underwent focal resections initially. Results are summarized in Table 22-4. There is a significant trend for patients who initially underwent invasive EEG monitoring to have a better outcome after reoperation than did patients whose initial surgical decision was based on interictal or ictal scalp EEG evaluations. Of 12 patients who had initial monitoring with strip electrodes, eight (66%) were seizure-free after reoperation. Only four of 12 patients (33%) who were evaluated initially with only ictal scalp EEG monitoring were seizure-free following reoperation. This trend is even more apparent if those patients who underwent surgeries on different lobes are removed from the sample. Under those circumstances, seven (86%) of eight strip-monitored patients were seizure-free after reoperation, whereas only two (22%) of nine of scalp-monitored patients were seizure-free. This is compatible with the fact

Table 22-1. Outcome from Second Focal Resection Following Initial Focal Resection or Stereotaxic Lesion

Operation	Outcome		
	Seizure Free	Significantly Improved	No Change
Temporal	12	5	6
Frontal	3	2	2
Other	0	1	1
Total	15 (48%)	8 (26%)	9 (29%)

Table 22-2. Outcome from Second Operation That Involved a Different Location than the First Operation

Patient	First Operation	Second Operation	Outcome
PH	Frontal lobe	Temporal lobe	Reduction
CH*	Frontal lobe	Temporal lobe	Seizure-free
CV*	Frontal lobe	Temporal lobe	Seizure-free
SW	Cingulotomies	Temporal lobe	No change
DW	Frontal lobe	Temporal lobe	No change
PP	Frontal lobe	Temporal lobe	No change
JM	Frontal lobe	Temporal lobe	No change

*Patients with structural lesions.

that invasive ictal monitoring is far more accurate in identifying the epileptogenic focus than is scalp monitoring [3–7].

In all nonlesional temporal lobe cases that have had a seizure-free outcome, the second surgery involved further resection of the hippocampus. In all these cases, the original pathology demonstrated typical mesial temporal sclerosis.

Corpus Callosotomy plus Focal Resections

Six patients had an anterior two thirds callosotomy followed by a focal resection at least 6 months later. The average age for this group was 21 years (range, 4–33 years), with the average age of onset at 6.5 years (range, 3–13 years) (Table 22-5). There was no morbidity or mortality in this group. One patient was rendered seizure-free, and one was significantly improved (greater than 75% reduction in seizure frequency) following the focal resection. Both patients had structural lesions that were removed during the second surgery, one a calcific astrocytoma of the temporal lobe and the other a porencephalic cyst in the occipital-temporal region. In both cases, these focal lesions could not be implicated as the epileptogenic focus during the initial presurgical evaluation. After the anterior corpus callosotomy, the seizures did not improve, and the subsequent EEG monitoring demonstrated that the majority of epileptiform activity was restricted to the hemisphere (but not necessarily the lobe) containing the lesion, thus making it more reasonable to assume the lesion was the seizure focus. Of the patients without structural lesions who underwent this combination of surgeries, only one demonstrated some additional improvement after focal resection (a right temporal lobectomy). The patient had both gelastic seizures and brief complex-partial seizures. The complex-partial seizures ceased after temporal lobectomy, but the gelastic seizures continued. The remaining three patients showed no seizure improvement following the corpus callostomy or the subsequent focal resection. Of these three

patients, one had a temporal lobectomy, one had a right frontal lobectomy, and one had a left frontal lobectomy. The three patients who did not improve after focal resection did not have invasive monitoring at any time during either of their evaluations.

One of the most important reasons for evaluating the outcome of repeat epilepsy surgery is to clarify the reasons for failure of the initial surgery. With that information we might be able to improve either the initial criteria for patient selection or the initial operative procedures. The optimal outcome for epilepsy surgery is complete freedom from seizures, which is most likely following a cortical resection rather than a corpus callosotomy. The most obvious causes of continued seizures after focal cortical resection are (a) a resection that was too conservative; (b) imprecise localization of the primary zone of epileptogenesis; (c) removal of the wrong cortical region, leaving the original focus; or (d) incorrect diagnosis of focal epilepsy.

First, consider the case for a focal resection that was too conservative. Most previous literature on reoperation has dealt primarily with temporal lobe surgery. Penfield and Jasper [8] were among the first to mention reoperation. They wrote, "A remaining zone of epileptogenic activity has been found in the hippocampus and complete hippocampal removal, either right or left, has sometimes converted failure into what promises to become success." Green and Sidell [9] have stated that ". . . failures of operative resection, related to excisions of only the restricted focus of lowest seizure threshold, may frequently be converted to successes with reoperation and complete excision of the epileptogenic area." Probably the largest series of reoperated patients comes from follow-up of Penfield's work as reported by Rasmussen [10]. From 1928 through 1971, 129 patients with nontumoral lesions had undergone reoperation, and adequate follow-up data for 2–39 years were available for 115 of them. Of the 115 patients, 29 (25%) became seizure-free and 31 (27%) were significantly helped with reoperation. Thus, 60 patients (52%) were helped with a second or third surgery. The cause

Table 22-3. Outcome from Second Operation That Involved a Structural Lesion

Patient	First Operation	Second Operation	Outcome*	Pathology
JH	Frontal lobe	Frontal lobe	SF	Cortical dysplasia
CH	Frontal lobe	Temporal lobe	SF	Oligodendroglioma
CK	Frontal lobe	Frontal lobe	SF	Oligodendroglioma
RM	Frontal lobe	Frontal lobe	NC	Tuberous sclerosis
SN	Temporal lobe	Temporal lobe	SF	Old hematoma cavity
BT	Frontal lobe	Frontal lobe	SF	Cortical dysplasia
CV	Frontal lobe	Temporal lobe	SF	Large cortical infarct

SF = seizure-free; NC = no change.

for failure of initial surgery was not completely clear, other than "follow-up studies, however, have indicated that success in stopping the seizures is correlated with the completeness of the removal of epileptogenic cortex, and excisions limited to restricted foci of lowest seizure threshold have usually failed to provide a satisfactory reduction in seizure tendency" [10]. This explanation is frustrating in that it does not clarify how the initial operation might be improved on to prevent or limit failures. Because temporal lobectomy is the most commonly performed epilepsy surgery, it must be assumed that the previously cited work is based primarily on temporal lobe surgery, although that is not stated.

With respect to reoperation of temporal lobe cases only, Olivier et al. [11] reported a series of 425 temporal lobectomies, of which 20 patients underwent reoperation with the following results: six patients (30%) became seizure-free, three patients (15%) had a marked reduction in seizures, and seven patients (35%) had a "worthwhile" improvement. At the time of first operation, 65% of these patients had no resection of the hippocampus, and 35% had only limited anterior resection of the hippocampus. In all cases the second operation involved a more radical hippocampal resection than the first. Thus, it is clear that *some* (but not all) of the temporal lobe failures are due to inadequate hippocampal resection.

The concept therefore emerges that the presurgical evaluation did not define in great enough detail the location of the epileptogenic focus, or "primary zone of epileptogenesis." Spencer et al. [12] have emphasized this hypothesis and feel that as many as 20% of hippocampal foci reside posterior to the usual limits of a standard resection. They have tested this hypothesis by implanting depth electrodes in a trajectory from the occipital pole anteriorly so that the electrode contacts travel the length of the hippocampus rather than recording from isolated points in the anterior hippocampus. When they find a posteriorly residing focus, they propose a modified temporal lobectomy with removal of the posterior hippocampus, similar in extent to Wieser and Yasergil's selective amygdalohippocampectomy [18]. Therefore, much of Olivier's data indirectly support Spencer's contention.

Are some failed operations due to faulty initial localization of the epileptogenic focus? In our series of 23 reoperations involving the temporal lobe, 12 patients (52%) were rendered seizure-free, and six patients (26%) showed no improvement. In one of the six failures, the original operation had been a stereotaxic lesion thought to be bilateral cingulotomies. In another four of the six failures, the original operation was a frontal lobe resection. In all six patients who had failed reoperation, their initial work-ups did not include invasive monitoring, so the accuracy of the initial decision remains unanswered. In comparison, 10 of the 12 patients rendered

Table 22-4. Outcome from Second Operation for 24 Patients Without Structural Lesions Who Were Initially Monitored with Subdural Strip Electrodes (Strips) or Scalp EEG (Scalp)*

	Outcome	
	Seizure-Free	Not Seizure-Free
Strips	8*	4***
Scalp	4**	8*

*The number of asterisks indicates the number of patients in each group who had undergone reoperation on a different lobe than the first surgery.

Table 22-5. Outcome from a Focal Resection after Initial Anterior Corpus Callosotomy

Patient	Resection	Outcome
KH	Right temporal	No change
BH	Left temporal	Significant reduction
AS	Left frontal	No change
BW	Right temporal	Improved
MG	Right occipital	Seizure-free
JH	Right frontal	No change

seizure-free after reoperation had been evaluated before the initial operation with subdural strip electrodes [13,14].

Of all data evaluated preoperatively, most surgeons rely most heavily on EEG data to determine which lobe should be resected. Many, but not all, surgeons require invasive ictal EEG monitoring to localize epileptogenic foci [15]. Until 1986 my colleagues and I reserved the use of invasive EEG monitoring for only those patients with difficult-to-interpret scalp EEG monitoring results. Recently, we [7] compared the relative accuracy with which scalp- and subdural-recorded EEG localized epileptogenic foci. We found that both interictal and ictal scalp recordings had a false localization and lateralization rate of close to 30% when identifying unilateral epileptogenic foci. We also found that 77% of patients operated on after invasive monitoring had seizure-free outcomes (including auras), whereas only 59% of patients operated on after only scalp monitoring had similar outcomes. Thus, it seems reasonable to assume that some of the poorer outcomes in patients who had only scalp EEG monitoring are due to insufficient or inaccurate localization of the epileptogenic focus. In fact, we found this to be true in a few cases. One patient had a frontal lobe resection based on scalp EEG monitoring. Four years later an evaluation at our center found her focus to be in the temporal lobe of the same hemisphere, where she had an oligodendroglioma. In two other cases, localization by scalp monitoring led to a corpus callosotomy when both patients had cortical foci that were subsequently removed.

The above cases primarily involved temporal lobe resections. Our growing experience with frontal lobe resections yields very similar conclusions, especially in those cases with incompletely removed structural lesions. For example, in two of our cases the original lesion was congenital cortical dysplasia that was incompletely resected at the first operation. In both cases, reoperation resulted in a seizure-free outcome.

In many cases, results of initial surgery apparently can be improved with more precise preoperative localization of the cortical focus. Because scalp recording has an inherent error rate for false localization and lateralization, improvement could come from increased use of invasive EEG monitoring preoperatively. However, foci of some patients will still be difficult to localize. More often than not, these foci reside outside the temporal lobes, and commonly within the frontal lobes. Purves et al. [16] have suggested that some cases of complex-partial seizures that cannot be localized with monitoring can first be treated with an anterior corpus callosotomy. The rationale is that if this initial surgery does not reduce

seizures to an acceptable frequency, callosal sectioning may decrease interictal and ictal epileptiform EEG spike propagation sufficiently to allow localization of the epileptogenic focus. The focus can thus be localized and removed in a subsequent resection. We have attempted this approach in six cases. In two cases structural lesions were involved, and reevaluation after anterior corpus callosotomy did localize the epileptogenic cortex to those lesions, which were removed with a good result. When now presented with similar cases we operate on the structural lesion rather than proceed with an anterior corpus callosotomy. In only one nonlesional case that was initially subjected to corpus callosotomy and was later followed by focal resection has the result been a reduction in seizure frequency, and even then it did not result in a seizure-free outcome. In the other three cases, the patients showed no further improvement after the focal resection. It is difficult to judge the merit of this approach because of several confounding variables. First, two of the three patients who failed to improve had focal frontal lobe resections, and in general the results of frontal resections are not as good as temporal resections. Second, the patients who did not do well had only scalp monitoring during both presurgical evaluations.

In summary, our experience has generated the following biases. First, even in initial cases, the scalp-recorded EEG can falsely localize and lateralize the epileptogenic focus [7,17]. From our experience, the scalp EEG is even more inaccurate after either a focal cortical resection or corpus callosotomy. In our experience, long-term EEG monitoring of a patient who has failed initial surgery does little to help localize the focus or determine if the initial surgical decision was correct. In fact, remonitoring has led us subsequently to remove an adjacent lobe without benefit. Consequently, we have come to the conclusion that the patient's initial evaluation is the most important for obtaining absolute accurate localization of the epileptogenic focus. For this reason, we advocate invasive ictal monitoring during the patient's initial surgical evaluation for all cases of nonlesional complex-partial seizures. Then, if the initial surgery does not yield a satisfactory result, the second surgery should be an enlargement of the original surgical site rather than removal of an adjacent lobe. One should only consider removing an adjacent lobe if it is involved with a structural lesion incompletely removed at first operation. If the operation involves the temporal lobe, further resection of hippocampus to the level of the superior colliculus should be considered. Finally, our results with focal resection after anterior corpus callosotomy have not been encouraging, and we have therefore abandoned this strategy.

References

1. Wyler AR, Hermann BP, Richey ET. Results of reoperation for failed epilepsy surgery. *J Neurosurg* 1989; 71:815–9.
2. Wood CC, Spencer DD, Allison T, McCarthy G, Williamson PD, Goff WR. Localization of human sensorimotor cortex during surgery by cortical surface recording of somatosensory evoked potentials. *J Neurosurg* 1988;68:99–111.
3. Engel J Jr, Crandall PH. Intensive neurodiagnostic monitoring with intracranial electrodes. *Adv Neurol* 1987;46:85–106.
4. Lieb JP, Engel J Jr, Gevins A, Crandall PH. Surface and deep EEG correlates of surgical outcome in temporal lobe epilepsy. *Epilepsia* 1981;22:515–38.
5. Spencer SS, Williamson PD, Bridgers SL, Mattson RH, Cicchetti DV, Spencer DD. Reliability and accuracy of localization by scalp ictal EEG. *Neurology* 1985;35: 1567–75.
6. Spencer SS. Depth electroencephalography in selection of refractory epilepsy for surgery. *Ann Neurol* 1981; 9:207–14.
7. Wyler AR, Richey ET, Hermann BP. Comparison of scalp to subdural recordings for localizing epileptogenic foci. *J Epilepsy* 1989;2:91–6.
8. Penfield W, Jasper H. *Epilepsy and the functional anatomy of the human brain,* Boston: Little, Brown, 1954.
9. Green JR, Sidell AD. Neurosurgical aspects of epilepsy in children and adolescents. In: Youmans JR, ed. *Neurological surgery.* Philadelphia: WB Saunders, 1982: 3858–909.
10. Rasmussen T. Surgical treatment of patients with complex partial seizures. In: Purpura DP, Penry JK, Walter RD, eds. *Advances in neurology.* New York: Raven Press, 1975:415–49.
11. Olivier A, Tanaka T, Andermann F. Reoperations in temporal lobe epilepsy (abstract). *Epilepsia* 1989; 29:678.
12. Spencer DD, Spencer SS, Mattson RH, Novelly RA, Williamson PD. Access to the posterior temporal lobe structures in the surgical treatment of temporal lobe epilepsy. *Neurosurgery* 1984;15:667–71.
13. Wyler AR, Walker G, Richey ET, Hermann BP. Chronic subdural strip electrode recordings for difficult epileptic problems. *J Epilepsy* 1988;1:71–8.
14. Wyler AR, Ojemann GA, Lettich E, Ward AA Jr. Subdural strip electrodes for localizing epileptogenic foci. *J Neurosurg* 1984;60:1195–1200.
15. Engel J Jr. Approaches to localization of the epileptogenic lesion. In: Engel J Jr, ed. *Surgical treatment of the epilepsies* New York: Raven Press, 1987:75–95.
16. Purves SJ, Wada JA, Woodhurst WB, et al. Results of anterior corpus callosum section in 24 patients with medically intractable seizures. *Neurology* 1988;38: 1194–1201.
17. Engel J Jr, Crandall PH. Falsely localizing ictal onsets with depth EEG telemetry during anticonvulsant withdrawal. *Epilepsia* 1983;24:344–55.
18. Wieser HG, and Yasergil H. Selective amygdalohippocampectomy as a surgical treatment of mediobasal lymbic epilepsy. *Surg Neurol* 1984;17:445–57.

APPENDIXES

Appendix A

Questionnaire for Seizure Patients

NAME OF PATIENT _____ DATE _____

DATE OF BIRTH _____ SEX _____ EDUCATION _____

OCCUPATION(S) _____ MARITAL STATUS _____

HANDEDNESS _____

ASSISTED BY: _____ RELATIONSHIP _____ AGE _____

EDUCATION _____

IF COMPLETED BY SOMEONE ELSE, GIVE:

NAME _____ RELATIONSHIP _____ AGE _____

EDUCATION _____

Please answer the following questions as precisely as possible. If you do not understand a question, place a question mark (?) beside it. You may use the back of the pages or additional sheets if there is not enough space for your answers.

Some of the questions can best be answered by a close relative or friend. Please get the appropriate assistance to complete the questionnaire.

---

1. At what age did your seizures begin?
   Minor seizures: Major seizures:

2. Describe any marked change in the severity of the seizure disorder over the years.

3. What may have caused the seizures (birth injury, febrile convulsions, head injury, etc.)?

4. List your present and previous medications.
   Medications—present: previous:

5. How often (per day, week, month, or year) do your minor and major seizures occur?
   Minor seizures: Major seizures:
      maximum frequency: maximum frequency:
      minimum frequency: minimum frequency:
      average frequency: average frequency:

6. What, if anything, may bring about a seizure?

7. Describe any changes occurring regularly for hours (or days) before the seizures.

   Indicate the duration of the experience:

8. What do you remember about your seizures?
   (Include a detailed description of any aura or warning you may have.)

   Indicate variation of the experience:

   Indicate duration of the experience:

9. What do others observe at the time of a seizure?

   Indicate variation of the observation:

   Indicate duration of the observed seizure:

10. Describe the aftermath of the seizure:

    Indicate duration of the aftermath:

11. List other medical problems you may have:

    _____

12. Your years of education:

13. What type of work did you wish to pursue?

14. Your work experience:

    When did you work last:

15. Your present living situation:

16. Your marital history:

17. Has sex been important in your life?

18. What effect has epilepsy had on your sex life?

    Since about when?

19. Do you have many close friends?

20. What effect has epilepsy had on your social life?

21. Briefly list your hobbies and other things you enjoy doing:

    _____

22. Your physical and emotional health before onset of epilepsy:
    (List any counseling, psychiatric treatment, medication, hospital stay.)

23. Describe the effects of epilepsy on your emotional life:
    (List any counseling, psychiatric treatment, medication, hospital stay.)

24. Do you have frequent depressive moods?
    Since about when?

25. Do you often lack energy?
    Since about when?

26. Do you have trouble with your sleep?
    Since about when?

27. Do you have many aches and pains?
    Since about when?

28. Do you have moods of great happiness?
    Since about when?

29. Do your moods often change unpredictably?
    Since about when?

30. Are you often very irritable? With outbursts of temper?
    Since about when?

31. Do you often mistrust others or imagine things?
    Since about when?

32. Do you sometimes hear or see things that are not there?
    Since about when?

33. Do you have frequent anxieties?
    Since about when?

34. Do you have fears of certain situations?
    Since about when?

35. Do you have periods of confusion or loss of memory, even without a seizure?
    Since about when?

36. Do you tend to be very good-natured and conscientious?
    Since about when?

37. Do you tend to be very orderly, strong on details, persistent in your actions? Please circle which one(s)
    apply to you and explain.
    Since about when?

38. Have you ever suffered from a drug or alcohol addiction?
    About when?

39. What are your religious (spiritual) beliefs and practices?
    Since about when?

40. List family members who have suffered from:
    Epilepsy
    Migraine
    Stuttering
    Neurologic disorder
    Psychiatric disorder

To be completed by Examiner:
Establish frequency of arousal (#18).
Establish polarity, rate and duration of mood swings (#29).
Establish nature and frequency of irritability (#30).
Establish a family tree (with occupations, illnesses, and exceptional traits of first- and second-degree relatives).

Examiner _____
Date _____

Appendix B

Postoperative Questionnaire (____ months postop)

Name of Patient _____ Date _____ Next-of-Kin _____

1. How often have you suffered seizures since your surgery (or last follow-up):
   None:
   Major:
   Minor:
   Aura without loss of consciousness:

2. What do you remember about your seizure?

3. What do others observe at the time of a seizure?

4. Describe the aftermath of a seizure:

5. Your present medications:

6. Your present employment, if any:

7. Your present living situation:

8. Any changes in your sexual interests and activities:

9. Any changes in your social life or pastimes?

10. Any changes in your religious (spiritual) beliefs or practices?

11. Have you had any counseling or psychiatric treatment?

12. Have you been on any medication for your nerves?

13. Have you been hospitalized for a nervous condition?

14. Do you have frequent depressive moods?
    Since about when?

15. Do you often lack energy?
    Since about when?

16. Do you have trouble with your sleep?
    Since about when?

17. Do you have many aches and pain?
    Since about when?

18. Do you have moods of great happiness?
    Since about when?

19. Do your moods often change unpredictably?
    Since about when?

20. Are you often very irritable?
    With outbursts of temper?
    Since about when?

21. Do you tend to be very good-natured and conscientious?

22. Do you often mistrust others or imagine things?
    Since about when?

23. Do you sometimes hear or see things that are not there?
    Since about when?

24. Do you have frequent anxieties?
    Since about when?

253

25. Do you have fears of certain situations?
    Since about when?

26. Do you have periods of confusion or loss of
    memory, even without a seizure?
    Since about when?

27. Describe any other changes you have experi-
    enced since the operation (or last follow-up).

To be completed by Examiner:
Establish frequency of arousal (#8).
Establish polarity, rate and duration of mood swings (#19).
Establish nature and frequency of irritability (#20).

Examiner _____

Date _____

Appendix C
Neurobehavior Inventory for Next-of-Kin

INSTRUCTIONS

On the following pages there are statements about personal habits, preferences, feelings, and beliefs. For each statement, please indicate whether the statement seems more true or more false about the person you are describing.

On the basis of your experiences with the patient, please give your first and most honest response to each item, *leaving no blanks*. There are no right or wrong answers—no ratings for better or worse—so please be guided by your memory and your impressions.

We appreciate your sincere cooperation in completing the Survey. Please fill in:

_____

Name of the Person You Are Describing

_____

Your Name

_____

Your Relation to the Patient

_____

Your Sex

_____

Your Age

_____

Highest Grade You Completed at School

_____

Number of Years You Have Known Patient

_____

Date

	True	False

A. Writing Tendency

1. Believes it would make good sense to keep a detailed diary.   ( )   ( )
2. Writes poetry, stories, or biography.   ( )   ( )
3. Writes down many things, copies passages from books, and so forth.   ( )   ( )
4. Records details about personal experiences and thinking.   ( )   ( )
5. Speaks about or is writing a book.   ( )   ( )

B. Sense of Law and Order

6. Personally very upset when people disobey the law.   ( )   ( )
7. Often believes he or she is the only one who is right.   ( )   ( )
8. Infuriated by cases where justice has not been done.   ( )   ( )
9. Goes out of the way to make sure the law is followed.   ( )   ( )
10. Detests people who try to break the rules.   ( )   ( )

C. Religious Convictions

11. Religious beliefs have become very important.   ( )   ( )
12. Believes the Bible has special meaning which he or she can understand.   ( )   ( )
13. Has had some very intense religious experiences.   ( )   ( )
14. Very religious (more than most people) in own way.   ( )   ( )
15. Religion and God are more personal experiences than for most people.   ( )   ( )

D. Anger and Temper

16. Little things make him or her angrier than they used to.   ( )   ( )
17. Gets into trouble because of temper.   ( )   ( )
18. Loses control of temper more frequently.   ( )   ( )
19. When angry, often explodes.   ( )   ( )
20. Often said to be hotheaded.   ( )   ( )

E. Orderliness

21. Has a habit of counting things or memorizing numbers.   ( )   ( )
22. Seems more sensitive to distractions than most people.   ( )   ( )
23. Becomes upset if things are not just right.   ( )   ( )
24. Mind gets stuck on so many different ideas that he or she cannot make a decision or do anything.   ( )   ( )
25. Tends to get bogged down with the fine points of a situation.   ( )   ( )

F. Feelings About Sex

26. Sex is less important than most people believe.   ( )   ( )
27. Hardly ever preoccupied with thoughts about sex.   ( )   ( )
28. Sexual activity has decreased.   ( )   ( )
29. Can do easily without sexual activity.   ( )   ( )
30. Has trouble becoming sexually aroused.   ( )   ( )

G. Fearfulness

31. Is very worried about hurting other people's feelings.   ( )   ( )
32. May become fearful of being alone.   ( )   ( )
33. Often feels suddenly fearful without apparent reason.   ( )   ( )
34. Tends to avoid crowds.   ( )   ( )
35. Is more afraid of doing the wrong thing than most people.   ( )   ( )

	True	False

H. Feelings of Guilt

	True	False
36. Can never forgive himself or herself for some of the things he or she has done.	( )	( )
37. Much of the time feels as if he or she has done something wrong or harmful.	( )	( )
38. Believes he or she has not lived the right kind of life.	( )	( )
39. After accidentally hurting someone's feelings cannot forgive himself or herself for a long time.	( )	( )
40. Really suffers after even a small mistake.	( )	( )

I. Seriousness

41. Finds few things really funny.	( )	( )
42. People do not seem to appreciate his or her jokes.	( )	( )
43. Feels that people should think about the point of many jokes more carefully instead of just laughing at them.	( )	( )
44. Feels that most jokes are not funny.	( )	( )
45. Says that there is too much foolishness in the world these days.	( )	( )

J. Sadness

46. Has had periods of days or weeks when he or she could not get going at all.	( )	( )
47. Feels that life is a strain much of the time.	( )	( )
48. Really down in the dumps most of the time.	( )	( )
49. Has often felt close to ending his or her life.	( )	( )
50. May feel suddenly that the future is hopeless.	( )	( )

K. Emotions

51. Feelings may suddenly take the place of thinking.	( )	( )
52. Almost everything triggers some emotional reaction.	( )	( )
53. Emotions control his or her life.	( )	( )
54. Subject to big shifts in mood.	( )	( )
55. Emotions have been so powerful that they have caused trouble.	( )	( )

L. Suspicion

56. Feels that fate is working against him or her.	( )	( )
57. Open to attack from many sides.	( )	( )
58. Believes that people tend to take advantage of him or her.	( )	( )
59. Sometimes may hear sounds or see things that are not really there.	( )	( )
60. At times may believe in something that in fact is not taking place.	( )	( )

M. Interest in Details

61. Sometimes gets terribly confused by little details.	( )	( )
62. Rarely tells people something without giving them all the details.	( )	( )
63. Needs to know every detail before making a decision.	( )	( )
64. Needs more details than most people to understand something.	( )	( )
65. Has trouble getting to the point because of all the details.	( )	( )

N. Cosmic Interests

66. Believes that nothing is more important than trying to understand the forces that govern this world.	( )	( )
67. Spends a lot of time thinking about the origins of the world and life.	( )	( )
68. Believes that powerful forces beyond control are working with his or her life.	( )	( )

	True	False
69. Believes he or she understands the real meaning or nature of this world.	( )	( )
70. More preoccupied than most people with the order and purpose of life.	( )	( )

O. Sense of Personal Destiny

	True	False
71. Feels people would learn a lot from the story of his or her life.	( )	( )
72. Thinks that he or she serves a supreme purpose in life.	( )	( )
73. Believes that powerful forces are acting through him or her.	( )	( )
74. Seems sure there is a significant meaning behind personal suffering.	( )	( )
75. Feels that the illness has been given so that he or she would meet certain people at the right time.	( )	( )

P. Persistence and Repetitiveness

	True	False
76. Cannot get off the point sometimes.	( )	( )
77. Sometimes get stuck on one idea so that he or she cannot make a decision or do anything.	( )	( )
78. When talking to someone, has trouble breaking off.	( )	( )
79. Sometimes keeps at a thing so long that others may lose their patience.	( )	( )
80. Is bothered for days by the same thoughts.	( )	( )

Q. Hatred and Revenge

	True	False
81. Has a tendency to break things or hurt people when infuriated.	( )	( )
82. Feelings of hatred can be very intense.	( )	( )
83. Talks about ripping some people to shreds.	( )	( )
84. Preoccupied with thoughts of revenge.	( )	( )
85. Infuriated by some of the things people have done to him or her.	( )	( )

R. Dependency

	True	False
86. Feels like a pawn in the hands of others.	( )	( )
87. Has gotten people angry by asking them to do so much.	( )	( )
88. Seems to depend on other people for many things.	( )	( )
89. Sometimes feels so helpless that he or she wants people to do everything.	( )	( )
90. Feels fortunate to receive so much help from people.	( )	( )

S. Happiness

	True	False
91. Has at times feeling of blissful joy.	( )	( )
92. Often does foolish things while in a good mood.	( )	( )
93. Sometimes feels so good that ideas come into mind faster than he or she can handle them.	( )	( )
94. Has had periods so full of pep that sleep did not seem necessary for several days.	( )	( )
95. Sometimes feels excitedly happy, on top of the world, without any reason or even when things are going wrong.	( )	( )

T. Physical Well-being

	True	False
96. Frequently has trouble getting a good night's sleep.	( )	( )
97. Is often bothered by severe headaches or other troublesome aches and pain.	( )	( )
98. Suffers from frequent periods of exhaustion or fatigue.	( )	( )
99. Worries often about his or her physical health.	( )	( )
100. Off and on is bothered by various odd bodily sensations.	( )	( )

Appendix D
Comprehensive Scoring Sheet

Patient _____ Date _____ NBI Scores _____

Self-Report _____ Preop. _____ Next-of-Kin _____ Postop. (_____ mo.)

	Potentially major clinical findings			
	NBI*		Clinical**	Global**
	SR	NK		
Depression				
Sadness	_____	_____	_____	_____
Physical Well-being	_____	_____	_____	_____
Happiness	_____	_____	_____	_____
Irritability				
Anger	_____	_____	_____	_____
Hatred	_____	_____	_____	_____
Suspicion	_____	_____	_____	_____
Fearfulness	_____	_____	_____	_____
Other (list)			_____	_____
			_____	_____

	Subtle emotional and behavioral findings			
	NBI*		Clinical**	Global**
	SR	NK		
Emotional intensity				
Emotions	_____	_____	_____	_____
Seriousness	_____	_____	_____	_____
Writing	_____	_____	_____	_____
Viscosity				
Orderliness	_____	_____	_____	_____
Details	_____	_____	_____	_____
Persistence	_____	_____	_____	_____
Conscience				
Law & order	_____	_____	_____	_____
Guilt	_____	_____	_____	_____
Transcendent trends				
Religion	_____	_____	_____	_____
Cosmic interests	_____	_____	_____	_____
Sense of destiny	_____	_____	_____	_____
Sexual feelings	_____	_____	_____	_____
Dependency	_____	_____	_____	_____

*0–5   **0 = None   1 = Mild   3 = Moderate   5 = Marked   NBI = Neurobehavior inventory   SR = Self report
NK = Next-of-Kin

259

Appendix E
WADA Evaluation

Name: _____ MCG: _____ Date: _____

Age: _____ Sex: _____ Handedness: _____ Rater: _____

INJECTION: Right Left Dose (mg) _____   Flaccid Hemiparesis Y N
Time Test Started: _____   **Running Time**

Initial Expressive Language (Counting)   0 1 2 3 4   __0 sec__

     (0 = normal, slowed or brief pause; 1 = counting perseveration with normal sequencing; 2 = sequencing errors;
     3 = single number or word perseveration; 4 = arrest)

Lateral Gaze Palsy <u>None</u> <u>R</u> <u>L</u>   0=normal, 1=mild
    Spontaneous ___ ___ ___   0 1 2 3   2=moderate, 3=severe
    Command ___ ___ ___   0 1 2 3 N/A

RECEPTIVE LANGUAGE (Initial-Simple):   0 1 2 3   Time _____

Modified Glasgow Coma Scale   If ptosis, note severity: 0 1 2 3 (0 = normal)
   <u>Motor</u> (ipsilateral and   If akinesia, note severity: 0 1 2 3
   contralateral arm):   Eye Opening: <u>Eye Movements:</u>

	Ipsi	Contra				
spontaneous	6	6	spontaneous	4	follows objects well	4
localizes	5	5	to loud noise	3	follows objects variably	3
withdraws	4	4	to pain	2	orients to loud noise	
abnormal flexion	3	3	nil	1	and light	2
extensor response	2	2			nil	1
nil	1	1				

                                                          Time

EARLY ITEM PRESENTATION: Begin   _____
                                           End   _____

COMPREHENSION (Delayed-Token card):   0 1 2 3   _____
    (0 = normal, 1 = mild, 2 = moderate, 3 = severe)
EXPRESSIVE LANGUAGE:
    Naming
        (A:screwdriver, pipe)   (errors) 0 1 2
        (B:comb, spoon)   _____
        Responses _____
    Repetition
        (A:Mary had a little lamb)   0 1 2 3 N/A
        (B:Jack and Jill went up the hill)
    Dysarthria   0 1 2 3 N/A
    Reading
        (A:The car backed over the curb.)   0 1 2 3 N/A
        (B:The rabbit hopped down the lane.)
VISUOSPATIAL DISCRIMINATION: Time _____
                             (errors) 0 1 2   FP _____
RECALL OF PRE-INJECTION ITEMS:
    Cup   Y N   Shoe   Y N   Sentence   Y N

Name: _____ Injection: R L   Date: _____

RECOGNITION/NAMING

Set A: lamp _____   pen _____   cup _____   Recognition _____ /2

    pear _____   shoe _____   broom _____   FP _____

Set B: paint brush_   hat _____   cup _____   Naming

    pie _____   book _____   shoe _____   _____ /6

RETEST:

Strength _____   Time _____

Language   errors

    Repetition (No ifs ands or buts)   0 1 2 3

    _____

    Comprehension   0 1 2 3

Time at which strength and language normal   Time _____

EARLY OBJECT RECOGNITION:

                           Time _____

_____	Y N	_____	Y N	_____	Y N
_____	Y N	_____	Y N	_____	Y N
_____	Y N	_____	Y N	_____	Y N
_____	Y N	_____	Y N	_____	Y N
_____	Y N	_____	Y N	_____	Y N
_____	Y N	_____	Y N	_____	Y N
_____	Y N	_____	Y N	_____	Y N	/8
_____	Y N	_____	Y N	_____	Y N	FP

Targets
List A: shark, helicopter, ball, car, boat, tongs, quarter, eraser
List B: clothespin, scrub pad, bowl, pizza cutter, battery, shell, toothbrush, rope

LATE ITEM MEMORY:

Recall of Postinjection Items   (Postrecovery)   Time _____

    Rhyme Free Recall   Y N   FP _____

    Rhyme Recognition   Y N   N/A   FP _____

List A: A = Old Mother Hubbard went to the cupboard
        B = Mary had a little lamb
        C = Mary, Mary quite contrary
        D = Three blind mice, Three blind mice

List B: A = Peter, Peter, Pumpkin Eater
        B = Jack be nimble, Jack be quick
        C = Jack and Jill went up the hill
        D = Humpty Dumpty sat on a wall

    Object Free Recall   (errors) 0 1 2   FP _____
    Object Recognition   (errors) 0 1 2   N/A
    (A:key, pipe, hammer, paper clip, screwdriver)   FP _____
    (B:watch, knife, comb, scissors, spoon)

Name: _____ Injection: R L   Date: _____

Visuospatial Recognition   (errors) 0 1 2   FP _____
Recall for Read Sentence   Y N   FP _____
Recognition of Read Sentence   Y N   N/A   FP _____

A: 1. The car came to a sudden stop.
    2. The boat sailed across the lake.
    3. The car backed over the curb.
    4. The airplane rose above the clouds.

B: 1. The elephant ate all the peanuts.
    2. The rabbit hopped down the lane.
    3. The possum hung from the tree.
    4. The rabbit hid in the briar patch.

Card Free Recall   number correct: _____   FP _____

        Recalled: _____

Card Recognition
Set A: telephone __   Y N   bird _____   Y N
                sword ____   Y N   piano _____   Y N
                apple _____   Y N   bed _____   Y N
                lamp _____   <u>Y</u> N   pear _____   <u>Y</u> N   Correct:____ /4
                cow _____   Y N   bridge _____   Y N
                pen _____   <u>Y</u> N   broom _____   <u>Y</u> N   FP _____

Set B: corn _____   Y N   glass _____   Y N
                fly _____   Y N   pie _____   <u>Y</u> N
                cake _____   Y N   bugle _____   Y N
                paint brush _ <u>Y</u> N   bird cage _____   Y N   Correct:____ /4
                wagon wheel _ Y N   book _____   <u>Y</u> N
                hat _____   <u>Y</u> N   ladder _____   Y N   FP _____

Comments: _____

_____

_____

                        Time Completed: _____

Denial/Anosognosia:
Affect Change:
Response Perseveration:
Paraphasic Errors:
Attentional Deficits:
Ptosis:
Angiography:

Impression:

Index

The abbreviations t and f denote tables and figures, respectively.

Absence epilepsy
childhood, 13–15, 14f–15f
juvenile, 20t, 20–21
myoclonic, 15
Acetazolamide
indications for, 28
for juvenile absence epilepsy, 21
Acquired epileptic aphasia, 17–18, 18f
Acquired immunodeficiency syndrome, 132, 141
ACTH. *See* Adrenocorticotropic hormone
Acute cortical stimulation, during anterior temporal lobectomy, 132–133
Adhesive paste, for electrode placement, 52
Adolescence, epileptic syndromes in, 19–21
Adrenocorticotropic hormone, for infantile spasms, 11
AEDs (antiepileptic drugs). *See* Anticonvulsant(s)
Affective seizures, benign partial epilepsy with, 17
Afterdischarges. *See* Epileptiform afterdischarges
Age
at amygdalohippocampectomy, and clinical outcome, 161, 162t
at operation, 28–29
at seizure onset
and clinical outcome from amygdalohippocampectomy, 160–161, 161t
and cognitive impairment, 172
and postoperative neuropsychological outcome, 84–85
and prognosis for seizure control, 83
and psychiatric morbidity, 219
Aggressive behavior
and childhood epilepsy, 172–173
postoperative improvement in, 220, 222
AHE. *See* Amygdalohippocampectomy
AI. *See* Asymmetry indices
AIDS. *See* Acquired immunodeficiency syndrome
Air embolism, with corpus callosotomy, 141, 144
Ammon's horn sclerosis, 91
Amnesia, 92
Amnestic syndrome, postoperative, prediction of, 99–105
Amobarbital, epileptic focus activation with, 42–45, 46f–47f, 47–48
Amobarbital (Wada) test. *See also* Intracarotid amobarbital (Wada) test
posterior cerebral artery, 104–105
selective temporal lobectomy, 168
Amygdala, 130
complex partial seizure origin in, 155, 156f
role in memory function, 166
Amygdalohippocampectomy, 131, 155–170, 189

anticonvulsant therapy after, 164–165, 165t–166t, 169
causal, 155, 168
vs. palliative, 155, 156t, 162t, 164
complications of, 168
indications for, 155
operative technique for, 155–159, 158f–159f, 168
outcome from
clinical, 159–161, 160f
neuropathologic, 159–160, 160t
neuropsychological, 166–167, 166f–167f, 167t
and patient characteristics, 160–161, 161t–162t
psychosocial, 167–168
seizure, 161–169, 162t, 163f
vs. anterior temporal lobectomy, 162–163, 164f–165f
palliative, 155, 168
and reoperation outcome, 244
stereotaxic, MRI-guided, 114
Amytal. *See* Amobarbital
Ancef. *See* Cefazolin sodium
Anesthesia. *See also* General anesthesia; Local anesthesia
for corpus callosotomy, 141
interference with epileptiform activity, 191
for language mapping, 193–194
narcotic, contraindications to, 141
Anesthetic agents. *See also specific agent*
assessment with, 41–42, 97
Anterior temporal electrodes, 52, 52f, 59
Anterior temporal lobectomy, 129–138, 189
acute cortical stimulation during, 132–133
afterdischarge threshold determination for, 134
anesthesia for, choice of, 131–133
central sulcus identification for, 133–134
complications of, 136–137
electrocorticography during, 134–135
general considerations, 129–132
language outcome from, 133, 208, 210–213
in children, 214–215
postoperative testing only, 210–211
preoperative-to-postoperative assessments, 211–213, 212t
operative technique for, 135–136
postoperative care for, 136
preoperative care for, 132
preoperative evaluation for, 131
seizure outcome from, 136–137
with respect to frequency, 200–202, 202t
factors influencing, 201–202
vs. amygdalohippocampectomy, 162–163, 164f–165f
selection criteria for, 131
surgical techniques for, 131–132
Antibiotics, prophylactic, 132

265